ESSENTIALS of
STRATEGIC
PLANNING
in HEALTHCARE

JEFFREY P. HARRISON

ESSENTIALS of STRATEGIC PLANNING

in HEALTHCARE

SECOND EDITION

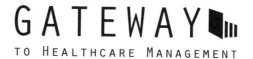

GATEWAY
TO HEALTHCARE MANAGEMENT

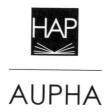

AUPHA

Health Administration Press, Chicago, Illinois
Association of University Programs in Health Administration, Arlington, Virginia

Your board, staff, or clients may also benefit from this book's insight. For more information on quantity discounts, contact the Health Administration Press Marketing Manager at (312) 424-9450.

20   19   18   17   16   5   4   3   2   1

Library of Congress Cataloging-in-Publication Data

Names: Harrison, Jeffrey P. (Jeffrey Paul), 1951–
Title: Essentials of strategic planning in healthcare / Jeffrey P. Harrison.
Description: Second edition. | Chicago, Illinois : Health Administration Press, [2016] | Includes bibliographical
    references and index.
Identifiers: LCCN 2015041795 (print) | LCCN 2015042611 (ebook) | ISBN 9781567937916 (alk. paper) |
    ISBN 9781567937947 (mobi) | ISBN 9781567937930 (epub) | ISBN 9781567937954 (xml)
Subjects: LCSH: Health services administration--Planning. | Strategic planning. | Health planning.
Classification: LCC RA971 .H296 2016 (print) | LCC RA971 (ebook) | DDC
    362.1068–dc23
LC record available at http://lccn.loc.gov/2015041795

The paper used in this publication meets the minimum requirements of American National Standard for Information Sciences—Permanence of Paper for Printed Library Materials, ANSI Z39.48-1984. ∞™

Acquisitions editor: Tulie O'Connor; Project manager: Theresa L. Rothschadl; Cover designer: James Slate; Layout: Cepheus Edmondson

Found an error or a typo? We want to know! Please e-mail it to hapbooks@ache.org, noting the book title and putting "Book Error" in the subject line.

For photocopying and copyright information, please contact Copyright Clearance Center at www.copyright.com or (978) 750-8400.

Health Administration Press
A division of the Foundation
    of the American College of
    Healthcare Executives
One North Franklin Street
Suite 1700
Chicago, IL 60606-3529
(312) 424-2800

Association of University Programs
    in Health Administration
2000 14th Street North
Suite 780
Arlington, VA 22201
(703) 894-0940

BRIEF CONTENTS

Preface xiii

Acknowledgments xvii

Coastal Medical Center Comprehensive Case Study 1

Chapter 1 Leadership, Mission, Vision, and Culture: The Foundation for Strategic Planning 29

Chapter 2 Transformational Leadership Maximizes Strategic Planning 61

Chapter 3 Fundamentals of Strategic Planning 77

Chapter 4 Strategic Planning and SWOT Analysis 100

Chapter 5 Healthcare Marketing 114

Chapter 6 Strategic Planning and Health Information Technology 128

Chapter 7 Strategic Planning and the Healthcare Business Plan 149

Chapter 8 Communicating the Strategic Plan 168

Chapter 9 Accountable Care Organizations and Physician Joint Ventures 178

Chapter 10 Strategic Planning and Post-acute Care Services 197

Chapter 11   Strategic Planning in Health Systems 213

Chapter 12   Pay for Performance and the Healthcare Value Paradigm 226

Chapter 13   The Future of Healthcare 248

Epilogue 263

Glossary 267

Index 277

About the Author 295

About the Contributors 297

DETAILED CONTENTS

Preface xiii

Acknowledgments xvii

Coastal Medical Center Comprehensive Case Study.......................... 1

    Introduction 1

    Healthcare Costs... 1

    The Competition 2

    Highlights of Coastal Medical Center 2

    Historical Perspective.. 4

    Board of Trustees.. 5

    Parent Corporation... 6

    Medical Staff... 7

    Subsidiary Companies 9

    Executives and Middle Management 11

    Corporate Staff 11

    Duplication of Functions.. 12

    Service and Professional Contracts.. 12

    Materials Management 13

    Special Projects 13

    New CEO 13

    General Conditions 15

    New Business Initiatives 16

Value-Based Purchasing... 17
Inpatient Data and Case-Mix Index.. 17
Conclusion 17
Exercises 17
Endnote... 18
Appendix A. Population and Household Data 18
Appendix B. Coastal Medical Center: Income Statement by Calendar
        Year (January 1–December 31)..................................... 20
Appendix C. Coastal Medical Center: Hospital Consumer Assessment
        of Healthcare Providers and Systems Scores................. 20
Appendix D. Coastal Medical Center: Balance Sheet 21
Appendix E. Coastal Medical Center: Financial Ratios 21
Appendix F. Coastal Medical Center: Leadership Survey 24
Appendix G. Coastal Medical Center: Value-Based Purchasing 25
Appendix H. Coastal Medical Center: Inpatient Data 27

Chapter 1   Leadership, Mission, Vision, and Culture: The Foundation for
        Strategic Planning.. 29
Learning Objectives 29
Key Terms and Concepts.. 30
Introduction 30
Definition of Leadership 32
Other Key Leadership Roles... 38
Physician Involvement in Healthcare Strategic Planning................. 41
Managed Care Organizations... 42
The Impact of Mission, Vision, and Culture on Profits and
        Strategic Planning.. 44
Strategic Planning... 50
The Impact of Ownership on Profits and the Strategic Planning
        Process.. 53
Implementing Organizational Change 55
Summary 55
Exercises 56
References... 58

Chapter 2   Transformational Leadership Maximizes Strategic Planning.............. 61
Learning Objectives 61
Key Terms and Concepts.. 62
Introduction 62
The Concept of Transformational Leadership 64

Why Is Transformational Leadership Important to Study? 68
Ethics as a Foundation for Leadership and Strategic Planning........................ 68
The Role of Transformational Leaders in Managing the
      Strategic Planning Process 69
Summary 74
Exercises 74
References... 75

Chapter 3 Fundamentals of Strategic Planning.. 77
Learning Objectives 77
Key Terms and Concepts... 78
Introduction 78
Definition 78
Analysis of the Environment Inside the Organization 79
Analysis of the Environment Outside the Organization 81
Gap Analysis.. 83
Planning Areas 86
Evaluation of Performance.. 91
Planning at the Local, Regional, and National Levels..................... 93
Endnotes 95
Summary 95
Exercises 96
References.. 97

Chapter 4 Strategic Planning and SWOT Analysis....................................... 100
Learning Objectives 100
Key Terms and Concepts... 101
Introduction 101
Definition... 101
Steps in SWOT Analysis... 102
SWOT Analysis: Internal and External Perspective........................ 106
Force Field Analysis 106
Gap Analysis 108
Downstream Revenue 109
Summary 110
Exercises 110
References... 112

Chapter 5 Healthcare Marketing... 114
Learning Objectives 114
Key Terms and Concepts... 115
Introduction 115

Definition.. 116
Strategic Healthcare Marketing.. 116
Marketing Media in the Current Environment.. 118
Healthcare Marketing at the Local and Regional Levels 123
Summary 124
Exercises 124
References... 125

Chapter 6   Strategic Planning and Health Information Technology.................. 128
Learning Objectives.. 128
Key Terms and Concepts.. 129
Introduction 129
Meaningful Use 131
E-Health... 132
Strategic Health Information Technology Initiatives 134
Strategic Planning for Health Information Technology 137
The Growing HIT Workforce 139
Healthcare Information Resources 140
Summary 144
Exercises 145
References... 146

Chapter 7   Strategic Planning and the Healthcare Business Plan 149
Learning Objectives.. 149
Key Terms and Concepts.. 150
Introduction 150
Definition... 150
Healthcare Business Plan 151
Planning Tools 162
Summary 163
Exercises 164
References... 166

Chapter 8   Communicating the Strategic Plan 168
Learning Objectives.. 168
Key Terms and Concepts.. 169
Introduction 169
Presentation of the Strategic Plan... 169
Summary 175
Exercises 175
References... 176

Chapter 9   Accountable Care Organizations and Physician Joint Ventures 178

   Learning Objectives 178

   Key Terms and Concepts 179

   Introduction 179

   Clinical Integration 179

   Patient-Centered Medical Home 180

   Potential Structures for Physician–Hospital Integration 183

   Physician Engagement in Strategic Planning 190

   Summary 190

   Exercises 191

   References 194

Chapter 10   Strategic Planning and Post-acute Care Services 197

   Learning Objectives 197

   Key Terms and Concepts 198

   Introduction 198

   Definitions 199

   Healthcare and US Population Demographics 200

   Inpatient Rehabilitation Facilities 201

   Skilled-Nursing Facilities 203

   Hospice 205

   Adult Health Day Care Centers 208

   Summary 209

   Exercises 209

   References 210

Chapter 11   Strategic Planning in Health Systems 213

   Learning Objectives 213

   Key Terms and Concepts 214

   Introduction 214

   Hospital Mergers and Acquisitions 214

   Integrated Delivery Systems 216

   Strategic Planning at the Health System Level 218

   Summary 222

   Exercises 222

   References 223

Chapter 12   Pay for Performance and the Healthcare Value Paradigm 226

   Learning Objectives 226

   Key Terms and Concepts 227

   Introduction 227

Medicare Pay-for-Performance Initiatives 229

Additional Initiatives in Pay for Performance... 231

Physicians' Attitudes Regarding Pay for Performance................................... 233

Incorporating Pay for Performance into a Strategic Plan 233

Quality Metrics... 236

Other Quality Considerations.. 240

Summary 242

Exercises 243

References.. 244

Chapter 13   The Future of Healthcare.. 248

Learning Objectives... 248

Key Terms and Concepts.. 249

Introduction 249

The New Healthcare Value Paradigm 250

Strategic Planning for Healthcare Value... 257

Summary 257

Exercises 258

References.. 259

Epilogue... 263

Glossary 267

Index 277

About the Author... 295

About the Contributors... 297

PREFACE

Essentials of Strategic Planning in Healthcare is intended to be the primary textbook for introductory courses in healthcare strategic planning. The book includes a comprehensive case study that students can use to work through the entire strategic planning process. Study questions and realistic exercises in each chapter are linked to the case study and give students an opportunity to work with healthcare data.

Healthcare research shows that the most successful organizations create a culture that fosters creativity, innovation, and transformational leadership. Effective strategic planning depends on leaders' commitment to creating an organizational culture that supports change. The first part of the book includes Chapter 1, "Leadership, Mission, Vision, and Culture: The Foundation for Strategic Planning," and Chapter 2, "Transformational Leadership Maximizes Strategic Planning." These chapters show leadership's important role in strategic planning and in creating an organizational culture that fosters successful strategic planning.

The second part of the book demonstrates essential strategic planning techniques for the healthcare field. It emphasizes the importance of positioning the healthcare organization relative to its environment to achieve its objectives and ensure its survival. Chapter 3, "Fundamentals of Strategic Planning," explains how to begin the strategic planning process with an analysis of the external environment and organizational factors critical to strategic planning. Chapter 4, "Strategic Planning and SWOT Analysis," focuses on the strengths, weaknesses, opportunities, and threats facing healthcare organizations and their importance in developing strategic plans. Chapter 5, "Healthcare Marketing," is new with this second edition because marketing is such an integral component of putting the strategic plan into action. In addition, with the growth of health systems, marketing is shifting from the local level to the regional or national level for some organizations.

The third part of the book focuses on the data that must be collected before a strategic plan can be developed, analytical tools that support strategic planning, and essential components of a strategic plan. Chapter 6, "Strategic Planning and Health Information Technology," identifies key data sources available to strategic planners in healthcare. Chapter 7, "Strategic Planning and the Healthcare Business Plan," discusses financial tools used to inform healthcare strategic planning. Finally, Chapter 8, "Communicating the Strategic Plan," emphasizes the importance of effectively communicating the strategic plan to multiple stakeholder groups.

The fourth part focuses on the development of strategic planning initiatives across the continuum of healthcare services. These developments include business initiatives in physician group management, long-term care, and other joint venture projects. Chapter 9, "Accountable Care Organizations and Physician Joint Ventures," stresses the impact of the Affordable Care Act of 2010 on kick-starting accountable care organizations and the strategic advantage hospitals can achieve through linking with physicians. Chapter 10, "Strategic Planning and Post-acute Care Services," explores strategic planning opportunities in inpatient rehabilitation, skilled nursing, hospice, and other post-acute care services.

The fifth part is written from a futurist perspective and discusses new developments in healthcare strategic planning. Chapter 11, "Strategic Planning in Health Systems," discusses the growth of national and international health systems and the increasing rate of integration among healthcare organizations. Chapter 12, "Pay for Performance and the Healthcare Value Paradigm," addresses the importance of pay-for-performance initiatives in maximizing an organization's income and quality of care. Finally, Chapter 13, "The Future of Healthcare," emphasizes high-quality healthcare at low cost as the healthcare value consumers are seeking today.

Each chapter of the book includes definitions of key terms, and the reference list included at the end of the chapters can also serve as a list of recommended readings. Chapters 9 through 13 are modular, enabling the instructor to exclude chapters or change their order according to individual preference or classroom requirements.

I hope you find that *Essentials of Strategic Planning in Healthcare* provides the knowledge and tools necessary for future organizational success.

Jeffrey P. Harrison
Jacksonville, Florida

INSTRUCTOR RESOURCES

This book's Instructor Resources include Power Point slides, HAP Course Lesson Plans, and other teaching tools.

For the most up-to-date information about this book and its Instructor Resources, go to ache.org/HAP and browse for the book's title or author name.

This book's Instructor Resources are available to instructors who adopt this book for use in their course. For access information, please e- mail hapbooks@ache.org.

HAP Course Lesson Plans are designed to promote an active classroom. Use the lesson plans to set up a new course or adapt your current syllabus to this edition of the text. Activities have been designed to enhance critical-thinking and problem-solving skills, as well as information retention and retrieval capacity. Designed for either an online or on-ground environment.

ACKNOWLEDGMENTS

I gratefully acknowledge the help of those who assisted me in this endeavor. I thank my children—Christopher, Stacey, Shannon, and Craig—who have supported my research and always challenged me to present my findings in a clear and understandable manner.

I want to thank my coauthors in the textbook. One of these is Dr. Debra Harrison, who is the chief nursing officer at the Mayo Clinic in Florida and an assistant professor of nursing in the Mayo College of Medicine. In addition, I want to thank Art Layne, MHA, a former healthcare CEO, for his contributions on healthcare marketing.

I also acknowledge the behind-the-scenes work necessary to publishing a book. I thank my mother, Gloria Harrison, who helped edit the initial drafts of each chapter. Finally, I thank the staff at Health Administration Press. They were a pleasure to work with and were there every step of the way.

COASTAL MEDICAL CENTER COMPREHENSIVE CASE STUDY

INTRODUCTION

This comprehensive case study serves as a basis for the exercises included throughout the book.

Coastal Medical Center (CMC) is a licensed, 450-bed regional referral hospital providing a full range of services. The primary service area is a coastal city and three counties, with a total population greater than 995,000, located in the Sunbelt. This tricounty area has had one of the fastest population growth rates in the country for the past five years. According to the local health planning council, the tricounty population is projected to increase by 15 percent from 2015 to 2020. Appendix A, at the end of this case study, provides detailed population statistics for the city and tricounty area.

The population growth rate for households (families) has been 1 to 2 percentage points higher than the overall population growth. The growth rate of the population under age 44 shows a young and growing community. Per capita (i.e., per person) income in the tricounty area is high and increasing. As the population of the tricounty area increases, the need for healthcare services is anticipated to increase. The area's economy is largely supported by manufacturing, with service companies and agriculture accounting for another 35 percent. Unemployment is typically 6 percent. The overall poverty rate is 12.4 percent. A recent study revealed that 40,000 city residents are below 125 percent of the established federal poverty level.

HEALTHCARE COSTS

Healthcare costs in the region are high in comparison to healthcare costs in most other areas in the state. In response to what they feel are excessively high healthcare costs, county businesses recently formed a business coalition, hired a full-time executive, and publicly stated their intent to achieve reduction in healthcare costs. The local press has expressed its concern about the high cost of healthcare in the local community and consistently bashes the area's hospitals and physicians. The coalition refused to allow the three major medical centers in the area to join, despite the fact that each is a major employer.

THE COMPETITION

CMC has two major competitors. Johnson Medical Center (JMC) is the larger of a two-hospital for-profit healthcare system, and Lutheran Medical Center (LMC) is the larger of a two-hospital, faith-based not-for-profit healthcare system.

JMC is located less than two miles from CMC and is a 430-bed tertiary care facility. JMC owns four nursing homes, two assisted living facilities, a durable medical equipment company, a wellness center, an ambulance service, and an industrial medicine business. These facilities are located in the tricounty area and are within a 30-minute drive of the main CMC facility. JMC's parent company, Johnson Health System, also owns one small hospital in the region.

Full-time equivalent (FTE)
Total number of full-time and part-time employees, which is expressed as an equivalent number of full-time employees.

JMC has 1,920 **full-time equivalents (FTEs)**, which translates to 5.2 FTEs per **adjusted occupied bed**. JMC recently used a consultant to reduce its FTEs, flatten its structure, broaden its control, and improve its operations in general.

JMC has been averaging an occupancy rate of 74 percent. Outpatient revenues are 40 percent of total revenues and have grown about 6 percent per year for the past two years. JMC had a bottom line (i.e., net income) of $15 million last year. Bottom lines for the two previous years were $11 million and $14 million. **Profit margins** have exceeded 5 percent for the past three years. In essence, JMC is a major strong competitor for CMC. The organization is reported to have a "war chest" of reserves exceeding $70 million.

Adjusted occupied bed
Number of inpatient occupied beds, adjusted (increased) to account for the bed occupancy attributed to outpatient services, partial hospitalization, and home services.

LMC is a 310-bed acute care hospital located outside the city limits but within the tricounty area. It does not offer tertiary, intensive services to the extent that CMC and JMC do, but it is a highly regarded general hospital that enjoys an occupancy rate of 75 percent. It is especially strong in obstetrics, pediatrics, general medicine, and ambulatory care. It attracts well-insured patients from the affluent suburban area.

LMC has 1,180 FTEs and typically operates at 6.1 FTEs per adjusted occupied bed. LMC provides a great deal of indigent care and, in accordance with the philosophy of the church, its budgets are set to generate only a 2 percent annual profit margin.

Profit margin
Difference between how much money the hospital brings in and how much it spends.

HIGHLIGHTS OF COASTAL MEDICAL CENTER

As a referral center, CMC offers almost every level of care, including a number of tertiary care services, with the exception of neonatology and severe burn–unit services. Many of its patients require high-intensity services. For this reason, its costs are the second highest in the entire state. The average length of stay of a patient at CMC is 9.2 days, compared to a statewide average of 6.4 days at hospitals of similar size and services. This difference is probably attributable to the intensity of services CMC offers. CMC's expenses per patient day are also the highest in the state, with the exception of two large university-affiliated teaching medical centers. Its FTEs per adjusted occupied bed (7.5), paid hours per adjusted patient day (35.2), and paid hours per patient discharge (238.5) all greatly exceed those of competitors and the norms of comparable facilities. CMC is currently authorized for 2,240 positions but actually employs 2,259 FTEs. Salary expenses per adjusted discharge and adjusted patient day are $2,760 and $491, respectively.

A recent one-year market share analysis for the broader eight-county region revealed the data presented in Exhibit Case.1.

CMC has market advantage in substance abuse, psychiatrics, pediatrics, and obstetrics. JMC has market advantage in adult medical and surgical care. At a recent administrative meeting, the following CMC utilization figures for the year were reviewed:

◆   Admissions are down 14 percent.

◆   Medicaid admissions are up 11 percent.

◆   Ambulatory care visits are down 10 percent.

◆   Surgical admissions are down 6.7 percent.

A recent auditor's report included the following notes:

◆   A significant adjustment was required at year-end to correctly reflect contractual allowance expense (i.e., the amount of money spent in hiring

EXHIBIT CASE.1
One-Year Market Share Analysis

Facility	Discharges	Percentage of Total
CMC	7,819	18
JMC	8,989	21
LMC	6,820	16
All others	19,546	45
Total	43,174	100

outside contractors). The data used at the beginning of the year to estimate contractual allowance expense were grossly inaccurate.

◆ Insurers were not billed for services by certain hospital-based employed specialists ($7 million for the past year) as a result of neglect on the part of the hospital billing staff.

◆ A total of $1.7 million in Medicaid reimbursement was not authorized. No follow-ups were done, and no claims were resubmitted.

HISTORICAL PERSPECTIVE

CMC was founded just after World War II using a Hill-Burton grant (see Highlight Case.1) and funds raised locally. From a modest beginning with 100 beds and a limited range of acute care service offerings, the medical center has grown to its present size of 450 beds and now offers a full range of services. Credit for the major growth and past success of CMC has been given to Don Wilson, who served as chief executive officer (CEO) from 1990 until his retirement in early 2012. Mr. Wilson was a visionary and successfully transformed the medical center to its present status as a tertiary care facility offering high-intensity care, including open-heart surgery and liver and kidney transplantation.

✳ HIGHLIGHT CASE.1
Hill-Burton Act

In the mid-1940s, many hospitals in the United States were becoming obsolete because they did not have money to invest in their facilities after the Great Depression and World War II. To combat this lack of capital and help states meet the healthcare needs of their populations, Senators Lister Hill and Harold Burton proposed the Hospital Survey and Construction Act, also known as the Hill-Burton Act. This act provided federal grant money to build or modernize healthcare facilities. In exchange, hospitals receiving the grant were obligated to provide uncompensated (free) care to those who needed care but could not pay for it.

The Hill-Burton Act expired in 1974, but in 1975 Congress passed Title XVI of the Public Health Service Act. Title XVI continues the Hill-Burton program by providing federal grant money for healthcare facility construction and renovation but more clearly defines the requirements for the facilities. For example, facilities receiving grant money must prove they are providing a certain amount of uncompensated care to populations that meet particular eligibility requirements.

Mr. Wilson's successor was Ron Henderson. For three years, Mr. Henderson practiced a loose, informal style of management. He seemed to sit back and enjoy himself while others ran the medical center. He was often characterized as a caretaker. The medical center made $52.5 million in 2012 following Mr. Wilson's retirement (the result of an excellent revenue stream and a strong balance sheet), so Mr. Henderson was not pressed to make major changes. He encouraged the board of trustees, the medical staff, and his administrative staff to submit new ideas for improving community healthcare services using CMC as the focal point for delivery. An avalanche of ideas was submitted during the first two years of Mr. Henderson's tenure. He moved quickly on these ideas and established himself as a person who made swift decisions on new ventures and kept things rolling. He simply let other executives "do their thing" and neither discouraged nor evaluated their work. His strategy was apparently rapid growth and diversity in new businesses. He made major fund commitments to new ideas but did little to evaluate the compatibility of those ideas with CMC's mission and its strategic direction, and he usually did not consider the financial implications of these ventures. His approach was simply "let's do it."

Before 2012, CMC was in excellent financial shape and faced few financial problems. By 2015, expenses began to skyrocket while utilization and revenues failed to keep pace. In addition, a hospital census indicated that, on average, 58 percent of CMC's patients were Medicare patients and 18 percent were Medicaid patients. As a result, the medical center suffered from reductions in reimbursement. Notable among CMC's excessive costs were labor, material, and purchased services. The chief financial officer (CFO) was convinced that a major part of this problem was the presence of three unions, including unionized employees in support services and unionized nursing services. Added to this cost burden was the more than $5 million being transferred to subsidize other CMC subsidiary companies.

During the second year of his tenure, Mr. Henderson began to receive criticism from the board of trustees. He had added 127 new positions despite solid evidence that utilization was experiencing a steep decline. His reasoning was that the declines were temporary and that business would soon be back to normal.

In 2015, the medical center suffered a net loss of $16 million (see Appendix B). Surprised by this major loss, the board of trustees fired Mr. Henderson. They contended that he should have informed them of these serious problems. They felt that a better strategic planning process should have been in place for the selection of projects, on which millions of dollars had been spent. The board of trustees could not understand how overall corporate net income could drop to a loss of $16 million when $7.3 million in profit had been made the previous year.

BOARD OF TRUSTEES

CMC's governing board has 27 members. All of its trustees are prominent, influential, and generally wealthy members of the community. The board is self-perpetuating, meaning its members have continued their positions beyond the normal limits without any external intervention. The same chair has served for ten years. Average tenure on the board is 17 years. Committees of the board are detailed in Exhibit Case.2.

Committee	Size	Meeting Frequency
Ambulatory care	11	Monthly
Audit	9	Quarterly
Budget	18	Quarterly
Construction	13	Monthly
Executive	16	Monthly
Executive compensation	9	Annually
Finance	13	Monthly
Joint conference	24	Monthly
Material and equipment	11	Monthly
Patient care	11	Monthly
Personnel	11	Monthly
Public relations	9	Monthly
Quality assurance	9	Monthly
Strategic planning	16	Monthly

One physician-at-large is included on the board. The chief of staff and the CEO attend all board meetings but are not allowed to vote on board decisions. There are no minority members despite the fact that racial minorities account for 12 percent of the service area population. Only one of the 27 members of the board is a woman. The average age of the trustees is 66.

PARENT CORPORATION

The parent corporation of CMC is Coastal Healthcare Incorporated. A parent board was created through corporate restructuring several years ago, but its role has never been clear. This board is made up of friends of the most powerful trustees of the CMC board. In essence, when corporate restructuring was the "in" thing to do, this holding company was formed. By appointing a few CMC trustees to also sit on the parent board and by appointing friends of present CMC trustees, it was believed the two boards would function as one happy family. However, there has been constant conflict from the beginning regarding the relative powers and roles of the two boards.

The parent board has 19 members, all of whom are white and male. The backgrounds of the parent board trustees mirror those of the CMC trustees in that they are prominent and mostly wealthy. Membership includes bankers, attorneys, business executives, business owners, developers, and prominent retired people.

Committees of the Coastal Healthcare Inc. (parent) board are detailed in Exhibit Case.3.

The following are some of the conflicts that have occurred between these two boards over the years:

- The parent board refused to approve the appointment of a new hospital CEO selected by the CMC board.

- In 2013, the two boards hired separate consultants to develop a long-range strategic plan. Two plans were produced but were never integrated and never really implemented.

- Committees from the parent board often request information about functions of the medical center, creating conflict because the parent board has a tendency to micromanage CMC's routine operations.

- Separate committees of both boards spent more than two years trying to revise CMC's mission statement.

MEDICAL STAFF

The medical staff at CMC has historically had difficulty cooperating with the board and administration. Patient length of stay is excessively high in most specialties, yet the physicians refuse to be educated on reimbursement and the need to reduce length of stay, excessive

Committee	Size	Meeting Frequency
Executive	11	Monthly
Finance	11	Monthly
Strategic planning	11	Quarterly

EXHIBIT CASE.3
Committees of the Coastal Healthcare Inc. (Parent) Board

tests, and so on. Approximately 90 percent of the medical staff also has privileges at one or more competing hospitals in town. Further, medical staff members have set up their own diagnostic services, especially the radiologists and neurologists, despite the fact that they were granted exclusive service contracts at CMC.

In recent years, the specialists, who represent the majority of the medical staff, have been increasingly dissatisfied. They complain that their referrals are decreasing or remaining flat and that CMC is not doing enough to help them establish and maintain a sufficient number. Hospital admissions for specialty services are declining drastically. To compound the problem, the competing medical centers are courting these specialists aggressively with attractive offers, such as priority scheduling in surgery and other special arrangements, all of which are legal.

The medical staff also rated various aspects of medical center operations as unsatisfactory in a recent survey. The subjects of their complaints ran the gamut and included the following:

- ◆ Nursing services, and especially the nurses' attitudes, are not satisfactory. Nurses have formed themselves into shared governance councils and are taking issue with both physicians and administration regarding their autonomy.

- ◆ Excessive delays exist in every aspect of operations. Surgical procedures start late, supplies or equipment are lacking when needed, and processes for admitting patients take too long.

- ◆ CMC's recent Hospital Consumer Assessment of Healthcare Providers and Systems (HCAHPS) scores confirm doctors' perception, with satisfaction with nurses' communication rated only 74 percent (Appendix C). Patient satisfaction with physicians' communication was even lower at 72 percent.

- ◆ Medical staff members think they should have more voice in both financial and operational matters, especially in capital budgeting. They believe they are asked to provide free services too frequently (e.g., by committees), and many have refused to serve without compensation to offset the practice income they have lost.

There are also quality problems. Two physicians should probably have their privileges revoked, three apparently have substance abuse problems, and several have not kept up with current practices and should be asked to retire. Persuading physicians to hold elected offices and accept committee responsibility has also been difficult. Payment of honoraria has helped, but few are still willing to serve. More than $200,000 has already been paid out to entice doctors to serve on committees.

SUBSIDIARY COMPANIES

Including CMC, Coastal Healthcare Inc. comprises 24 subsidiary corporations:

- **Medical Enterprises** is a for-profit joint venture with physicians. The company is developing computers that enhance imaging services. Thus far, CMC has invested $18 million in this company. No cash flow is expected for three to four years.

- **Three nursing homes**. These long-term care facilities are collectively losing almost $1 million annually. **Debt service** on two of them is very high. Only one is within patient transfer distance of CMC. The second is 70 miles away, and the third is 82 miles away. All three have unions. Almost all of the residents of the two facilities losing the greatest amount are Medicaid patients; there are only a few self-pay patients.

- **CMC Management Services** was formed to sell management and consulting services. The company lost $360,000 last year, which was its third year of operation.

- **Regional Neuroimaging** is a joint venture with physicians. The company lost $920,000 in its first year of operation. Capital invested by the hospital to date totals $9 million.

- **American Ambulance** is a local ambulance company. Financially, it just breaks even, but it does increase admissions to CMC, especially through trauma pickups.

- **Home Health Inc.** provides home health care services in an eight-county area. Its operating loss last year was $290,000. The company has considerable difficulty attracting and retaining professional personnel, especially nurses and physical therapists.

- **Industrial Services Inc.** provides health services to industrial companies throughout the state. Only one of the six operating locations is close enough to CMC to generate referrals. None of the operating sites is making a profit, though the company is five years old.

- **MRI Enterprises** is a successful mobile magnetic resonance imaging joint venture with a physician group. It has a consistently positive bottom line.

- **Textile Enterprises** is a large, high-tech laundry completed three years ago. It was intended to serve the medical center and many other companies in the region. Because of its debt service, union wages, and remote location, the

Debt service
Cash required over a given period for the repayment of interest and principal on a debt.

laundry has yet to break even. After three years, it still does not have its first non-CMC service contract.

- **Caroleen Hospital** (60 beds), **Grant Hospital** (74 beds), and **Ellenboro Hospital** (90 beds) are all small, rural hospitals purchased to feed patients to CMC. All are unprofitable. Collectively, the three require $2.5 million in subsidies annually.

- **HMO Care** is a health maintenance organization joint venture with 20,000 subscribers. After three years of operation, its costs are still rising. Last year, it required $2 million in subsidies.

- **Northeast Clinic** is a large multispecialty group of 11 physicians who were fed up with government red tape and sold out to CMC last year. CMC now employs these physicians and is responsible for all medical group operations. It is too early to determine whether this venture will succeed.

- **Imaging Venture** is a recently formed radiology joint venture. Until it becomes successful—if it does—it will cost just under $1 million in debt service annually.

- **North Rehabilitation**, a 60-bed inpatient rehabilitation facility, was just opened. It is expected to succeed because CMC will refer all of its rehabilitation patients here, and there is no other rehabilitation facility in the region.

- **Center for Pain** has been a successful outpatient facility and is expected to remain successful. Its space is leased, overhead is kept low, and the physicians are salaried.

- **Coastal Wellness**, a fitness and wellness center, was developed five years ago at a cost of $10 million. It is located in a coastal community and is intended to attract those from wealthy areas. A significant number of CMC employees and their family members use Coastal Wellness at a lower monthly rate, with the rest subsidized by CMC. Coastal Wellness is currently underutilized, so CMC subsidizes it with $220,000 annually.

- **Central Billing** was formed to attract patient billing contracts from health facilities and physician groups. It has been moderately successful and reached the break-even point this past year.

- **City Contractors**, a separate, small general contracting company, was just formed. It will require about $200,000 annually in subsidy.

- **Bay Enterprises** is a land acquisition and holding company.

EXECUTIVES AND MIDDLE MANAGEMENT

CMC employs 20 executives (defined as positions above the administrative director level). Total annual executive compensation is $6.2 million. Each executive has an executive secretary whose average compensation is $35,000, which amounts to an executive-level support cost of $700,000.

Each of the other 23 subsidiary companies employs executives and executive support personnel in addition to regular employees. This executive overhead is a drain on CMC because many of the subsidiary companies do not break even and thus must be subsidized.

CMC employs 15 administrative directors, who function in the hierarchy between department vice presidents and department directors. Their principal purpose is to handle problems at the department level so that these problems do not escalate to the department vice president.

There are 67 director-level positions in the organization. Directors are responsible for a particular department or function. Managers are the next level down the line of supervision. There are 31 managers. Collectively, these managers have 68 supervisors working for them.

The compensation and benefits policy of CMC deviates substantially from industry norms in terms of range. For example, the directors' annual salaries range from $85,000 to more than $170,000. Annual salaries for directors in the United States typically fall between $115,000 and $140,000.[1]

CORPORATE STAFF

Coastal Healthcare Inc. consists of the following offices:

- ◆ Office of the CEO, who has five assistants to the president (i.e., administration, board, ethics, community, and staff assistants)

- ◆ Office of the senior vice president for finance (three people)

- ◆ Office of the senior vice president for corporate affairs (four people)

- ◆ Office of the senior vice president for corporate development (three people)

- ◆ Office of the vice president for legal affairs (five people)

- ◆ Office of the vice president for medical affairs (two people)

- ◆ Office of the vice president for marketing (two people)

- ◆ Office of the vice president for strategic planning (two people)

These corporate staff members serve as advisers and coordinators; oversee their functional areas at CMC; and, where needed, oversee the various subsidiary companies.

The parent company corporate staff comprises 26 total FTEs. The total costs of corporate overhead are $2.3 million annually. In addition, during the past year, the corporate officers purchased the consulting services listed in Exhibit Case.4.

DUPLICATION OF FUNCTIONS

Throughout CMC, functions have been duplicated as the organization has grown. For example, there are three education departments and three transportation departments. There is both an inpatient and an outpatient pharmacy, each with its own director. CMC and 12 of the larger subsidiary companies have separate human resources management functions.

There are 24 boards, one for each subsidiary company, and each board has a large number of committees. Executives from CMC and the parent corporation sit on these boards and their committees.

SERVICE AND PROFESSIONAL CONTRACTS

CMC contracts with many service providers. Service contracts include housekeeping, food service, record transcription, biomedical maintenance, security, and many others. These contracts are renewed regularly with the same firms. CMC also contracts with countless health professionals. For example, CMC contracts with two physicians to cover CMC's pediatrics clinic at an annual cost of $380,000, and CMC furnishes the facilities as well as

EXHIBIT CASE.4
Consulting Services Purchased by the Parent Corporation

Consultant Purpose	Cost
Conduct board retreat	$35,000
Prepare restructuring recommendations	$65,000
Write organization history	$60,000
Provide policy advice	$25,000
Lobby	$50,000
Undertake compensation (wage/salary) study	$72,000
Conduct labor negotiations	$120,000
Advise on management development	$90,000
Conduct managed care study	$47,000
Total	**$564,000**

professional and support personnel. Numerous physicians have negotiated arrangements through which they regularly receive checks for committee service, advice, and so on. Many of these negotiations are not documented in written contracts.

The hospital-based specialists' contracts are based on a percentage of gross earnings, with no provision for any type of adjustments to the gross amount. Several of these arrangements are long-standing but not documented in writing.

MATERIALS MANAGEMENT

CMC is organized traditionally, meaning there is no centralized materials management function. Purchasing is done throughout the organization from a large number of vendors. The pharmacy, laboratory, and other services do their own ordering, arrange contracts, and handle other supply and equipment matters. For example, the laboratory recently purchased a large computer software package without the knowledge of the purchasing agent or the information services department.

Large stores of inventory can be found throughout the facility. CMC also owns excessive and obsolete equipment. Central storage occupies a huge amount of space and carries what appears to be an overabundance of many items.

SPECIAL PROJECTS

Fifty-three "special projects" at various stages of progress are under way at CMC, ranging from the addition of a new education center to renovation of the food service department. A large number of start-ups are also under development. For example, CMC is considering a joint venture with physicians to build an ambulatory surgery center offering the latest robotic surgery technology. Analysis of the projected costs of these projects, and of the working capital many of them will need before they become profitable (if they ever do), has revealed that the organization will suffer severe financial distress if these projects continue. Moreover, the financial feasibility of many of them is uncertain. Finally, these projects have not been centrally coordinated, nor has their potential impact on the organization's mission and strategic direction been discussed. These projects were simply developed on the basis of individual interests of various executives and managers. By his inaction and lack of leadership, Mr. Henderson gave everyone free rein to do their own thing—and they did.

NEW CEO

CMC hired an executive search firm specializing in healthcare to look for a new CEO. After a nationwide search, the board of trustees decided to hire Richard Reynolds. Mr. Reynolds appeared to be a no-nonsense CEO who had the knowledge and skills needed to determine the problems at CMC and resolve them. During his first few weeks in the new position, he did an exhaustive analysis of CMC with the assistance of a transition consultant and the executives and managers of the organization. The following list highlights his findings:

◆ Compared to national personnel standards, many of the departments at CMC are grossly overstaffed. More than 100 new positions were added during the most recent fiscal year, despite the fact that utilization did not justify these positions. The overall administrative structure is top-heavy.

◆ CMC has 58 general contracts, many of which are standing contracts with consultants who appear to be receiving large monthly retainers but are not providing services. In addition, CMC has 121 contracts with physicians. Again, these physicians appear to be providing few services. The previous CEO apparently made numerous agreements to subsidize various physicians and pay them large sums for performing administrative services that are normally done on a voluntary basis by members of the medical staff.

◆ CMC has 53 major new service projects in the planning or construction phase. The analysis indicated they will require more than $100 million in future commitments, and Mr. Reynolds is not sure that CMC will be able to service the necessary debt. No project priorities exist and no feasibility studies have been done for most of the projects, so there is no way to forecast the financial impact of these "innovative ideas" on the organization.

◆ CMC has a large number of duplicate departments. Mr. Reynolds pinpointed many departments and services that could be consolidated.

◆ CMC has 66 "special" programs, collectively accounting for a $6 million outflow of cash. These programs are not directly related to CMC's tertiary care mission. CMC seems to have developed every type of program conceivable, from one end of the care continuum to the other, without considering whether the programs support its mission or generate a positive cash flow.

◆ In materials management, Mr. Reynolds found nearly $8 million in "unofficial" inventory stored throughout various facilities of the medical center and a declining inventory turnover rate of 42 percent. There is no centralized materials management system for the purchasing, storage, distribution, and accountability of materials.

◆ While the median operating margin for medical centers of similar size and service was about 2.5 percent during the past year, CMC experienced a multimillion-dollar loss and a –13.6 percent operating margin. In addition, the medical center's return on equity was a major problem. The number of **days accounts receivable** in other medical centers averaged 48 days during the past year; CMC's days accounts receivable were far greater at 58 days. Most alarming, CMC's cash on hand at any given time represented only 17.2 operating days. Finally, the hospital's major bond issue has been recently

Days accounts receivable
Average number of days an organization takes to collect payments on goods sold and services provided, calculated as follows: Average accounts payable (in dollars) × 365 (days per year) ÷ Sales revenue.

downgraded to the lowest credit rating, and the age of CMC's physical plant is 13 years, which is older than the average not-for-profit facility age of 11 years and the average for-profit facility of 7 years. (Days accounts receivable is the average number of days it takes to collect payments that clients owe to the organization The "normal" range is 40 to 50 days. A number significantly greater than 50 indicates the organization is having difficulty collecting payments from its clients; a number significantly lower than 40 indicates that the organization has overly strict credit policies that might be preventing it from taking in higher sales revenue.)

- ◆ Medicare has just notified the CFO that recovery of $4 million is forthcoming as a result of past errors in the Medicare cost report.

- ◆ The business coalition is becoming well established and intends to aggressively pursue discounted services through direct contracting.

- ◆ Coastal Healthcare Inc. is neither structured nor functions as a local healthcare system. Clinical services and administrative support are not integrated. For this reason, Coastal Healthcare Inc. does not meet the classic definition of a healthcare system provider.

- ◆ Nationally, capitation payment arrangements have not been successful for many hospitals. CMC is not in a favorable position to become an accountable care organization. To become an accountable health plan, CMC would have to partner with primary care and specialty physicians to meet the total healthcare needs of a defined patient population.

- ◆ No value-oriented efforts (e.g., continuous quality improvement, benchmarking) have been initiated at CMC.

- ◆ No leadership development is available for the board of trustees, medical staff, and administration.

- ◆ No formal strategic planning process is in place at either the CMC or the Coastal Healthcare Inc. level.

- ◆ No physician–hospital organizational arrangements exist.

GENERAL CONDITIONS

Mr. Reynolds quickly learned that he had taken a position in an organization with a governing board that is generally content to approve anything the CEO recommends. The medical staff appears no better in that they were principally focused on their own self-interest and show little interest in the affairs of the medical center.

Control systems are lacking, and CMC does not have a comprehensive information system. Moreover, the quality of care appears low, and a large number of legal cases against the medical center are pending. With respect to materials management, several suppliers have refused to deliver supplies because of delays in accounts payable.

Mr. Reynolds summed up the medical center's situation to the board by reporting that there is an immediate cash flow problem, people-related expenses are far too high, material-related expenses are well above those expected, plant-related expenses are excessive, contract amounts are excessive, and accounts receivable are too high. He also remarked that CMC seems to have no sense of direction or overall corporate strategy.

With the help of his transition consultant, Mr. Reynolds surveyed and interviewed his department heads. Given the financial situation and the results of the survey, Mr. Reynolds knows he faces a difficult challenge.

Mr. Reynolds concluded that the prior CEO had followed the one-man rule concept and had failed to build necessary knowledge and management skills among the vice presidents. Thus, when difficulties occurred in the organization, inertia set in. The reactions of his executives and managers are characterized by indecisiveness and unwillingness to take risks for fear of compromising their job security. In addition, he found an excessive number of administrative positions.

An examination of CMC's balance sheet (see Appendix D), financial ratios (Appendix E), and structure led Mr. Reynolds to conclude that the corporation is overexpanded, overleveraged, and overdependent on a narrow market. The organization is too expensive to operate, bloated with bureaucracy, inefficient in its services, and unimaginative in its approach to strategic planning and change.

From his discussion with the leadership team and other hospital staff, Mr. Reynolds believed CMC's leaders are considerably dissatisfied. To confirm his beliefs, he had the transition consultant administer a brief leadership survey, which included detailed questions about corporate culture and job satisfaction (Appendix F). Mr. Reynolds has decided to do a similar survey of all hospital staff within the next six months to obtain more baseline data on the organization's corporate culture and its ability to deal with the changes he knows are coming.

NEW BUSINESS INITIATIVES

To expand its physician staff, CMC has constructed a hospital-owned medical office building in a growing community five miles from the hospital. This effort has been successful and has attracted a prominent group of orthopedic physicians who now refer their surgical procedures to the hospital. As part of this expansion, and because the orthopedic workload has grown, CMC is exploring the financial feasibility of opening a physical therapy clinic at this new location. On the basis of current physician referral patterns, CMC anticipates $250,000 in outpatient physical therapy net income at the new location during the upcoming 12 months.

VALUE-BASED PURCHASING

Medicare value-based purchasing is a combined effect of efficiency and quality metrics. Value-based performance metrics have been identified at CMC in areas such as clinical processes; patient satisfaction; outcomes; readmission rates for heart attack, heart failure, pneumonia, chronic obstructive pulmonary disease, and hip or knee surgery; and hospital-acquired infections and conditions (Appendix G). The fact that CMC has a negative payment adjustment following each of these value-based purchasing metrics reflects the percentage reduction in Medicare reimbursement for the most current year.

INPATIENT DATA AND CASE-MIX INDEX

CMC had a case-mix index of 1.666 in 2015 (Appendix H). This index, which reflects the level of complexity for inpatient services, declined significantly since 2012, when it was 1.729. Given that the average case-mix index for an acute care hospital in the United States was 1.32 in 2015, CMC is more clinically complex than the average acute care hospital in the United States, but the level of complexity declined over the past four years. A major reason for this decline was the changing medical/surgical mix of the inpatients at CMC from 2012 to 2015 (Appendix H). Specifically, CMC's medical volume increased from 65 percent in 2012 to 66.26 percent in 2015. Conversely, CMC's surgical volume decreased from 35 percent in 2012 to 33.74 percent in 2015. This decline in surgical volume led to a reduction in volume in the overall case mix as well as an overall decline in profitability.

CONCLUSION

As Mr. Reynolds now ponders the many problems he has uncovered at CMC, he wonders what other problems lie beneath the surface. Every day he encounters additional major problems. At this point, Mr. Reynolds is so overwhelmed that he is unsure how to proceed. He does know, however, that priorities need to be set, the deteriorating situation needs to be turned around, and a strategic plan needs to be developed to chart the future of the organization.

EXERCISES

Assume you are Mr. Reynolds. Being new to the position, you are faced with major challenges. The questions and exercises at the end of each chapter in this book provide an opportunity to gain leadership experience in managing change in a healthcare organization. Most important, you will gain experience in developing a strategic plan.

ENDNOTE

1. Annual salary statistics found at salary.com, 2015, "Critical Care Director Salaries," accessed August 2, www1.salary.com/Critical-Care-Director-Salary.html; salary.com, 2015, "Emergency Services Director Salaries," accessed August 2, www1.salary.com/Emergency-Services-Director-Salary.html.

APPENDIX A. POPULATION AND HOUSEHOLD DATA

	Riverside County	Metro City	Rural County	Ocean County
POPULATION AND HOUSEHOLD				
Square miles	609	775	601	485
Population density per square mile	214	1,028	245	111
Population 2010	83,829	672,971	105,986	28,701
Population 2015	129,832	794,569	146,739	53,506
Population 2020 (forecast)	148,289	842,179	163,082	63,543
% Population growth 2010–2015	54.88%	18.08%	38.45%	86.43%
% Population growth forecast 2015–2020	14.22%	5.10%	11.14%	18.76%
Households 2010	33,431	256,772	36,664	11,882
No. of households 2015	52,322	310,603	52,448	22,904
No. of households 2020 (forecast)	59,895	331,539	58,623	27,305
% Household growth 2010–2015	56.5%	20.97%	43.05%	92.76%
% Household growth forecast 2015–2020	14.5%	6.75%	11.77%	19.21%
Average household size	2.48	2.57	2.80	2.34
No. of families	35,793	205,123	40,907	16,766
% Urban population	56.5%	98.7%	59.6%	59.9%
% Rural population	43.5%	1.5%	40.4%	40.1%
% Female population	51.2%	51.5%	50.7%	51.5%
% Male population	48.8%	48.7%	49.3%	48.5%
% White population	91.1%	67.4%	88.6%	87.9%
% Black population	6.5%	28.5%	7.3%	9.5%
% Asian population	1.4%	3.8%	3.0%	1.6%
% Hispanic origin population	2.7%	4.3%	4.4%	5.2%
% Other population	1.4%	2.1%	3.1%	2.3%
% Population aged 0–5 years	6.5%	8.7%	8.0%	4.9%
% Population aged 6–11 years	8.1%	9.1%	9.6%	6.0%
% Population aged 12–17 years	8.2%	8.7%	10.2%	6.7%
% Population aged 18–24 years	6.4%	8.9%	7.2%	4.4%
% Population aged 25–34 years	9.7%	14.4%	11.6%	7.3%

% Population aged 35–44 years	17.8%	18.1%	18.7%	12.9%
% Population aged 45–54 years	17.0%	14.6%	15.9%	14.3%
% Population aged 55–64 years	10.2%	7.7%	8.9%	14.4%
% Population aged 65–74 years	8.8%	5.7%	5.6%	17.2%
% Population aged 75 years or older	7.3%	5.1%	4.3%	11.9%
Median age	41.3	35.5	36.8	50.5
INCOME AND EDUCATION				
Total household income	$5,145,536,895	$20,994,962,608	$3,656,788,183	$1,650,526,132
Median household income	$49,103	$41,410	$49,270	$42,975
Per capita income	$39,632	$26,423	$24,920	$30,847
Average income > $200,00	$474,930	$430,207	$348,177	$450,993
Education—% less than high school (age 25+)	11.2%	13.6%	11.5%	12.6%
Education—% high school graduate (age 25+)	31.6%	33.9%	35.4%	36.6%
Education—% some college (age 25+)	25.5%	26.9%	29.9%	27.1%
Education—% college graduate (age 25+)	22.1%	19.3%	16.8%	15.4%
Education—% graduate degree (age 25+)	9.6%	6.4%	6.5%	8.3%
EMPLOYMENT AND OCCUPATION				
Males employed (age 16+)	35,604	201,461	40,722	12,093
Females employed (age 16+)	29,337	169,863	30,949	9,654
Total employees (age 16+)	64,941	371,324	71,671	21,747
% White-collar occupations	62.9%	63.1%	61.8%	57.3%
% Blue-collar occupations	22.8%	23.6%	25.9%	27.5%
% Service occupations	14.3%	13.3%	12.4%	15.2%
% Local government workers	7.6%	7.0%	7.4%	7.7%
% State government workers	3.2%	2.4%	2.2%	1.6%
% Federal government workers	1.8%	3.5%	6.3%	0.9%
% Self-employed workers	9.0%	5.2%	6.3%	9.2%
CONSUMER EXPENDITURES				
Annual expenditures per capita ($US)	$18,211.60	$16,580.10	$16,226.00	$18,322.00
Healthcare expenditures per capita ($US)	$2,347.20	$2,183.90	$2,105.70	$2,390.30
Healthcare insurance expenditures per capita ($US)	$428.00	$385.00	$370.00	$482.20
COST OF LIVING				
Consumer Price Index	147.1	147.1	147.1	147.1
Medical care Consumer Price Index	211.3	211.3	211.3	211.3

Appendix B. Coastal Medical Center: Income Statement by Calendar Year (January 1–December 31)

	2015	2014	2013	2012
Inpatient revenue	719,329,916	755,618,849	784,412,051	827,231,608
Outpatient revenue	476,770,514	557,698,826	598,747,225	625,466,528
Total patient revenue	1,196,100,430	1,313,317,675	1,383,159,276	1,452,698,136
Contractual allowance (discounts)	809,575,220	912,970,880	970,156,446	1,062,616,080
Net patient revenues	386,525,210	400,346,795	413,002,830	390,082,056
Operating expense	416,531,087	421,383,586	411,066,597	356,255,182
Depreciation expense	22,616,659	17,701,123	21,479,371	21,412,330
Operating income	**−52,622,536**	**−38,737,914**	**−19,543,138**	**12,414,544**
Other income (contributions, bequests, other)	0	0	0	0
Income from investments	0	0	0	0
Governmental appropriations	0	0	0	0
Miscellaneous nonpatient revenue	36,527,105	47,063,315	37,025,334	40,113,376
Total nonpatient revenue	36,527,105	47,063,315	37,025,334	40,113,376
Total other expenses	0	944,991	0	0
Net income (loss)	**−16,095,431**	**7,380,410**	**17,482,196**	**52,527,920**

Note: Data are annualized for periods other than 12 months.

Appendix C. Coastal Medical Center: Hospital Consumer Assessment of Healthcare Providers and Systems Scores

	CMC	JMC	LMC	State Average	National Average
HCAHPS scores					
Patients who reported that nurses "Always" communicated well	74%	76%	83%	75%	79%
Patients who reported that doctors "Always" communicated well	72%	76%	85%	78%	82%
Patients "Always" received help as soon as they wanted	55%	63%	71%	62%	68%
Patients who reported that their pain was "Always" well controlled	66%	69%	75%	68%	71%
Staff "Always" explained about medicine before giving it to them	56%	60%	67%	60%	64%
Patients reported their room and bathroom were "Always" clean	65%	72%	80%	70%	74%
Reported area around their room was "Always" quiet at night	57%	60%	70%	58%	61%
Given info about what to do during their recovery at home	83%	85%	90%	83%	86%
"Strongly Agree" they understood their care when they left the hospital	43%	51%	65%	48%	51%
Gave their hospital a rating of 9 or 10 (0 [lowest] to 10 [highest])	62%	74%	90%	67%	71%
Patients reported YES, definitely recommend the hospital	63%	80%	92%	69%	71%

APPENDIX D. COASTAL MEDICAL CENTER: BALANCE SHEET

	2015	2014	2013	2012
Assets	339,055,010	347,278,187	384,551,932	403,459,670
Current assets	110,521,790	118,237,279	113,813,971	92,255,629
Fixed assets	143,848,624	132,031,268	141,037,047	130,904,980
Other assets	84,684,596	97,009,640	129,700,914	180,299,061
Liabilities and fund balances	339,055,010	347,278,187	384,551,932	403,459,670
Liabilities	289,863,632	268,244,657	296,496,775	295,606,794
Current liabilities	48,603,946	72,234,880	75,507,585	53,932,358
Long-term liabilities	241,259,686	196,009,777	220,989,190	241,674,436
Fund balances	49,191,378	79,033,530	88,055,157	107,852,876

APPENDIX E. COASTAL MEDICAL CENTER: FINANCIAL RATIOS

	2015	2014	2013	2012
PROFITABILITY RATIOS				
EBITDAR (earnings before interest, taxes, depreciation, amortization, and rent)	$6,521,228	$30,150,947	$38,961,567	$73,940,250
Definition: Net income + Interest + Depreciation and amortization + Lease cost				
Net income (before taxes)	–$16,095,431.00	$7,380,410.00	$17,482,196.00	$52,527,920.00
Interest expense	$0.00	$5,069,414.00	$0.00	$0.00
Depreciation and amortization expense	$22,616,659.00	$17,701,123.00	$21,479,371.00	$21,412,330.00
Lease cost	$0.00	$0.00	$0.00	$0.00
Operating margin	–13.60%	–9.70%	–4.70%	3.20%
*Definition: (Total operating revenue – Total operating expense) / Total operating revenue * 100*				
Total operating revenue (net patient revenue)	$386,525,210.00	$400,346,795.00	$413,002,830.00	$390,082,056.00
Total operating expense	$439,147,746.00	$439,084,709.00	$432,545,968.00	$377,667,512.00
Excess margin	–3.80%	1.90%	3.90%	12.20%
*Definition: (Total operating revenue – Total operating expenses + Nonoperating revenue) / (Total operating revenue + Nonoperating revenue) * 100*				
Total operating revenue (net patient revenue)	$386,525,210.00	$400,346,795.00	$413,002,830.00	$390,082,056.00
Total operating expense	$439,147,746.00	$439,084,709.00	$432,545,968.00	$377,667,512.00
Nonoperating revenue (nonpatient revenue)	$36,527,105.00	$47,063,315.00	$37,025,334.00	$40,113,376.00
Return on equity	–32.70%	9.30%	19.90%	48.70%
*Definition: (Total assets – Total liabilities) * 100*				
Net income (before taxes)	–$16,095,431.00	$7,380,410.00	$17,482,196.00	$52,527,920.00

(continued)

(continued from previous page)

Total assets (general fund only)	$339,055,010.00	$347,278,187.00	$384,551,932.00	$403,459,670.00
Total liabilities (general fund only)	$289,863,632.00	$268,244,657.00	$296,496,775.00	$295,606,794.00
Return on assets (ROA)	−4.70%	2.10%	4.50%	13.00%
*Definition: Net income / Total assets * 100*				
Net income (before taxes)	−$16,095,431.00	$7,380,410.00	$17,482,196.00	$52,527,920.00
Total assets (general fund only)	$339,055,010.00	$347,278,187.00	$384,551,932.00	$403,459,670.00

LIQUIDITY RATIOS

Current ratio	2.3	1.6	1.5	1.7
Definition: Total current assets / Total current liabilities				
Total current assets (general fund only)	$110,521,790.00	$118,237,279.00	$113,813,971.00	$92,255,629.00
Total current liabilities (general fund only)	$48,603,946.00	$72,234,880.00	$75,507,585.00	$53,932,358.00
Quick ratio	2.1	1.5	1.4	1.6
Definition: (Total current assets – Inventory) / Total current liabilities				
Total current assets (general fund only)	$110,521,790.00	$118,237,279.00	$113,813,971.00	$92,255,629.00
Inventory (general fund only)	$10,018,876.00	$6,729,591.00	$6,962,951.00	$7,474,424.00
Total current liabilities (general fund only)	$48,603,946.00	$72,234,880.00	$75,507,585.00	$53,932,358.00
Days cash on hand	17.2	27.9	15.6	7.1
Definition: (Cash on hand + Market securities) / (Total operating expenses – Depreciation) /365				
Cash on hand (general fund only)	$19,681,648.00	$32,156,613.00	$17,610,303.00	$6,918,137.00
Market securities (temporary investments) (general fund only)	$0.00	$0.00	$0.00	$0.00
Total operating expense	$439,147,746.00	$439,084,709.00	$432,545,968.00	$377,667,512.00
Depreciation expense	$22,616,659.00	$17,701,123.00	$21,479,371.00	$21,412,330.00
Days cash on hand, all sources	63.4	81.3	101.7	160.0
Definition: (Cash on hand + Market securities + Investments) / (Total operating expenses – depreciation expenses) /365				
Cash on hand (general fund only)	$19,681,648.00	$32,156,613.00	$17,610,303.00	$6,918,137.00
Market securities (temporary investments) (general fund only)	$0.00	$0.00	$0.00	$0.00
Investments (general fund only)	$52,629,288.00	$61,748,147.00	$96,899,834.00	$149,230,656.00
Total operating expense	$439,147,746.00	$439,084,709.00	$432,545,968.00	$377,667,512.00
Depreciation expense	$22,616,659.00	$17,701,123.00	$21,479,371.00	$21,412,330.00
Days in net patient accounts receivable	47.6	41.7	48.2	44.6
Definition: (Accounts receivable – Allowances for uncollectible) / (Total operating revenue /365)				
Accounts receivable (general fund only)	$183,116,459.00	$208,154,053.00	$234,270,934.00	$221,427,548.00

Allowances for uncollectible (general fund only)	$132,664,535.00	$162,430,546.00	$179,696,832.00	$173,782,393.00
Total operating revenue (net patient revenue)	$386,525,210.00	$400,346,795.00	$413,002,830.00	$390,082,056.00
Days in net total receivable	58.8	51.4	57.1	50.2

Definition: (Accounts receivable + Notes receivable + Other receivables – Allowances for uncollectible) / (Total operating revenue / 365)

Accounts receivable (general fund only)	$183,116,459.00	$208,154,053.00	$234,270,934.00	$221,427,548.00
Notes receivable (general fund only)	$0.00	$0.00	$0.00	$0.00
Other receivables (general fund only)	$11,846,498.00	$10,605,372.00	$10,022,079.00	$6,055,862.00
Allowances for uncollectible (general fund only)	$132,664,535.00	$162,430,546.00	$179,696,832.00	$173,782,393.00
Total operating revenue (net patient revenue)	$386,525,210.00	$400,346,795.00	$413,002,830.00	$390,082,056.00
Average payment period (days)	42.6	62.4	67.0	55.3

Definition: Total current liabilities / (Total operating expenses + Total other expenses – Depreciation) / 365

Total current liabilities (general fund only)	$48,603,946.00	$72,234,880.00	$75,507,585.00	$53,932,358.00
Total operating expense	$439,147,746.00	$439,084,709.00	$432,545,968.00	$377,667,512.00
Total other expense	$0.00	$944,991.00	$0.00	$0.00
Depreciation expense	$22,616,659.00	$17,701,123.00	$21,479,371.00	$21,412,330.00

ACTIVITY RATIOS

Inventory turnover	42.2	66.5	64.6	57.6

Definition: (Total operating revenue + Nonoperating revenue) / Inventory

Total operating revenue (net patient revenue)	$386,525,210.00	$400,346,795.00	$413,002,830.00	$390,082,056.00
Nonoperating revenue (nonpatient revenue)	$36,527,105.00	$47,063,315.00	$37,025,334.00	$40,113,376.00
Inventory (general fund only)	$10,018,876.00	$6,729,591.00	$6,962,951.00	$7,474,424.00
Total asset turnover	1.2	1.3	1.2	1.1

Definition: (Total operating revenue + Nonoperating revenue) / Total assets

Total operating revenue (net patient revenue)	$386,525,210.00	$400,346,795.00	$413,002,830.00	$390,082,056.00
Nonoperating revenue (nonpatient revenue)	$36,527,105.00	$47,063,315.00	$37,025,334.00	$40,113,376.00
Total assets (general fund only)	$339,055,010.00	$347,278,187.00	$384,551,932.00	$403,459,670.00
Average age of plant	13.8	18.3	15.5	6.6

Definition: Accumulated depreciation / Depreciation expense

Accumulated depreciation	$312,510,684.00	$323,110,889.00	$333,323,022.00	$141,225,357.00

(continued)

(continued from previous page)

Depreciation expense	$22,616,659.00	$17,701,123.00	$21,479,371.00	$21,412,330.00
Personnel expense as a percent of total operating revenue	41.90%	42.30%	39.90%	45.80%

*Definition: (Salary expense + Contract labor + Fringe benefits) / Total operating revenue * 100*

Salary expense	$116,760,383.00	$117,450,538.00	$116,029,482.00	$114,008,926.00
Contract labor	$37,853,003.00	$42,326,811.00	$45,261,139.00	$56,208,185.00
Fringe benefits	$7,444,288.00	$9,742,577.00	$3,653,311.00	$8,620,180.00
Total operating revenue (net patient revenue)	$386,525,210.00	$400,346,795.00	$413,002,830.00	$390,082,056.00

CAPITAL RATIOS

Long-term debt to net assets	4.90	2.48	2.51	2.24

Definition: Total long-term liabilities / (Total assets − Total liabilities)

Total long-term liabilities (general fund only)	$241,259,686.00	$196,009,777.00	$220,989,190.00	$241,674,436.00
Total assets (general fund only)	$339,055,010.00	$347,278,187.00	$384,551,932.00	$403,459,670.00
Total liabilities (general fund only)	$289,863,632.00	$268,244,657.00	$296,496,775.00	$295,606,794.00
Total debt to net assets	5.89	3.39	3.37	2.74

Definition: Total liabilities / (Total assets − Total liabilities)

Total assets (general fund only)	$339,055,010.00	$347,278,187.00	$384,551,932.00	$403,459,670.00
Total liabilities (general fund only)	$289,863,632.00	$268,244,657.00	$296,496,775.00	$295,606,794.00

APPENDIX F. COASTAL MEDICAL CENTER: LEADERSHIP SURVEY

PERCEIVED CORPORATE CULTURE

Item	Positive %	Neutral %	Negative %
1. Leadership	28	9	63
2. Structure	22	14	64
3. Control	66	20	14
4. Accountability	20	7	73
5. Teamwork	26	7	67
6. Organization identity	31	17	52
7. Work climate	17	17	66
8. Risk taking	15	9	76
9. Conflict management	24	24	52
10. Perceived autonomy	51	12	37
11. Results oriented	29	20	51
12. Mutual trust	36	8	56
13. Communication	24	7	69
14. Team spirit	7	21	72
15. Attitudes	21	22	57
16. Vision	19	5	76
17. Reward system	36	27	37
18. Group interaction	20	45	35
19. Value of meetings	26	7	67
20. Faith in organization	28	6	66

SELF-EVALUATION OF POSITION

Item	True %	Partly True %	Not True %
1. Sufficient decision-making authority	34	50	16
2. Clear understanding of role	43	30	27
3. Clear understanding of performance expectations	26	44	30
4. Fully use training and experience	27	33	40
5. Mix of management and routine is correct	33	30	37
6. Amount of work is reasonable	28	32	40
7. Work offers challenge, satisfaction, and growth	30	30	40
8. Performance is recognized	38	32	30
9. Compensation is satisfactory	45	35	20
10. Quality work is recognized and rewarded	29	41	30
11. Upward communication is effective	21	40	39
12. Downward communication is effective	17	50	33
13. Cross communication is effective	15	55	30
14. Operations problem solving is timely and thorough	17	43	40
15. Strategic decisions are timely and effective	26	30	44

APPENDIX G. COASTAL MEDICAL CENTER: VALUE-BASED PURCHASING

	CMC	JMC	LMC	State Average	National Average
Accreditation	Yes	Yes	Yes		
EmergencyService	Yes	Yes	Yes		
EmergencyVolume	High	Very high	Medium		
AverageTimePatientsSpentinEDBeforeAdmitted asInpatient	624 min.	338 min.	247 min.	282 min.	272 min.
AverageTimePatientsSpentinEDAfterAdmitOrder BeforeinaBed	277 min.	132 min.	92 min.	108 min.	97 min.
AverageTimePatientsSpentinEDBeforeBeingSent Home	226 min.	151 min.	145 min.	143 min.	133 min.
AverageTimePatientsSpentinEDBeforeSeenby HealthProfessional	55 min.	35 min.	33 min.	23 min.	24 min.
AverageTimePatientsSpentinEDWithBrokenBones BeforePainMed	84 min.	72 min.	57 min.	56 min.	55 min.
%ofPatientsLeftWithoutBeingSeen	8%	4%	1%	2%	2%
HeartAttackPatientsGivenAspirinatDischarge	99%	99%	100%	99%	99%
HeartAttackPatientsGivenStatinPrescriptionat Discharge	97%	99%	100%	99%	98%
HeartAttackPatientsGivenPCIWithin90Minutesof Arrival	88%	95%	95%	97%	96%
HeartFailurePatientsGivenACEInhibitororARBfor LeftVentric	95%	96%	98%	98%	97%
HeartFailurePatientsGivenanEvaluationofLVS Function	99%	100%	100%	100%	99%

(continued)

(continued from previous page)

HeartFailurePatientsGivenDischargeInstructions	80%	92%	94%	96%	95%
PneumoniaPatientsGiventheMostAppropriateInitial Antibiotic	90%	95%	92%	98%	96%
SurgeryPatientsWhoReceivedPreventative AntibioticsOneHou	97%	99%	99%	99%	99%
SurgeryPatientsWhosePreventativeAntibioticsare StoppedWi	92%	98%	98%	99%	98%
SurgeryPatientsTakingBetaBlockersRemainon BetaBlockers	98%	98%	98%	99%	98%
SurgeryPatientsGiventheRightAntibioticAfter Surgery	96%	98%	99%	99%	99%
HeartSurgeryPatientsWhoseBloodSugarKeptin Control24H	90%	98%	100%	96%	94%
SurgeryPatientsWhoseUrinaryCathetersRemoved FirstorSecondDay	93%	95%	98%	98%	98%
PatientsHavingSurgeryWarmedinORorNormal TempatEndofSurg	99%	100%	100%	100%	100%
IschemicStrokePatientsWhoReceivedMedtoBreak UpClotsWi3Hrs	N/A	62%	89%	81%	73%
IschemicStrokePatientsWhoReceivedMedtoPrevent ComplicWi2Da	95%	98%	100%	98%	98%
StrokePatientsReceivingBloodThinnersWi2Days	95%	99%	99%	97%	95%

Healthcare-Associated Infections	Comparison to National Benchmark		
	CMC	JMC	LMC
Central line–associated bloodstream infections	No different	No different	Better
Catheter-associated urinary tract infections	Worse	Worse	No different
Surgical-site infections from colon surgery	No different	No different	Better
Surgical site infections from hysterectomy	Worse	No different	No different
Methicillin-resistant *Staph. aureus* (MRSA)	Worse	No different	No different
Clostridium difficile (*C.diff.*)	Worse	No different	Better

APPENDIX H. COASTAL MEDICAL CENTER: INPATIENT DATA

Trend Report

Inpatient Utilization Statistics	2015	2014	2013	2012
Case-mix index	1.666	1.692	1.713	1.729
Medical MS-DRGs	66.26%	65.57%	65.00%	65.38%
Surgical MS-DRGs	33.74%	34.43%	35.00%	34.62%
Routine discharges to home	5,729	5,343	5,110	5,092
Discharges to other acute care hospitals	85	94	94	81
Discharges to skilled nursing facilities	1,360	1,346	1,238	1,305
Deaths	404	289	330	314
Other discharges	2,120	2,171	1,962	1,661
Total discharges	9,698	9,243	8,734	8,453
Psychiatric discharges (DPU, included in total)	493	508	451	443
Rehabilitation discharges (DPU, included in total)	139	171	141	166
Medicare Advantage (HMO) discharges (not included in total)	942	1,872	2,308	2,518

2015 Statistics for the Top 20 Base MS-DRGs

Base MS-DRG Description	Base MS-DRG	IPPS Cases	ALOS	Average Charges ($)	Average Payment ($)	Average Cost ($)	Case-Mix Index	CC/MCC Rate (%)	MCC Rate (%)
Percutaneous cardiovascular proc with drug-eluting stent	247-246	625	2.5	74,651	15,101	18,173	2.181	16.3	16.3
Septicemia or severe sepsis without MV, 96+ hours	872-871	372	5.7	37,703	12,184	10,773	1.750	83.3	83.3
Circulatory disorders except AMI, with cardiac catheter	287-286	369	2.9	29,818	8,016	6,933	1.192	12.2	0.1
Psychoses	885	358	11.4	32,643	9,090	15,899	.954	0.0	0.0
Major joint replacement or reattachment of lower extremity	470-469	341	2.7	51,019	15,705	14,908	2.165	5.3	5.3
Heart failure and shock	293-292-291	321	4.9	22,240	8,064	7,189	1.161	84.7	40.5
Cardiac arrhythmia and conduction disorders	310-309-308	235	3.8	18,250	5,860	5,572	.846	66.8	28.9
Simple pneumonia and pleurisy	195-194-193	201	4.3	21,561	8,363	6,482	1.171	88.6	41.8
Renal failure	684-683-682	195	4.7	26,116	8,336	7,983	1.192	90.3	39.0
Chronic obstructive pulmonary disease	192-191-190	194	4.0	19,327	7,055	5,795	1.020	82.0	47.9
Intracranial hemorrhage or cerebral infarction	066-065-064	175	4.2	27,743	9,202	8,564	1.333	80.0	37.1
Rehabilitation	946-945	161	12.5	58,027	18,985	25,646	1.302	73.3	0.0
Chest pain	313	151	2.0	13,040	3,075	3,498	.562	0.0	0.0

(continued)

(continued from previous page)

Esophagitis, gastroenterological, and miscellaneous digestive disorders	392-391	143	3.7	22,967	5,629	6,152	.839	22.4	22.4
Gastrointestinal hemorrhage	379-378-377	130	4.1	27,877	8,333	8,311	1.202	95.4	26.2
Extracranial procedures	039-038-037	127	2.1	37,900	9,886	8,455	1.315	29.1	7.9
Kidney and urinary tract infections	690-689	114	4.2	20,054	6,347	6,036	.945	41.2	41.2
Other vascular procedures	254-253-252	113	5.0	63,355	17,428	16,646	2.342	62.8	31.0
Permanent cardiac pacemaker implant	244-243-242	108	4.2	62,635	19,251	13,980	2.681	61.1	25.0
Acute myocardial infarction, discharged alive	282-281-280	105	4.8	37,112	10,517	10,275	1.422	84.8	53.3
All other base MS-DRGs		3,915	5.4	54,080	14,658	14,758	2.058		
TOTAL		8,453	5.0	45,557	12,506	12,827	1.729		

2015 Statistics by Medical Service

	Number Medicare Inpatients	Average Length of Stay	Average Charges ($)	Average Cost ($)	Medicare CMI	CMI-Adjusted Average Cost ($)
Cardiology	1,513	3.6	23,498	6,550	1.030	6,362
Cardiovascular surgery	1,123	3.9	86,224	21,103	2.909	7,255
Gynecology	38	2.1	36,756	8,613	1.084	7,944
Medicine	1,691	5.3	33,073	10,221	1.283	7,967
Neurology	502	4.3	27,248	8,378	1.200	6,982
Neurosurgery	42	9.5	114,058	30,272	3.492	8,669
Obstetrics	12	5.2	20,415	9,146	.687	13,324
Oncology	101	5.5	39,450	11,021	1.638	6,729
Orthopedic surgery	795	3.8	61,015	17,228	2.369	7,271
Orthopedics	145	4.1	23,034	7,127	1.060	6,725
Psychiatry	459	10.5	30,824	14,766	.924	15,989
Pulmonology	796	4.9	32,695	9,258	1.419	6,522
Surgery	513	8.8	100,849	27,114	3.858	7,027
Surgery for malignancy	37	6.9	89,678	22,285	2.138	10,425
Urology	420	4.5	27,637	8,082	1.199	6,742
Vascular surgery	265	3.7	52,825	13,205	1.886	7,002
TOTAL	8,453	4.98	45,557	12,827	1.729	7,421

LEADERSHIP, MISSION, VISION, AND CULTURE: THE FOUNDATION FOR STRATEGIC PLANNING

Leadership is the capacity to translate vision into reality.

—Warren Bennis

Innovation distinguishes between a leader and a follower.

—Steve Jobs

LEARNING OBJECTIVES

After you have studied this chapter, you should be able to

➤ develop an understanding of the healthcare system and its organizational complexity, including the role of healthcare leaders as they make decisions and formulate strategy;

➤ understand the importance of board and medical staff leadership;

➤ understand the role and importance of organizational structure and governance;

➤ discuss complex issues in the healthcare industry from the perspective of previous leadership literature;

➤ apply leadership and managerial principles to organizational and systemwide problems in healthcare;

➤ understand the importance of an organization's mission, vision, and values in healthcare strategic planning;

➤ discuss leadership's role in developing an organizational culture of ethics and professionalism; and

➤ compare systems and techniques to measure an organization's own performance and the performance of other organizations.

KEY TERMS AND CONCEPTS

➤ Board of directors

➤ Chief executive officer

➤ Chief financial officer

➤ Chief information officer

➤ Chief medical officer

➤ Chief nursing officer

➤ Credentialing

➤ Culture

➤ Fiduciary

➤ For-profit hospital

➤ Goals

➤ Health information technology

➤ Incentive

➤ Infrastructure

➤ Internal data

➤ Joint venture

➤ Leadership

➤ Magnet hospital designation

➤ Medical staff

➤ Mission

➤ Not-for-profit hospital

➤ Organizational culture

➤ Senior marketing executive

➤ Servant leadership

➤ Stakeholder

➤ Systems approach

➤ Values

➤ Vision

INTRODUCTION

Healthcare spending in the United States reached $2.9 trillion in 2013 (CMS 2014). This figure was up from $2.1 trillion in 2006—a 38 percent increase (Catlin et al. 2008). It represents an expenditure of $7,026 per person in 2006, climbing to $9,255 per person in 2013. As a percentage of the US economy, healthcare spending was 16 percent of the gross domestic product (GDP) in 2006 and 17.4 percent of the GDP in 2013. During 2013, the largest component of healthcare expenditures was hospital care, which increased 4.3 percent from the prior year, to $936.9 billion. The second largest component was physician services, which in 2013 increased 3.8 percent to $586.7 billion. The third largest component was prescription drugs—$271.1 billion in 2013. Nursing care facilities ranked fourth at $155.8 billion.

Healthcare costs are increasing at a significant rate, and the industry needs leaders who can allocate resources more efficiently. Research shows that, taken as a group, hospitals are one of the largest employers in the country, and they are critical to attracting new business to a geographic area. Healthcare also contributes to the United States' economic and social well-being; 18.5 million Americans were employed in healthcare in 2015 (BLS 2015). The US hospital industry comprises a wide range of hospitals of varying size (see Exhibits 1.1 and 1.2).

Organizations, like people, have personalities. This personality develops over time and is shaped by the organization's history, the environment in which it operates, and the beliefs of its key individuals. These factors are reflected in the organization's mission, vision, and culture.

The healthcare field changes constantly. As a result, healthcare organizations, like individuals, must continually adapt to survive and prosper. They must develop a culture that supports change and periodically evaluate their mission, vision, and values to make sure they are relevant in the current environment. This evaluation provides a foundation for the strategic planning process.

Growth is important to an organization's future success. It helps the organization recruit physicians and provides greater economies of scale (see Highlight 1.1), which can result in increased profitability. To grow, organizations need effective **infrastructures**, high-performance work processes, and skilled personnel, and they must provide their employees with appropriate **incentives**. Most important to growth is good strategy development, which is a product of excellent leadership and diversity of individuals and expertise. Strategic planning is an effective way for organizations to improve their allocation of resources (see Highlight 1.2). Resources need to be allocated in a way that allows organizations to provide healthcare services as efficiently as possible. Research has shown that the efficient allocation of healthcare resources in the production process is linked to improved quality (Vigen, Duncan, and Coughlin 2013). The following section discusses the role of hospital leaders, particularly their function in strategic planning.

Infrastructure
Underlying foundation or basic framework.

Incentive
Reward that motivates someone to take action or perform, such as a bonus payment awarded for achieving a goal.

Exhibit 1.1
US Hospitals by Category, 2005 to 2014

Type	2005	2014	Change (no.)	Change (%)
Government, federal	229	210	−19	−8
Government, nonfederal	1,435	1,294	−141	−9.8
Not-for-profit	3,204	3,118	−86	−2.7
For-profit	1,480	1,661	181	12.2
Total	**6,348**	**6,283**	−65	−1

Source: Data from AHA (2005, 2014).

EXHIBIT 1.2
US Hospitals
by Bed Size,
Category, and Year

	2005	2014	Change (no.)	Change (%)
Bed size 0–99				
Government, federal	100	94	–6	–6
Government, nonfederal	879	832	–47	–5
Not-for-profit	1,393	1,429	36	2.5
For-profit	948	1,040	92	9.7
Bed size 100–199				
Government, federal	45	45	0	0
Government, nonfederal	256	181	–75	–29
Not-for-profit	743	655	–88	–12
For-profit	340	335	–5	–1.5
Bed size 200–299				
Government, federal	31	33	2	6.4
Government, nonfederal	117	110	–7	–6
Not-for-profit	456	405	–51	–11
For-profit	119	120	1	0.8
Bed size 300–399				
Government, federal	20	17	–3	–15
Government, nonfederal	74	54	–20	–27
Not-for-profit	279	245	–34	–12
For-profit	45	56	11	24.4
Bed size 400+				
Government, federal	33	21	–12	–36
Government, nonfederal	109	117	8	7.3
Not-for-profit	333	384	51	15
For-profit	28	110	82	293
Total				
Government, federal	229	210	–19	–8
Government, nonfederal	1,435	1,294	–141	–9.8
Not-for-profit	3,204	3,118	–86	–2.7
For-profit	1,480	1,661	181	12.2
Overall total	6,328	6,283	45	–0.7

Source: Data from AHA (2005, 2014).

DEFINITION OF LEADERSHIP

At the most basic level, **leadership** is the ability to guide, influence, and inspire individuals to meet goals (for the purposes of this book, organizational goals). Competency models that focus on leadership in the healthcare environment have been developed by many organizations, including the Healthcare Leadership Alliance (HLA) and the National Center for Healthcare Leadership (NCHL; see Highlight 1.3). Based on the most current research, these models identify behaviors and technical skills (competencies) that characterize outstanding leadership performance.

Leadership
Ability to guide,
influence, and inspire
individuals to meet
organizational goals.

HIGHLIGHT 1.1 Economies of Scale

The principle of *economies of scale* is based on the premise that an organization will be able to achieve greater savings if it is providing for a large number of patients (and employing a large number of providers) rather than just a few. A larger number of patients creates a need for a higher volume of supplies. As the volume of supplies in an organization increases, it becomes possible to buy those supplies in bulk instead of individually. When an organization buys in bulk, the average cost it has to pay per unit usually decreases. For an everyday example, you experience economies of scale if you buy your soda in a 12-pack rather than individually—you might spend $4.99 for 12 cans (or $0.42 each) rather than $1 for one can in a vending machine.

 HIGHLIGHT 1.2 Allocation of Resources

Allocation of resources is how an organization plans to spend its money as well as how it will focus the efforts of its employees and use its other resources. Because the resources of every organization are limited, the leadership team must decide which projects are most important and which are not important enough to invest in. For example, a hospital might have to choose between implementing an electronic health record system (going paperless) and buying new equipment for the imaging department.

Stakeholder
One who is involved in or affected by an organization's actions.

Board of directors
Governing body appointed to hold fiduciary responsibility for the organization.

Chief executive officer (CEO)
Highest-ranking executive in an organization, responsible for strategic planning, hiring senior leadership, and managing operations.

Fiduciary
An individual or a group who acts for and on behalf of another in a relationship of trust and confidence.

In the rapidly changing healthcare environment, strategic planning is becoming increasingly important to overall organizational success. Strategic planning involves the development of organizational objectives (i.e., what the organization wants to accomplish), the management of action plans, and the measurement of ongoing performance. An important part of strategic planning is the development of relationships with **stakeholders**, which include the board of directors, the leadership team, hospital staff, physicians, patients, local employers, insurers, community groups, and government agencies.

In healthcare organizations, the **board of directors** and the **chief executive officer (CEO)** are at the top of the leadership structure. The *board of directors* is the governing body appointed to hold **fiduciary** responsibility for the organization. (Piedmont Healthcare's board of directors is illustrated in Exhibit 1.3. Piedmont Healthcare is a large, not-for-profit health system based in Atlanta, Georgia.) As part of this responsibility, the board makes policy decisions, which guide the future of the organization. An essential area of

HIGHLIGHT 1.3 The Healthcare Leadership Alliance and the National Center for Healthcare Leadership

The HLA is a consortium of the nation's premier professional healthcare administration associations, representing more than 140,000 healthcare management professionals. The goal of the alliance is to pursue common interests and advance the healthcare management profession. It uses the combined knowledge and experience of its members to improve the field of healthcare management. These organizations are

- the American College of Healthcare Executives,

- the American Organization of Nurse Executives,

- the Healthcare Financial Management Association,

- the Healthcare Information and Management Systems Society, and

- the Medical Group Management Association.

The HLA (2013) categorizes key competencies under five domains: communication and relationship management, leadership, professionalism, knowledge of the healthcare environment, and business knowledge.

The NCHL is a nonprofit organization dedicated to ensuring high-quality, relevant, and accountable leadership for healthcare organizations in the twenty-first century. This is accomplished by using competency-based leadership models, benchmarking against best-in-class organizations, and establishing standards of best practice. It also supports evidence-based research, innovation, and quality improvement. The NCHL (2015) strives to improve the abilities of healthcare leaders to improve healthcare in the United States through research, publications, benchmarking, and formation of leadership networks.

Health information technology
Information and communication technology in healthcare, such as electronic health records, clinical alerts and reminders, and decision support systems.

the board of directors' responsibility is the development of a strategic plan consistent with the organization's mission and vision.

Many believe that an organizational culture that embraces continuous quality improvement (CQI; see Highlight 1.4) is necessary for long-term success and that the board of directors should focus on measuring performance to ensure healthcare quality. The Institute of Medicine (IOM; see Highlight 1.5) believes that improving healthcare will require changes to the structure and processes of the delivery system as well as a focus on coordination of care across all services. In addition, successful delivery of healthcare in the future will depend on the use of **health information technology**, such as electronic health records.

EXHIBIT 1.3
Sample Board
of Directors
(Piedmont
Healthcare,
Atlanta, Georgia)

Board of Directors	Number
Physician directors	6
Chief executive officer	1
Community directors	8
Treasurer (chief financial officer), ex officio	1
Government, federal	1

The *CEO* is the highest-ranking executive in an organization and is responsible for strategic planning, hiring senior leadership, and managing operations. The CEO is often a member of the board of directors and is an important interface between the board and operations. The CEO also represents the organization to key stakeholders, including regulatory authorities and community groups. A competent CEO emphasizes organizational

---

✱ HIGHLIGHT 1.4 Continuous Quality Improvement

The idea behind CQI is that no process or service is perfect and that an organization must continually strive to eliminate errors from its system to get closer and closer to perfection. The study and championing of CQI have taken many forms in many industries and have become an important aspect of healthcare management.

Healthcare organizations often use CQI to measure their performance. A hospital may collect data about one of its processes and compare these data to the data of other hospitals in the area and around the country. For example, a hospital may keep track of how often its patients are given the wrong medicine or the wrong dose of a medicine and then compare its results to national standards. If the hospital has a higher frequency of errors than the national standard, the hospital might implement a CQI program to try to improve the statistic. Such a program would involve studying the processes that lead to errors, recommending changes to improve the processes, implementing the changes, and then collecting the data once again for measurement against the national standards to see if the improvement has been achieved. The main principle behind CQI is that quality should be constantly under investigation and, thus, that the organization is always working to improve.

HIGHLIGHT 1.5 Institute of Medicine

The IOM was founded in 1970 as a nongovernmental, nonprofit organization that would provide impartial information and advice about healthcare in the United States. It is part of the National Academies. The IOM's aim is to help those in government and the private sector make informed health decisions by providing reliable information. Many of the studies that the IOM undertakes begin as specific mandates from Congress; others are requested by federal agencies and independent organizations. The IOM (2015) also convenes a series of forums, roundtables, and standing committees, as well as other activities, to facilitate discussion, discovery, and critical thinking.

The IOM has published studies on the state of healthcare that have drawn a lot of attention; for example, in 2000 it disclosed the high number of medical errors occurring in hospitals in its report *To Err Is Human*, and in subsequent reports it continued to identify the health field's progress on quality. More recently, the IOM issued publications such as *Future Directions of Credentialing Research in Nursing*, *Research Priorities to Inform Public Health and Medical Practice for Ebola Virus Disease*, and *Investing in the Health and Well-Being of Young Adults*.

transformation by envisioning, energizing, and fostering change. Analytical and innovative thinking, a community orientation, and strategic planning are essential to this focus. At the execution level, CEOs must demonstrate an ability to communicate, manage change, influence staff, and measure performance. They also need to possess excellent people skills; they must build relationships, uphold professional ethics, develop talent, and lead teams. Most important, CEOs should focus on organizational values, direction, and performance expectations.

THE BOARD OF DIRECTORS' ROLE IN STRATEGIC PLANNING

Hospitals with a high-functioning board of directors perform better and are more profitable (Collum et al. 2014). In particular, outstanding hospital boards are composed of external members who are committed to the strategic planning process. Also important is the board's relationship to the community. A collaborative, community-oriented board stays in touch with the needs of the local population and develops new services to meet those needs. Such services can improve the health and well-being of the community as well as enhance the reputation of the healthcare organization.

Board participation in the strategic planning process helps build consensus among senior leadership and staff about the organization's future direction. Board members' involvement in subcommittees, board meetings, and strategic planning retreats can all increase the board's participation in strategic planning.

CEO succession is one of the board's most important responsibilities (Bowen 2014). Leadership development should be based on future needs of the organization as identified through the strategic planning process. Because the board plays an integral part in the strategic planning process and in defining the organization's mission, logic dictates that it be involved in leadership development to ensure future success. Additionally, the board should evaluate leadership's recommendations for new service lines (see Highlight 1.6) and monitor the quality of care provided by the organization.

THE CEO'S ROLE IN STRATEGIC PLANNING

A senior leadership team is an important asset to an organization and can give it a competitive advantage in the marketplace. High-performing senior leadership teams use formal management processes to improve efficiency and enhance quality. Research has found that these high-performance work processes result in better value in healthcare services (Harrison and Meyer 2014).

In 2006, the CEO turnover rate among US hospitals was 16 percent, resulting in approximately 700 CEO transitions annually (Cirillo 2006). However, the rate of hospital CEO turnover increased to 20 percent in 2013, which represented the highest rate of hospital CEO turnover since 1981 (Bowen 2014).

A competent CEO is critical to the future success of the organization, so the board should help a new CEO develop team-building skills and the financial knowledge necessary to support the strategic planning process. In addition to maximizing performance, effective team building ensures that everyone in the organization is on the same page and that transitions to new leadership are smooth. In 2015, the median compensation for a

---

(*) HIGHLIGHT 1.6 Service Lines

Service lines are specialty areas of care provided by a healthcare organization—for example, cardiology, oncology, orthopedics, or transplantation services. Organizations may provide full-service care, or they may specialize in just a few service lines and strive to excel in those areas. In general, some service lines—such as cardiology—are lucrative; other service lines—such as emergency departments in areas with a high uninsured population—may be unprofitable.

CEO in a freestanding hospital with total net revenue less than $250 million was $456,000 (ACHE 2015).

The CEO, in consultation with the board, is ultimately responsible for creating and implementing the strategic plan. The strategic planning process should also include physicians and other staff in the organization.

OTHER KEY LEADERSHIP ROLES
THE CHIEF FINANCIAL OFFICER

The **chief financial officer (CFO)** is responsible for planning, organizing, and directing all financial activities, including budgeting, cost accounting, patient accounting, payer relations (see Highlight 1.7), and investing. The CFO normally reports directly to the CEO. In 2015, the median compensation for a CFO in a freestanding hospital with total net revenue less than $250 million was $309,000 (ACHE 2015).

The CFO is critical to the development of the strategic plan because of his responsibility for projecting workload and providing financial data. Key data include growth projections, market share, departmental budgets, and performance measures. Thus, the CFO needs to understand financial modeling (see Highlight 1.8). Gathering and providing accurate and timely information are often the most difficult parts of the strategic planning process. In a small hospital, the CFO also often functions as the project manager for strategic planning.

THE CHIEF NURSING OFFICER

The **chief nursing officer (CNO)** is responsible for planning, organizing, and directing all nursing activities, including policy development, implementation of nurse staffing models

Chief financial officer (CFO)
Executive responsible for planning, organizing, and directing all financial activities.

Chief nursing officer (CNO)
Nurse executive responsible for planning, organizing, and directing all nursing activities.

(✳) HIGHLIGHT 1.7 Payer Relations

Healthcare in the United States is an unusual service industry in that a single transaction of care usually involves three parties: the person receiving the care (i.e., the patient), the person or the organization providing the care (i.e., the physician or nurse, or the hospital or physician practice), and the party paying for the care (i.e., the payer). The payer may be an insurance company, a health plan, or even the government (e.g., Medicare, Medicaid).

Payer relations is the term used to describe the interactions of the healthcare provider with the payer. The provider's activity can include negotiating contracts regarding the amounts to be paid for specific procedures, educating payers about new procedures, and building and maintaining good relationships with payers.

⊛ HIGHLIGHT 1.8 Financial Modeling

Financial modeling is the construction of a formula or program, either by computer or on paper, to predict what might happen if certain financial decisions are made. By plugging different numbers into the formula to see how they change the results, a financial modeler can better decide the best course of action for an organization.

For example, say the CFO of a hospital wants to know what the financial impact would be if the facility's surgical staff increased the number of operations it performed per week. The CFO would construct a financial model that takes into account the additional costs (more staff, more supplies, more wear and tear on the equipment, more patients in the recovery rooms) and the additional revenue (more operations and, therefore, more money collected). On the basis of the calculation, the CFO would be able to make an informed decision about whether increasing the number of operations would be profitable for the hospital.

(see Highlight 1.9), and ongoing quality improvement efforts. The CNO normally reports to the CEO. In 2015, the median compensation for a CNO in a hospital with total net revenue less than $250 million was $200,000 (ACHE 2015).

Nursing leaders are important participants in the organization's decision-making processes and should be involved in strategic planning. They can provide a valuable perspective on resource allocation, the marketing of new services, and quality enhancement. In 2011, the American Hospital Association (AHA) surveyed more than 1,000 hospital boards and found that 6 percent of board members were nurses; 20 percent were physicians (Hassmiller and Combes 2012). According to the IOM (2011) *Future of Nursing* report, "Public, private, and governmental health care decision makers at every level should include representation from nursing on boards, on executive management teams, and in other key leadership positions." To achieve **Magnet hospital designation**, hospitals must document the nurse executive's role in the senior leadership decision-making process.

Magnet hospital designation
Status awarded by the American Nurses Credentialing Center to hospitals whose nursing staff meets certain criteria based on quality and professional practice.

THE CHIEF INFORMATION OFFICER

The **chief information officer (CIO)** is responsible for planning, organizing, and directing all of the organization's information systems (e.g., enterprise information systems, clinical information systems, electronic health records) and often manages the organization's telecommunication systems. From a strategic planning perspective, the CIO has an important role in systems design and analysis. In some cases, the CIO reports to the CFO; however, the CIO may more appropriately report to the CEO. In 2015, the median compensation for a CIO in a hospital with total net revenue less than $250 million was $210,000 (ACHE 2015).

Chief information officer (CIO)
Executive responsible for planning, organizing, and directing all information systems in the organization.

HIGHLIGHT 1.9 Nurse Staffing Models

How many nurses are needed to staff a hospital unit? This question is tricky; the answer is not simply a ratio of patients to nurses. Nurse staffing models are guidelines a hospital unit uses to determine how many and what kind of nurses are needed to care for the patients on that unit. Nurse staffing models take into account

- the number of patients on the unit,

- how sick each patient is,

- what kind of technology and other aids are available to help the nurses perform their work, and

- the nurses' and other caregivers' level of training.

The mix of these factors affects how well patients recover from their illnesses. A mix that is deficient in some way can even cause hospitalized patients to become more ill. This potential illustrates the importance of a proper nurse staffing model.

The CIO's role is critical because the strategic planning process hinges on the management of information and the use of information systems. Data collection is essential to strategy development and includes gathering both internal and external information. Sources of external data include peer-reviewed articles, professional associations, healthcare websites, databases, community surveys, patient focus groups, interviews with community leaders, and physicians. **Internal data** from leaders, staff, and internal databases are important because they highlight an organization's strengths and weaknesses.

Internal data
Information and facts that can be gathered from sources within an organization.

THE SENIOR MARKETING EXECUTIVE

The **senior marketing executive** is responsible for developing, directing, and executing a comprehensive, systemwide marketing strategy. This strategy includes promoting new and existing programs and services, conducting market research, and advertising via various media. The senior marketing executive typically reports to the CEO. In 2015, the median compensation for a senior marketing executive in a hospital with total net revenue less than $250 million was $183,000 (ACHE 2015).

Senior marketing executive
Executive responsible for developing, directing, and executing a comprehensive, systemwide marketing strategy that includes advertising, market research, production, and sales.

CONSULTANTS

The healthcare environment is extremely complex. As a result, the need for highly skilled technical professionals is increasing. Many healthcare organizations fill this need through the use of consultants. Because consultants are external to the organization, they can review data objectively, challenge the status quo, conduct in-depth research on highly technical topics, and obtain candid opinions from stakeholders.

A wide range of stakeholders and other individuals are involved in strategic planning, and the use of an outside consultant to facilitate the strategic planning process may contribute to improved results. The outside consultant can provide a national perspective on the healthcare field as well as unbiased observations on issues associated with strategic planning. Consulting firms can aid in the strategic planning process and can participate in working groups in the organization that focus on key areas of operation.

On the negative side, consultants come and go, so the organization has access to their technical skills only for the period of their contract. For continuity and stability, many organizations decide to develop the skills of existing employees or recruit these consultants for permanent staff positions.

PHYSICIAN INVOLVEMENT IN HEALTHCARE STRATEGIC PLANNING
THE CHIEF MEDICAL OFFICER

The **chief medical officer (CMO)** is responsible for planning and implementing programs to improve the quality of patient care. The CMO also participates in **medical staff** meetings, **credentialing**, and medical staff recruitment. In larger hospitals, the CMO is usually a full-time employee who reports to the CEO. In 2015, the median compensation for a CMO in a freestanding hospital with total net revenue less than $250 million was $345,000 (ACHE 2015).

CMOs and other physician leaders (also called *clinical leaders*) develop strategic competencies by combining management theory and practical experience to address the healthcare challenges of the twenty-first century. They must be adept at strategic planning, allocating resources, and developing new clinical services. A primary goal is to create value for stakeholders. The most important competencies for physician executives include strong leadership skills, technical expertise, innovation, and a **systems approach** to problem solving.

Under the CMO's direction, senior clinical leaders can improve treatment outcomes by supporting innovation in clinical practice and interdisciplinary collaboration among members of the healthcare delivery team. Physicians are key stakeholders in the organization and play an essential role in developing and marketing new clinical services. Even more important, physicians should be part of the feedback loop in monitoring quality of care.

In response to persistent and systematic shortcomings in quality, the IOM published a landmark report in 2001, *Crossing the Quality Chasm: A New Health System for the 21st Century*, which called for fundamental change in healthcare. The report identified six aims for achieving high-quality care delivery—safety, effectiveness, efficiency, patient-centeredness, timeliness, and equitability—all of which are important to strategic planning. Effective physician leaders need competencies such as strategic planning, mentoring, and budgeting to support organizational goals, improve performance, and ensure efficiency and quality of care (Dubinsky, Feerasta, and Lash 2015).

Chief medical officer (CMO)
Executive responsible for planning and implementing programs to improve the quality of patient care.

Medical staff
Full- and part-time physicians and dentists who are approved and given privileges to provide healthcare to patients in a hospital or another healthcare facility; may be employed by the facility or granted admitting privileges to practice.

Credentialing
Process used to evaluate a physician's qualifications and practice history.

Systems approach
Management that emphasizes the interdependence of elements inside and outside an organization.

The Medical Staff

Physicians and hospital leaders are cofiduciaries for patients' welfare. To be a *fiduciary* for a patient means possessing the knowledge needed to promote the patient's well-being and being committed to using one's expertise for the patient's benefit. This healthcare concept of the cofiduciary draws on organizational ethics as well as a sense of morality.

The management of physician relationships is important and is becoming more complex as the healthcare system evolves. Physician managers must make strategic decisions regarding the employment of primary care physicians, hospitalist physicians, and clinical specialists. For example, hospital emergency departments need physician coverage, and trauma centers need on-call specialty physicians for support. Strategy decisions are also influenced by the increasing competition between hospitals and physician-sponsored outpatient services and other lucrative product lines.

Because physicians are major stakeholders in the healthcare system, they should be involved in business planning regarding the implementation of new clinical services. An outstanding physician reputation is fundamental to developing successful clinical service lines. Therefore, the strategic planning process should include physician input and foster physician support of the organization. To ensure medical staff support and long-term success, physicians should be involved in committees responsible for the review and approval of new business initiatives as well as in financial planning and medical staff development (Epstein 2014).

Unfortunately, as a result of increasing workload and administrative responsibilities, many physicians lack the time to participate in hospital-sponsored meetings, making physician participation in the strategic planning process problematic.

Managed Care Organizations

In the 1980s, conventional fee-for-service health insurance plans began to be replaced by health maintenance organizations (HMOs) and preferred provider organizations (PPOs). By the end of the 1990s, enrollment in HMOs and PPOs had skyrocketed. To attract these enrollees, hospitals needed to contract with these organizations. HMOs and PPOs used this dependency to their advantage and began to reduce the amounts they paid to hospitals for the services they provided. To offset this decrease in income, hospitals had to find ways to maintain their profit margins. They began to emphasize shorter hospital stays for inpatients. If an HMO was reimbursing them at a flat rate regardless of how long the patient stayed in the hospital, shorter stays equated to higher profits. For example, say the HMO was reimbursing the hospital $20,000 for a particular treatment. If a two-day inpatient stay for this treatment cost the hospital $10,000 and a three-day stay cost the hospital $15,000, the hospital would make $10,000 if it limited the patient stay to two days, but only $5,000 if the patient stayed for three days. This pressure to reduce length of stay was even greater for hospitals with low occupancy rates. Unable to adapt and maintain profits in this changing environment, many independent hospitals were forced into bankruptcy, closure, merger with more successful hospitals, or acquisition by another company.

The Affordable Care Act (ACA) of 2010 includes a Centers for Medicare & Medicaid Services proposal to create accountable care organizations (ACOs; see Highlight 1.10). Since that time, more than 360 Medicare ACOs have been established in 47 states, serving more than 5.6 million Medicare beneficiaries. ACOs represent one part of a comprehensive series of initiatives and programs in the ACA that are designed to lower costs and improve care by advancing three key strategies for improving care while investing dollars more wisely: incentives, tools, and information. ACOs in the Pioneer ACO Model and Medicare Shared Savings Program generated more than $372 million in total program savings. This encouraging news comes from preliminary quality and financial results from the second year of performance for 23 Pioneer ACOs and final results from the first year of performance for 220 Shared Savings Program ACOs. Meanwhile, the ACOs outperformed published benchmarks for quality and patient experience in 2013 and improved significantly on almost all measures of quality and patient experience in 2014 (HHS 2014).

Healthcare is produced at the local level, and maximizing the quality and efficiency of healthcare services provides ongoing benefits in these communities. As a result, it is important to put in place structures and processes that improve the delivery of healthcare

---

✱ HIGHLIGHT 1.10 Health Maintenance Organizations, Preferred Provider Organizations, and Accountable Care Organizations

HMOs, PPOs, and ACOs are managed care organizations—that is, insurance providers that are structured to control costs and improve care by using certain strategies, such as offering incentives to care providers who keep their costs of care down and prevent unnecessary treatments.

HMOs contract with hospitals, physicians, and other caregivers to provide care to their clients. In exchange for providing customers to the contracted providers, the HMO is assigned a group of providers who have agreed to abide by the HMO's treatment guidelines. To receive coverage, clients of HMOs must see providers who are part of that HMO's network. In 1973, the US government began to require all employers of at least 25 people to offer an HMO option to their employees.

Groups of providers contract with PPOs to provide care at reduced rates to the PPO's clients. Unlike HMOs, PPOs cover services rendered by out-of-network providers, but at a lower reimbursement rate than that offered for the services of an in-network provider.

Medicare ACOs are groups of doctors, hospitals, and other healthcare providers and suppliers who come together voluntarily to provide coordinated, high-quality care at lower costs to their Medicare patients (HHS 2014).

EXHIBIT 1.4
Healthcare Quality
and Efficiency
Model

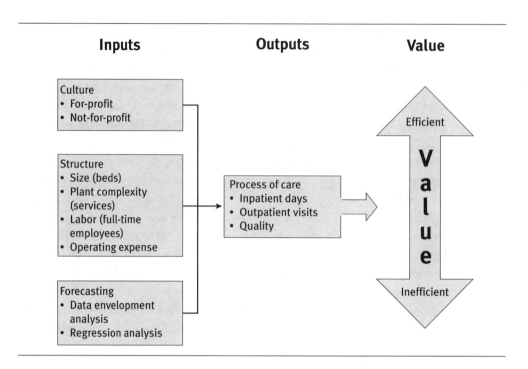

services. Within this context, federal healthcare policy attempts to enhance society's ability to allocate scarce healthcare resources most appropriately across the continuum of healthcare services (see Exhibit 1.4).

THE IMPACT OF MISSION, VISION, AND CULTURE ON PROFITS AND STRATEGIC PLANNING

MISSION

The **mission** of an organization is usually a one-sentence statement describing the fundamental purpose of the organization's existence. In healthcare, an organization's mission is partially determined by ownership status. A hospital may be a not-for-profit organization, a for-profit organization, a government-operated organization, or a joint venture, and this status will shape its mission. A mission statement will help guide decisions about priorities, actions, and responsibilities. Differences in mission reflect different motivations and **goals** and influence the type of strategic plan an organization develops.

Not-for-Profit Hospitals

Not-for-profit hospitals are considered 501(c)(3) organizations by the Internal Revenue Service (IRS; see Highlight 1.11). The 501(c)(3) designation identifies an organization as a corporation that is operated exclusively for religious, charitable, scientific, public safety, literary, or educational purposes. The promotion of health is considered a charitable activity that relieves the government of having to provide healthcare services. As a result,

Mission
Written statement
of an organization's
fundamental purpose.

Goals
Written objectives that
can be measured to
assess performance.

Not-for-profit hospital
Hospital designated as
a 501(c)(3) organization
by the Internal Revenue
Service and eligible for
tax-exempt status.

> ## (✻) HIGHLIGHT 1.11 Internal Revenue Service
>
> The IRS is the US government agency that collects taxes from citizens and corporations and enforces tax law. The IRS has been appointed by Congress to enforce the Internal Revenue Code, which includes complicated tax guidelines for citizens, for-profit corporations, and not-for-profit and charitable organizations.

not-for-profit hospitals receive favorable treatment from the government. They may apply for tax-exempt status, on the condition that they operate exclusively for the welfare of the public, do not have a profit motive, and provide appropriate levels of charity care. In addition to exemption from federal taxes, exemption from property tax, and exemption from tax on bond interest, 501(c)(3) organizations enjoy many benefits, including tax-deductible donations from benefactors. (See Highlight 1.12 for an explanation of these tax concepts.) Large, not-for-profit health systems in the United States include Ascension Health, Kaiser Permanente, and Mayo Clinic.

For-Profit Hospitals

For-profit hospitals are organizations owned by investors, or *shareholders* (for a detailed discussion, see Harrison, Spaulding, and Mouhalis 2015). In contrast to not-for-profit hospitals, their mission is to generate profits for their shareholders. For-profit healthcare organizations must pay federal and state corporate income taxes and local property taxes and should generate appropriate returns for stockholders.

For-profit hospital
Investor-owned hospital that must pay federal and state taxes on its profits.

The modern for-profit healthcare field was born in the late 1960s with the creation of Hospital Corporation of America (HCA) by Dr. Thomas Frist and Jack Massey. Today, HCA operates 178 hospitals in the United States and additional hospitals abroad.

One major advantage of for-profit health systems is their ability to make money through the sale of stock. As a result, they can more easily enact rapid expansion (build or acquire hospitals), renovate their facilities, and purchase new technology. Building or acquiring new hospitals creates economies of scale (see Highlight 1.1), which can improve efficiency and lead to lower costs. The four largest for-profit hospital chains in the United States in 2015 were Community Health Systems in Brentwood, Tennessee; HCA in Nashville, Tennessee; Tenet Healthcare Corporation in Dallas, Texas; and LifePoint Hospitals in Brentwood, Tennessee (Gamble 2014).

Government Hospitals

Government hospitals are operated by state, local, and federal governments to meet specific missions. For example, some states and municipalities operate acute care and psychiatric

> ✳ **HIGHLIGHT 1.12** Tax Exemption, Tax Deduction, Bond Interest, and Bad Debt Write-Off
>
> - *Tax exemption*: The hospital does not have to pay federal or property taxes because it is a charitable organization.
>
> - *Tax deduction*: Any money given to a charitable hospital can be deducted—that is, the donor can claim the contribution on his taxes, and the donated money is subtracted from that person's total taxable income for the year. Lower taxable income means that person pays less income tax. This arrangement motivates people to donate to the charitable hospital, and the hospital thus acquires money.
>
> - *Bond interest*: Buyers of bonds issued by a charitable organization do not have to pay taxes on the interest earned on those bonds. An organization might issue bonds if it wanted to raise funds for new construction or to fund new technology, for example. A bond is purchased for a certain price, and the purchaser receives regular interest payments from the amount invested. After a certain period, the purchaser receives the entire amount back, plus the interest he has been collecting over that period. The exemption from bond interest tax encourages people to purchase such bonds, and the charitable organization thus raises money.
>
> - *Bad debt write-off*: A hospital's *bad debt* is money that other organizations or individuals owe the hospital that will never be paid. The hospital is able to write off the amount of bad debt as an expense to the organization (rather than income as it was originally recorded).

hospitals for low-income patients. The US Department of Defense, Department of Veterans Affairs, Public Health Service, and Department of Justice all operate hospitals. Government hospitals are funded through a process that does not depend on the healthcare market (Harrison and Meyer 2014). Funding for the construction of government hospitals is exempt from many governmental regulations over healthcare, including the National Health Planning and Resources Development Act of 1974 and certificate-of-need review (CON; see Highlight 1.13).

Joint Ventures

Joint venture
Partnership formed between two or more organizations that draws on their combined resources to accomplish a specific purpose.

In healthcare, a **joint venture** is a partnership formed between two or more provider organizations with different missions for purposes of accomplishing a unified mission that draws on their individual strengths. Through joint ventures, healthcare organizations can

HIGHLIGHT 1.13 Regulations: National Health Planning and Resources Development Act of 1974 and Certificate-of-Need Review

These two regulations were created in response to the rising costs of the US health services system and the inequity of access to healthcare across the nation. Before these regulations, healthcare providers were reimbursed (by Medicare and other insurers) even for inefficient or failed care, so they had few incentives to keep costs down. Some areas of the country had too many hospitals and healthcare options, which resulted in duplicate costs (money was spent building and maintaining a hospital when there already was a facility a few blocks away) and uncoordinated care. Other areas (often rural) had no options for reasonably priced healthcare.

The National Health Planning and Resources Development Act was passed in 1974 to enforce more careful planning of health services. Among other things, the act created regional health services agencies and assigned them the responsibility of collecting data so that they could identify needs and deficiencies in the area, develop long-range plans to correct the deficiencies, and provide technical and financial assistance to implement the plans.

CON regulations, which require health services planners to obtain approval from state or federal government to build a new healthcare facility, were implemented to give a structure to the National Health Planning and Resources Development Act. Initially, all 50 states were required to develop a structure through which all new facility proposals had to pass to receive approval. The CON requirements are aimed at reducing healthcare costs and controlling the building of new, potentially unnecessary facilities. Although the mandate was repealed in 1987, 36 states still have a CON program, and the remaining 14 states have some type of regulation over duplication of services (NCSL 2015).

pool their resources (e.g., management expertise), attract new customers, adopt new technologies, spread costs and risks, or meet a community's need for a new healthcare service. Joint ventures also provide opportunities for improved relationships between hospitals and physician groups. Instead of competing with each other, hospitals and physician groups can combine their resources to produce mutually beneficial outcomes. Additionally, a joint venture may streamline the patient care experience. For example, say Physician Group A operates independently of Hospital B. A patient of Physician Group A has a need that it is not able to fulfill. Hospital B, however, has the resources to fulfill that need, so Physician Group A refers the patient to Hospital B. Physician Group A's record-keeping system is different from that of Hospital B, so the transfer of information between hospitals is unlikely to be smooth. Further, Physician Group A will not profit from referring a patient elsewhere. If Hospital B and Physician Group A formed a joint venture, they could adopt a mutual record-keeping system, allowing for seamless transfer of patient information. Further, Physician Group A would not have to direct its business elsewhere. As a partner with Hospital B, it, too, would profit from the services performed by Hospital B.

Joint ventures are located in communities that have more elderly patients, lower unemployment, and fewer HMOs. They also offer more clinical services and have a higher patient occupancy rate, a higher average patient length of stay, lower long-term debt, and a greater number of managed care contracts. Most important, joint ventures can have a positive financial impact on US hospitals; joint ventures provide an opportunity to implement new healthcare services in the local community while allowing the partners to combine their money, people, and facilities for the maximum benefit of all.

Specialty Hospitals

Not-for-profit hospitals, for-profit hospitals, government hospitals, and nongovernment hospitals can be further broken down by specialty, which affects their mission and, hence, strategic planning process. Exhibit 1.5 provides information on the types of specialty hospitals in the United States and the ownership of those hospitals.

VISION

Vision
Short, inspiring statement of what an organization intends to achieve in the future.

An organization's **vision** is a short, inspiring statement of what it intends to achieve in the future. A vision statement should be broad and forward thinking and should specify goals the organization wishes to accomplish over time. A hospital's senior leadership team should create a vision that is meaningful to staff and describes the state of affairs to which the organization aspires.

CULTURE

Culture
Collection of values and norms shared by a group of individuals.

Culture is a collection of **values** and norms shared by a group of people. Organizations have cultures composed of values, customs, and traditions that reflect their ethical beliefs. Senior leadership teams base their decisions on these tenets, and these decisions affect their organization's performance.

Values
Social principles, goals, and standards of an organization.

At the most basic level, society is composed of families who share genetic material and have developed similar values to cope with changes in their environment. Some species (such as *Tyrannosaurus rex*) have become extinct, and some societies (such as that of the Incas) have disappeared, suggesting that animals, humans, and even societies must adapt to survive. Like people, organizations progress through a life cycle that includes birth, growth, maturation, and regeneration or death. Their culture and values dictate how they deal with change as they move through this cycle. In a dynamic, complex industry such as healthcare, an organization's culture must support change if it is to successfully evolve over time.

Type	Government, Federal	Government, Nonfederal	Not-for-Profit	For-Profit	Total
Medical and surgical					
2005	205	1,132	2,762	732	4,831
2014	190	1,033	2,719	741	4,683
Change (no.)	−15	−99	−43	9	−148
Change (%)	−7.3	−9	−1.5	1.2	−3
Psychiatric					
2005	10	205	85	161	461
2014	11	191	99	229	530
Change (no.)	1	−14	14	68	69
Change (%)	10	−6.8	16.5	42	15
OB/GYN					
2005	0	1	9	9	19
2014	0	0	6	6	12
Change (no.)	0	−1	−3	−3	−7
Change (%)	0	−100	−33	−33	−37
Ear, nose, and throat					
2005	0	0	6	0	6
2014	0	0	4	0	4
Change (no.)	0	0	−2	0	−2
Change (%)	0	0	−33	0	−33
Rehabilitation					
2005	1	14	63	155	233
2014	2	8	53	196	259
Change (no.)	1	−6	−10	41	26
Change (%)	100	−43	−16	26	−33
Orthopedic					
2005	0	0	5	18	23
2014	0	1	6	25	32
Change (no.)	0	1	1	7	9
Change (%)	0	100	20	39	39
Children's					
2005	0	18	103	17	138
2014	0	12	107	22	141
Change (no.)	0	−6	4	5	3
Change (%)	0	−33	4	29	2
Other					
2005	8	68	135	424	635
2014	7	49	124	442	622
Change (no.)	−1	−19	−11	18	−13
Change (%)	−12.5	−28	−8	4	−2
All					
2005					6,346
2014					6,283
Change (no.)					−63
Change (%)					−1

EXHIBIT 1.5
US Hospitals by Specialty and Ownership

Source: Data from AHA (2005, 2014).

Organizational culture
Shared beliefs among individuals in an organization.

Organizational culture is an expression of shared beliefs among individuals in an organization. Culture is important because it ensures healthcare professionals are working toward common goals. The development of organizational policies and practices sets the achievement of these goals in motion. Furthermore, organizational culture should give staff members the authority they need to do their jobs and should hold them responsible for their actions. An empowering organizational culture is associated with improved team morale, enhanced healthcare quality, and higher levels of patient satisfaction.

Changing a healthcare organization's culture can improve patient safety (Wick et al. 2015). In particular, a cultural emphasis on quality can play a key role in improved clinical outcomes. Healthcare organizations should provide a positive working environment for clinical providers because physicians and other clinicians who are stressed or dissatisfied with their jobs have a greater incidence of providing suboptimal patient care.

The development of core behaviors that support a common purpose is crucial to achieving improved quality and clinical outcomes. Organizational culture needs to focus on improving clinical processes rather than blaming individuals for suboptimal care. When members of the healthcare team focus on the clinical process, they can clearly see their roles. When there is no confusion about roles, team members will communicate more effectively with each other. In addition, a focus on the clinical process instead of blame encourages the team to think from a position of curiosity and innovation rather than of fear and anxiety.

STRATEGIC PLANNING

Strategic planning is an ongoing process, not a onetime project, based on an organization's mission, vision, and values. In many healthcare organizations, this process begins with an off-site retreat during which the board of directors and senior leadership revisit the organization's mission, vision, and values to ensure they are still valid. The board retreat also serves as a forum in which senior leaders and other stakeholders build consensus on the action to be taken and clarify how they will contribute to and support the planning effort.

A hospital's mission, vision, and strategy must be in sync with the way it allocates its money. Healthcare organizations have limited financial resources, so a hospital's mission, vision, and strategy need to guide its investments. If an organization fails to link its strategic plan to its financial decisions, it may invest in inappropriate technology, equipment, or facilities and end up depleting its resources.

When organizations link their strategic plan to their spending behaviors, their investments benefit them over the long term. They may build new facilities, renovate existing ones, or invest in appropriate new information technology. Historically, many financial decisions were driven solely by physician requests. Unfortunately, many of these decisions had a short-term impact rather than a long-term, lasting effect on their organizations' development.

When an organization's vision lines up with its strategic plan, it maximizes its return on investment (ROI; see Highlight 1.14). By balancing its mission and its need to maintain

> **(✱) HIGHLIGHT 1.14** Return on Investment
>
> ROI is a performance measure used to evaluate the efficiency of an investment. To calculate the ROI, the benefit of the investment is divided by the cost of the investment and expressed as a percentage. A simple formula expresses it:
>
> ROI = (Money gained from investment − Money invested) ÷ Money invested.
>
> A positive result indicates a positive ROI; a negative result indicates a loss. For example, if you buy five lottery tickets at $1.00 each and win $15, the ROI would be ($15 − $5) ÷ $5 = 2 (i.e., 200%). You have a positive ROI. If, however, you win only $3, the ROI would be ($3 − $5) ÷ $5 = −0.4 (or −40%). The ROI is negative—you've lost money.

a competitive advantage, an organization can adjust its strategy (1) to ensure that profitable business initiatives are able to fund unprofitable mission-based activities and (2) to determine when to invest in new programs or close others. The mission, vision, and values statements of Piedmont Healthcare are shown in Exhibit 1.6.

An organization's mission, vision, and values should be the guideposts in assessing organizational performance, and compliance with the organization's values should be a factor in annual employee performance evaluations. In support of its values, the organization should have annual goals and objectives, and part of the performance measurement process should be based on the organization's progress toward their fulfillment.

According to the AHA (2015a) report *Engaging Trustees in the Redefinition of the H* (see Highlight 1.15), an organization's mission and vision should describe its commitment to the community. They should be documented and shared with leadership, physicians, and staff as well as with patients and their families. Organizational leaders should meet regularly with community partners to assess the delivery of healthcare in the community and, on the basis of their evaluation, plan initiatives to improve the community's health status.

An organization's mission in healthcare must include a commitment to quality and patient safety. The concept of **servant leadership** is crucial to this commitment. In a culture that embraces servant leadership, relationships are based on communication and listening. Leaders serve as mentors and teachers to ensure that their staff members become wiser and more autonomous. At the same time, these leaders are followers in that they continually learn from individuals in the organization. Servant leadership creates a culture in which employees are considered partners in the organization's mission, not a disposable resource.

Servant leadership
Culture in which employees become partners in fulfilling the organization's mission.

EXHIBIT 1.6
Sample Mission,
Vision, and Values
Statements
(Piedmont
Healthcare,
Atlanta, Georgia)

Vision
By 2020, Piedmont Healthcare will be nationally recognized as a Top 10 community healthcare system where patients want to go for a superior healthcare experience, dedicated professionals want to work, and the best physicians want to practice.

Mission
Healthcare marked by compassion and sustainable excellence in a progressive environment, guided by physicians, delivered by exceptional professionals, and inspired by the communities we serve

Values
- Compassion: Caring for every person every day with dignity and respect
- Commitment: Dedicating ourselves to improving the lives of others
- Service: Providing a safe and supportive environment to ask, learn, and heal
- Excellence: Leading in quality through expertise, innovation, and technology
- Balance: Using resources efficiently and effectively

 HIGHLIGHT 1.15 American Hospital Association

The AHA is a national association for hospitals and healthcare networks. Healthcare organizations as well as individuals can become members of the AHA.

The mission of the AHA is to advance the health of individuals and communities. The AHA (2015b) leads, represents, and serves hospitals, health systems, and related organizations that are accountable to their communities and committed to health improvement.

It meets this mission through the following:

1. *Advocacy*: The AHA represents and lobbies for the concerns of healthcare facilities in Washington, DC, whenever an issue comes up in Congress that will affect hospitals.
2. *Research*: The AHA researches healthcare trends and publishes its findings in many newsletters and periodicals.
3. *Information*: The AHA provides information about healthcare to providers and the public.

The AHA works with its members; state, regional, and metropolitan hospital associations; and other organizations to shape and influence federal legislation and regulation to improve the ability of its members to deliver quality healthcare.

THE IMPACT OF OWNERSHIP ON PROFITS AND THE STRATEGIC PLANNING PROCESS

Reduced operating margins affect a healthcare organization's ability to raise capital for replacement facilities, adopt new medical technology, and participate in joint ventures. As healthcare reimbursements decline and the requirement for costly healthcare technology grows, many healthcare organizations, driven by financial need, are using the strategic planning process to explore merger or acquisition, which could lead to a change in ownership status.

Research shows that healthcare organizations are improving efficiency and quality through consolidation and integration of services. Although health systems in the United States continue to acquire hospitals, not-for-profit health systems have reduced their acquisitions over the past decade, whereas for-profit health systems have been actively acquiring hospitals over the past decade (refer to Exhibit 1.1). These acquisitions are leading to significant growth in the for-profit hospital industry.

NOT-FOR-PROFIT STRATEGY

Historically, not-for-profits' strategic capital plans were primarily focused on physical assets (e.g., diagnostic and clinical equipment, real estate property, buildings). However, as all systems experience more complexity in patient care, changes in reimbursement policies, and the advent of ACOs, they need to focus on strategies such as physician acquisition, clinical information technology investments, and reengineering their ambulatory care approaches to transform care delivery models. Regardless of their tax status, hospitals and health systems face operating environments that include declining volumes and demand for inpatient services and limited revenue growth. They have also experienced the shift away from hospital-based care to more outpatient settings (Wong-Hammond and Damon 2013).

Given the undeniable stress on finances this shift has created, and in combination with the further pressures of value-based purchasing and the possibility of penalties for low-value care, routine maintenance and large capital expenditures for aging facilities are often delayed. However, they should not be delayed indefinitely; strategic capital plans can help find funding sources in support of mission-driven operational and growth initiatives. Ensuring that a health system's access to capital is sustained and available through multiple channels will allow for a more seamless execution of initiatives to meet long-term organizational needs and goals (Wong-Hammond and Damon 2013).

FOR-PROFIT STRATEGY

Although significantly smaller than the not-for-profit hospital sector, the for-profit hospital industry is rapidly growing in size and market penetration. A focus on new clinical services and an increasing presence in developing communities have prompted this growth. Additionally, many for-profit hospitals are evaluating the closure of duplicate, unprofitable clinical services as part of the strategic planning process.

Government Hospital Strategy

Although most government hospitals provide care to a predetermined population, they still need to participate in strategic planning to meet the changing needs of their patients and foster an organizational culture that supports change. In some northern communities, demand for inpatient services has decreased as a result of migration of the veteran population to the Sunbelt. Consequently, occupancy levels have decreased in the federal hospitals located in these communities. This development has made these facilities potential targets for closure. To prevent closure, the federal hospital system should explore ways these hospitals could use their excess hospital beds and resources. Services the federal government purchases from local markets, such as skilled nursing care and ambulatory care, could be provided by these facilities instead. For example, the Veterans Administration operates 171 medical centers, 350 outpatient clinics, 126 nursing home care units, and 35 domiciliary-care units for veterans. Similarly, the Department of Defense currently operates 59 hospitals worldwide (Harrison and Meyer 2014).

Research has shown that federal hospitals have become more efficient in providing both inpatient and outpatient services. Specifically, Harrison and Meyer (2014) used data envelopment analysis software to evaluate a panel of 165 federal hospitals in 2007 and 157 of the same hospitals again in 2011. Results indicated that overall efficiency in federal hospitals improved from 81 percent in 2007 to 86 percent in 2011.

Joint Venture Strategy

As shown in Exhibit 1.1 and documented further in Chapter 11, the number of freestanding (i.e., independent) hospitals is decreasing as more and more hospitals join multihospital systems. Many not-for-profit healthcare organizations are only marginally profitable, and their aging facilities need major renovations. As a result, they are considering joint ventures with for-profit companies as a method of acquiring additional financial resources.

From the perspective of a for-profit company, a joint venture with a not-for-profit organization is advantageous because (1) a not-for-profit organization is less expensive to purchase than another for-profit company, (2) the for-profit company can gain increased market share (i.e., the not-for-profit organization's customers will likely become customers of the new joint venture), and (3) the community will look favorably on the for-profit organization for partnering with a not-for-profit organization.

From the perspective of a not-for-profit organization, a joint venture with a for-profit organization is advantageous because (1) together, they have a greater pool of resources (financial and other) and (2) the not-for-profit organization will not have to give up all its power and will continue to have a say in operational decisions. At the health system level, joint ventures are one way a corporation can extend its network and gain resources. A lesser-known organization also can achieve instant recognition by joining with an organization whose products and services carry a trusted, well-known brand name.

In response to a rapidly changing healthcare environment, joint ventures are an opportunity for hospitals, physicians, and other healthcare organizations to work together to meet community healthcare needs. Faced with rising costs, decreasing reimbursement from insurers, and global competition, hospitals and physicians may use joint ventures to combine clinical and financial resources, claim a greater share of the market, and gain a better strategic position. To remain in a position of competitive advantage, organizations that pursue joint ventures must create a culture of trust between hospitals and physicians. In most cases, such a relationship requires a change of culture to see a joint venture as an opportunity rather than a threat. Physicians may view joint ventures as a threat because joint ventures often require them to give up their autonomy (e.g., the joint venture requires the physician to refer patients primarily to the joint venture, whereas previously the physician could refer patients to a wide range of providers). Despite the fact that joint ventures promise to benefit both partners' profit in the long run, some hospitals initially view joint ventures as a threat because joint ventures require them to share profits that they previously collected for themselves only.

One goal of physician–hospital joint ventures should be to increase the value of healthcare services to patients while providing a win–win situation for the hospital and physicians. When planning a joint venture, the two parties need to share information, develop a shared vision, and focus on improving efficiency in the delivery of healthcare. As a result, the joint venture will foster a sense of shared ownership.

IMPLEMENTING ORGANIZATIONAL CHANGE

The survival strategies discussed thus far require comprehensive organizational change. For change to occur smoothly and result in successful outcomes, everyone in the community needs to be involved in the strategic planning process, including the community's leaders, the organization's leaders and staff, and the organization's patients. The organization must share its mission, vision, and values with the community and encourage all stakeholders to develop alliances. Such an approach strengthens the organization's links with the external environment. Organizations whose culture emphasizes alliances, ongoing evaluation of change, wide participation from all stakeholders, and creativity are more likely to achieve successful outcomes. As will be discussed in Chapter 2, a transformational leadership approach that fosters a high level of staff involvement encourages innovation as part of the change process.

SUMMARY

In today's rapidly evolving healthcare environment, a leader is one who promotes change. The literature and organizational theory provide clear evidence that outstanding leadership is associated with increased organizational performance and future success. Effective leadership and strategic planning can significantly enhance the quality of patient care.

In the current environment of healthcare reform, healthcare leaders must uphold professional ethics and operate from a foundation of trust, honesty, and integrity in their dealings with patients and stakeholders. At all levels of the organization, leaders need to demonstrate ethics and honesty to gain employees' support.

Healthcare in the United States is experiencing a growing shortage of financial resources. An inability to adapt to the changing environment has forced many hospitals into bankruptcy, closure, merger with one or more hospitals, or acquisition by another company. To survive, many healthcare organizations are using strategic planning to position themselves for future success. Strategic planning is an ongoing process, not a onetime project, based on an organization's mission, vision, and values. These statements help organizations focus their investments, allocate their resources, and provide the foundation for implementing appropriate change.

An organization's mission, vision, and values are shaped by its ownership status. Organizations may be not-for-profit, for-profit, government operated, or joint ventures. Differences in mission reflect different motivations and goals, and these differences influence the type of strategic plan an organization develops.

Top organizations focus on their mission; monitor performance; participate in continuous quality improvement; and maintain relationships with patients, physicians, staff, and community stakeholders. Such organizations provide higher-quality care, have lower costs, are more profitable, and report higher rates of employee satisfaction.

EXERCISES

REVIEW QUESTIONS

1. Evaluate this statement: "The board of directors has fiduciary responsibility for organizational resources." Provide an example from your own experience that illustrates the impact a board can have on organizational performance.

2. In healthcare organizations' attempts to enhance their leadership, what are the roles of the board of directors, senior leaders, and physicians?

3. Adequate reimbursement levels are an important consideration in the strategic planning process. Discuss the recent trends in HMO, PPO, and ACO development and the impact they have on strategic planning.

4. An organization's mission is the fundamental purpose of its existence. Discuss the types of hospital ownership in the United States and how they may influence an organization's strategic plan.

5. Culture is a collection of values shared by a group of people. Discuss important attributes of organizational culture in healthcare.

COASTAL MEDICAL CENTER EXERCISE

On the basis of information provided in Chapter 1 and the CMC case, how effective has the board trustees been in providing oversight for the organization? From an operational perspective, how have the new CEO and senior leadership team provided the oversight necessary for CMC to move forward on a new road to success?

COASTAL MEDICAL CENTER QUESTIONS

1. Discuss the role of the board of trustees in providing oversight to CMC. Has the board met its fiduciary responsibility?
2. Does the CMC board regularly monitor performance? If so, how and how often?
3. Does the CMC board hold management accountable for achievement of the strategic plan? If so, how?
4. Recommend changes to the role of the board as well as types of members who should be appointed to the board.
5. CMC's past CEO Don Wilson provided leadership to a highly successful healthcare organization for more than 20 years and was considered a visionary. Develop a list of five areas in which you think Wilson's performance was particularly outstanding.
6. Does the quality of the new leadership at CMC set the stage for future success?

INDIVIDUAL EXERCISE: DEVELOPING A PERSONAL CAREER PLAN

Using the information discussed in Chapter 1, the specific hospital data provided in Exhibits 1.1, 1.2, and 1.5, and the following exercises, develop a personal career plan. The purpose of the career plan is to enable you to look at yourself in relation to your career with particular emphasis on the unique characteristics of the types of hospitals discussed. Think for some time before attempting to formulate your thoughts on paper. Your overall perception and analysis of the leadership team and its professional role will be important as you move forward in your career. If you have not chosen a specific career at this time, then identify a potential career of interest for this assignment. This report should represent your best academic efforts to date.

INDIVIDUAL QUESTIONS

1. Identify the organizational structure (e.g., for-profit, not-for-profit, federal) and specialty (e.g., medical and surgical, psychiatric, children's) of the hospital you are most interested in. Why does the mission, vision, and culture of that organization draw your interest?

2. What skills, education, qualifications, and experiences will be most important for your future success?
3. Project the next three years in terms of your selected career. What skills and qualifications are required for you to excel during this time? Which of these do you particularly need to strengthen?
4. Describe the basic qualities of leadership discussed in Chapter 1. What qualities do you think will contribute most to the success of individuals in supervisory or leadership positions? Do you think you possess some of the basic qualities necessary for future success in the same supervisory or leadership positions?

REFERENCES

American College of Healthcare Executives (ACHE). 2015. "Hospital Executive Salary Information: 2015." Accessed February 18, 2016. www.ache.org/newclub/career/SALARY.cfm.

American Hospital Association (AHA). 2015a. *Engaging Trustees in the Redefinition of the H.* Accessed August 2. www.aha.org/content/14/engaging_trustees_redefinition_H_tools_resources.pdf.

———. 2015b. "Vision and Mission." Accessed April 8. www.aha.org/about/mission/shtml.

———. 2014. *AHA Annual Survey Database 2014*. Chicago: American Hospital Association.

———. 2005. *AHA Annual Survey Database 2005*. Chicago: American Hospital Association.

Bowen, D. 2014. "The Growing Importance of Succession Planning." *Healthcare Executive* 29 (4): 8.

Catlin, A., C. Cowan, M. Hartman, S. Heffler, and the National Health Expenditure Accounts Team. 2008. "National Health Spending in 2006: A Year of Change for Prescription Drugs." *Health Affairs* 27 (1): 14–29.

Centers for Medicare & Medicaid Services (CMS). 2014. "National Healthcare Expenditures 2014 Highlights." Accessed December 22. www.cms.gov/Research-Statistics-Data-and-Systems/Statistics-Trends-and-Reports/NationalHealthExpendData/Downloads/highlights.pdf.

Cirillo, A. 2006. "Leadership Turnover: Don't Lose Sight of Market Strategy When a New CEO Takes the Helm of Your Healthcare Organization." *Health Care Strategic Management* 24 (9): 15–16.

Collum, T., N. Menachemi, M. Kilgore, and R. Weech-Maldonado. 2014. "Management Involvement on the Board of Directors and Hospital Financial Performance." *Journal of Healthcare Management* 59 (6): 429–45.

Dubinsky, I., N. Feerasta, and R. Lash. 2015. "A Model for Physician Leadership Development and Succession Planning." *Healthcare Quarterly* 18 (1): 38–42.

Epstein, J. 2014. "Fostering Hospital-Physician Relationships: 5 Strategies." *Managed Healthcare Executive*. Published October 10. http://managedhealthcareexecutive. modernmedicine.com/managed-healthcare-executive/news/fostering-hospital-physician-relationships-5-strategies.

Gamble, M. 2014. "13 Largest For-Profit Hospital Operators in 2014." *Becker's Hospital Review*. Published June 19. www.beckershospitalreview.com/lists/15-largest-for-profit-hospital-operators-2014.html.

Harrison, J., and S. Meyer. 2014. "Measuring Efficiency Among US Federal Hospitals." *Health Care Manager* 33 (2): 95–180.

Harrison, J., A. Spaulding, and P. Mouhalis. 2015. "The Efficiency Frontier of For-Profit Hospitals." *Journal of Health Care Finance* 41 (4): 1–23.

Hassmiller, S., and J. Combes. 2012. "Nurse Leaders in the Boardroom: A Fitting Choice." *Journal of Healthcare Management* 57 (1): 8–11.

Healthcare Leadership Alliance (HLA). 2013. "About the HLA Competency Directory." Accessed April 7, 2015. www.healthcareleadershipalliance.org/directory.htm.

Institute of Medicine (IOM). 2015. "About the IOM." Updated June 30. www.iom.edu/About-IOM.aspx.

————. 2011. *The Future of Nursing: Leading Change, Advancing Health.* Washington, DC: National Academies Press.

————. 2001. *Crossing the Quality Chasm: A New Health System for the 21st Century.* Washington, DC: National Academies Press.

National Center for Healthcare Leadership (NCHL). 2015. "About Us." Accessed April 7. www.nchl.org/static.asp?path=2887.

National Conference of State Legislatures (NCSL). 2015. "Certificate of Need: State Health Laws and Programs." Published September. www.ncsl.org/research/health/con-certificate-of-need-state-laws.aspx.

US Bureau of Labor Statistics (BLS). 2015. "Economic News Release: Employment Situation (Table B-1)." Accessed August 2. www.bls.gov/news.release/empsit.t17.htm.

US Department of Health & Human Services (HHS). 2014. "New Affordable Care Act Tools and Payment Models Deliver $372 Million in Savings, Improve Care." Published September 16. www.hhs.gov/news/press/2014pres/09/20140916a.html.

Vigen, G., I. Duncan, and S. Coughlin. 2013. *Measurement of Healthcare Quality and Efficiency: Resources for Healthcare Professionals.* Society of Actuaries. Accessed August 2, 2015. www.soa.org/research/research-projects/health/research-quality-report.aspx.

Wick, E. C., D. J. Galante, D. B. Hobson, A. R. Benson, K. H. K. Lee, S. M. Berenholtz, J. E. Efron, P. J. Pronovost, and C. L. Wu. 2015. "Organizational Culture Changes Result in Improvement in Patient-Centered Outcomes: Implementation of an Integrated Recovery Pathway for Surgical Patients." *Journal of the American College of Surgeons* 221 (3): 669–77.

Wong-Hammond, L., and L. Damon 2013. "Financing Strategic Plans for Not-for-Profits." *Healthcare Financial Management* 67 (7): 70–76.

CHAPTER 2

TRANSFORMATIONAL LEADERSHIP MAXIMIZES STRATEGIC PLANNING

Debra A. Harrison, Jeffrey P. Harrison

Transformational leaders don't start by denying the world around them. Instead, they describe a future they would like to create.

—Seth Godin

LEARNING OBJECTIVES

After you have studied this chapter, you should be able to

➤ identify, describe, and discuss the theoretical concepts of leadership in healthcare organizations;

➤ explain the importance of assessing the performance of healthcare organizations;

➤ describe the situational and environmental factors that influence effective decision making;

➤ identify and describe personal leadership orientation, styles, and strengths;

➤ describe, apply, and critique selected leadership skills essential to effective management of healthcare organizations;

➤ define and describe the concepts of team building and conflict resolution;

➤ analyze leadership's role in developing a strong ethical culture and nurturing a learning organization; and

➤ compare transactional leadership to transformational leadership and discuss where each falls on the hierarchy of leadership styles.

KEY TERMS AND CONCEPTS

➤ Charisma

➤ Code of ethics

➤ Ethics

➤ External rewards

➤ Groupthink

➤ High-performance work processes

➤ Internal rewards

➤ Magnet Recognition Program

➤ Management of change

➤ Morale

➤ Transactional leadership

➤ Transformational leadership

INTRODUCTION

Transactional leadership
Model of leadership that emphasizes giving rewards for good performance or taking corrective action for poor performance.

Transformational leadership
Model of leadership that emphasizes flexibility, selflessness, and interpersonal motivation to maximize individual and group potential.

At the time of this writing, a search of the term *leadership* in Google generated 490 million hits. An Amazon.com search for new books on leadership yielded 663 released in the past 90 days, with 216 coming soon. There is no shortage of information on leadership theories, qualities, skills, and styles. There are autocratic, participative, situational, transactional, and transformational theories of leadership, and more. This book focuses on the leadership needed in strategic planning and, more specifically, strategic planning in healthcare.

A conversation about healthcare nearly always includes the word *change*. Every aspect of healthcare has been affected by recent change, including reimbursement, quality, safety, and cost reduction (Delmatoff and Lazarus 2014). As our complex healthcare environment undergoes radical reform, its leaders will need to practice transformational leadership skills instead of rely on only traditional problem solving. Leaders must develop a process for embracing and directing change in a way that will allow organizations to grow and prosper. The key to this process is transforming both self and team, which positions an organization for extraordinary results (Chartrand 2010).

In recent literature on healthcare leadership, many authors compare and contrast **transactional leadership** with **transformational leadership** (see Exhibit 2.1). This chapter considers and elaborates on these two models and the question of which approach is the more suitable for leaders in healthcare. It also discusses the role of the leadership team in plan execution and engagement of staff in the planning process.

EXHIBIT 2.1

Two Contrasting
Leadership Models

Model Elements	Transactional	Transformational
Focus	Managerialism	Leadership and team
Main goals	Efficiency and increased productivity	Effectiveness and performance-driven metrics
Motivating questions	How can we do things right?	Should we be doing this at all?
Alignment	Policies and procedures	Mission, vision, and values
Sources of power	Control via organizational hierarchy	Relationships and team engagement
Tools	Reward and punishment	Inspiration and motivation of others
Approach	Linear thinking or status quo	Problem solving and innovation

The transactional leadership model emphasizes rewarding employees for successful completion of a task and taking corrective action for performance that does not meet expectations. It is sometimes called *managerial leadership* because it is focused on enforcing policy, not necessarily changing the future. This type of leadership is effective in emergency situations as well as for projects that need to be carried out in a specific way. It assumes that employees are motivated by self-interest or **external rewards**, such as money, or the threat of punishment.

The transactional approach is firmly integrated into healthcare. Traditionally, care has been provided in a hierarchical structure with physicians as the leaders, which gave them a level of control that superseded that of other healthcare providers and prevented a collaborative approach.

Transactional leadership in healthcare organizations is also well suited to the standardization of **high-performance work processes**—processes used to systematically pursue ever-higher levels of overall organizational and individual performance—to increase patient safety (Baldrige Performance Excellence Program 2015). Doing something the same way every time helps to prevent errors and harm to the patient. These processes allow for maximum efficiency and use technology to avoid duplication and reduce the chance for error. They result in a standardized outcome. In addition, specific policies and procedures must be followed consistently, such as those pertaining to confidentiality, human research subject protection, medication administration, universal protocol, and site marking for surgical procedures. In all these situations, a transactional approach is highly functional.

However, healthcare is complex and constantly changing—fertile ground for the transformational leadership style. Faced with rapidly changing technology and demographics, and

External rewards
Tangible incentives outside an individual that motivate that person to perform, such as money and gifts; the threat of punishment for nonperformance could also be a motivator.

High-performance work processes
Work processes used to systematically pursue ever-higher levels of overall organizational and individual performance (emphasizing, e.g., quality, productivity, innovation rate).

under pressure to improve clinical care, healthcare organizations need to plan strategically to move ahead. The healthcare field will need leaders capable of motivating employees, managing change, and unifying everyone in the organization through a common cause—dynamic people who inspire followers to pursue their visions. The real question in the future may not be which style of leadership is needed but rather at what time each style is most useful.

THE CONCEPT OF TRANSFORMATIONAL LEADERSHIP

The growing complexity of healthcare has increased the need for multidisciplinary teams composed of physicians, nurses, pharmacists, respiratory therapists, dietitians, and other professionals as well as managers, directors, and administrators. The transformational leadership model emphasizes a shared vision, motivating others to become the best they can be, and **internal rewards** such as the enjoyment that arises from the job itself. People will follow someone who inspires them, is enthusiastic, and leads with vision and values (Kumar 2013). A transformational leader is able to communicate the mission and vision of the organization, examine new perspectives, solve problems creatively, and develop and mentor employees. Transformational leaders are generally energetic, enthusiastic, and passionate. This style is often described as leading rather than managing.

The transformational leadership model was introduced by James MacGregor Burns in 1978. Burns described transformational leadership as a process in which leaders and followers (e.g., employees, volunteers) raise one another to higher levels of motivation (Burns 1978). Researcher Bernard M. Bass expanded on Burns's original ideas and published a book in 2005, *Transformational Leadership*, with coauthor Ronald E. Riggio. The theory expounded in the book is referred to as Bass's Transformational Leadership Theory and includes four components of transformational leadership: intellectual stimulation, individualized consideration, inspirational motivation, and idealized influence (for a fuller explanation, see Highlight 2.1).

The transformational leadership model uses transactions and interpersonal relationships to meet organizational goals necessary to achieve a vision (Rolfe 2011). John Paul Jones, Eleanor Roosevelt, Winston Churchill, Dr. Martin Luther King Jr., Lee Iacocca, John F. Kennedy, Ronald Reagan, and Barack Obama could all be considered leaders who used a transformational approach to prompt dramatic change. However, transformational leaders are not necessarily famous figures. The owner of the restaurant Zazie in San Francisco had been a waitress in the past and thus knew that her workers deserve to have careers and benefits as others do. She instituted a surcharge of $1.25 on all orders; transparently notifies customers of the charges; and uses that to pay for health, dental, and retirement benefits for her 35 employees. Many of them have been working for Zazie for more than 20 years. When asked if her profit margin is lower than other restaurants that do not offer benefits, she said that the mean profit margin is 5 percent for most competitor restaurants, while hers is 22 percent in a good year. She is a transformational leader. Her innovative approach—providing a full benefits package to historically underserved employees—has

Internal rewards
Feelings that arise out of performing an activity and that motivate an individual to perform, such as the enjoyment from creating a work of art or playing a sport.

✳ Highlight 2.1 Bass's Transformational Leadership Theory

Bass proposes a theory of transformational leadership that is measured in terms of the leader's effect on followers (Bass and Bass 2008). It describes four components of transformational leadership:

1. *Intellectual stimulation*: Transformational leaders challenge the status quo and encourage creativity among followers. They allow followers to learn, explore, and experiment. Transformational leaders increase their followers' awareness of problems, helping them to view the issues from a new perspective. This process of intellectual stimulation creates an environment that encourages innovation when faced with rapid "white-water" change.

2. *Individualized consideration*: Transformational leaders cultivate relationships by encouraging and supporting individual followers. They use social skills to foster the sharing of ideas, and they recognize contributions. They encourage their followers and provide them with developmental opportunities that often lead to enhanced team building and improved group dynamics.

3. *Inspirational motivation*: Transformational leaders have a clear vision and articulate it clearly to followers. They also motivate others to pursue goals with passion. This behavior is often called **charisma**—leadership charm that provokes strong emotions and loyalty in followers—and is linked to having a compelling vision.

4. *Idealized influence*: Transformational leaders serve as role models for followers. If a follower trusts and respects his leader, he will emulate this individual and internalize her ideals. Such leaders purposefully do what they want others to do, instead of just talking about it—sometimes called *walking the talk*. For transformational leaders, failing to walk the talk or to adhere to a professional code of ethics can have a negative impact on trust among followers.

Charisma
Leadership charm that provokes strong emotions and loyalty in followers.

yielded low turnover, motivated workers, and loyal customers (McFadden and Fieldstadt 2015).

How Transformational Leadership Works

Transformational leaders focus on linking their followers with goals and values by developing a common cause. When they do so successfully, they become motivators, facilitators, educators, and visionaries. Followers develop a high degree of confidence in their direction and a sense of loyalty. As discussed in Chapter 1, the organization's vision should be widely accepted throughout the organization and congruent with the leader's vision. Followers often internalize the leader's values and moral convictions and thereby perceive a need for change. As a result, they are motivated to pursue goals that are higher than they could accomplish individually.

Motivation differs among individuals and may stem from external or internal sources, which are often related to situational or organizational factors, values, and ideals. Common internal motivation techniques include the use of personal charisma, individual attention to the follower, intellectual stimulation through assignment of tasks, and emotional appeal. Several common attributes are seen in leaders who are transformational (see Exhibit 2.2).

Leadership styles could be considered a hierarchy (see Exhibit 2.3). Along the transactional–transformational continuum of leadership, there are a series of leadership styles. At the bottom of the hierarchy is the *directing leadership* style. Leaders who take a directive approach use authoritative command to communicate with and motivate their subordinates. The second level of the hierarchy is the *participating leadership* style. Leaders who take a participatory approach coach their subordinates and serve as role models. The next level up is the *delegating leadership* style. This leadership style affords subordinates some independence and self-direction, for the purpose of improving performance. At the top of the hierarchy is the *transformational leadership* style, which empowers the group and heightens subordinates' awareness of the organization's mission, vision, values, and goals, as wel as the role of these factors in the organization's strategy. Higher strategic awareness can lead to increased **morale**—positive emotions and a sense of common purpose among members of a group—and greater productivity.

Morale
Positive emotions and sense of common purpose among members of a group.

EXHIBIT 2.2
Attributes and Personality Characteristics of Transformational Leaders

Attributes and personality characteristics contributing to the success of transformational leaders include the following (Rolfe 2011):

Attributes
- Being visionary or futuristic
- Ability to catalyze followers
- Motivation
- Goal orientation
- Expertise
- Flexibility
- Excellent communication skills
- Invocation of group respect, shared vision, and improved culture

Personality characteristics
- Self-knowledge
- Self-confidence and positive self-image
- Authenticity
- Charisma
- Intelligence
- Ability to empathize with followers

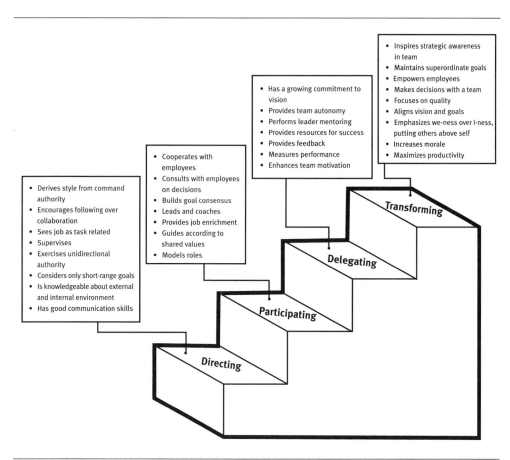

EXHIBIT 2.3
The Hierarchy of
Leadership Models

- Inspires strategic awareness in team
- Maintains superordinate goals
- Empowers employees
- Makes decisions with a team
- Focuses on quality
- Aligns vision and goals
- Emphasizes we-ness over I-ness, putting others above self
- Increases morale
- Maximizes productivity

- Has a growing commitment to vision
- Provides team autonomy
- Performs leader mentoring
- Provides resources for success
- Provides feedback
- Measures performance
- Enhances team motivation

- Cooperates with employees
- Consults with employees on decisions
- Builds goal consensus
- Leads and coaches
- Provides job enrichment
- Guides according to shared values
- Models roles

- Derives style from command authority
- Encourages following over collaboration
- Sees job as task related
- Supervises
- Exercises unidirectional authority
- Considers only short-range goals
- Is knowledgeable about external and internal environment
- Has good communication skills

Transforming

Delegating

Participating

Directing

The transformational leadership approach is considered highly effective in improving patient safety. In a descriptive correlational study conducted in 41 nursing departments across nine hospitals, a safety climate survey and multifactorial leadership questionnaire were completed by staff nurses. A transformational leadership style was demonstrated to be a positive contributor to a good safety climate and decreased a culture of blame. Leaders must concentrate on developing transformational leadership skills to not only improve relationships with their staff but also improve patient safety and promote continuous improvement (Merrill 2015). For situations—whether organizational, political, economic, or social—in which followers are frustrated, stressed, or unhappy with the current state of affairs, a transformational leader can use her skills to defuse the tension. If an individual is able to emerge from the group to represent its desires and needs in such situations, that individual is likely to become a leader. From this position of authority, the leader is able to influence the course and direction of events to bring about change, often with revolutionary results. Leaders such as Genghis Khan, Cyrus the Great of Persia, Gandhi, and the Roman Emperor Constantine I are examples of individuals who stepped up in this manner, won the hearts and minds of followers, and radically changed the world.

WHY IS TRANSFORMATIONAL LEADERSHIP IMPORTANT TO STUDY?

Transformational leadership is important to an executive's success and is a critical resource in an organization's ongoing strategic planning process. No well-known leader of our time has become successful or has led an organization to success without first understanding the principles of transformational leadership. At the core of all the attributes of a transformational leader is personal integrity and ability to maintain the public's trust (Manion 2011). Without integrity, there is no trust.

To thrive in the dynamic field of healthcare, organizations must engage in careful strategic planning. To bring about the goals in their strategic plans, organizations need to tap their greatest resource—people. Transformational leadership leverages this resource by motivating individuals to adopt goal-oriented behavior that supports the organization's mission, vision, and values.

ETHICS AS A FOUNDATION FOR LEADERSHIP AND STRATEGIC PLANNING

Ethics
Moral duty, values, and obligation.

Although a comprehensive discussion of **ethics** is beyond the scope of this book, it is important to note that ethics can be summarized as a sense of moral duty, values, and obligation. It is central to leadership, strategic planning, and motivating followers to accomplish mutual goals consistent with the organization's values. An organization's failure to uphold business ethics can lead to disastrous consequences, including bankruptcy or closure. In healthcare, examples of corporate ethical problems include HealthSouth's 2003 accounting scandal and American pharmaceutical giant Pfizer's kickbacks scandal (SEC 2003; see Highlight 2.2).

ETHICAL CONSIDERATIONS OF THE HEALTHCARE LEADER

Transformational leaders must be attuned to the organizational culture in which they function. Many ethical models exist, and the ethical model upheld by one culture may differ from the one upheld in another. For example, perspectives on healthcare issues such as abortion, genetic engineering, and euthanasia vary from organization to organization.

In an attempt to regulate corporate ethical behavior, the federal government and other organizations have enacted laws and established principles of ethical conduct. In 2002, Congress passed the Sarbanes-Oxley Act in reaction to a number of major fraud cases involving large US corporations. In healthcare, numerous professional organizations have established their own **codes of ethics**. For example, as part of its credentialing process, the American College of Healthcare Executives (ACHE) requires that healthcare executives maintain the highest level of ethical behavior. The Preamble to ACHE's *Code of Ethics*, which provides a guide to standards of behavior and ethical conduct for healthcare leaders, appears in Highlight 2.3.

Code of ethics
Guide to standards of behavior and ethical conduct.

Following the Preamble, the ACHE (2011) *Code of Ethics* provides healthcare executives with specific guidance on professional conduct and addresses the importance of honesty,

---

(✲) Highlight 2.2 When Corporate Ethics Lead to Harm

In 2003, the US Securities and Exchange Commission (SEC) announced that it was filing fraud charges against HealthSouth Corporation (HRC) of Birmingham, Alabama, and its CEO and chairman, Richard M. Scrushy. HRC is the nation's largest provider of out-patient surgery and diagnostic and rehabilitative healthcare services, with specialized rehabilitation hospitals in 33 states and Puerto Rico. Shortly after HRC became publicly traded in 1986, at Scrushy's instruction, the company began to artificially inflate its earnings to match Wall Street analysts' expectations and maintain the market price for HRC's stock. Between 1999 and the second quarter of 2002, HRC intentionally over-stated its earnings by at least $1.4 billion in reports filed with the SEC. Scrushy person-ally profited from the artificially inflated earnings. He sold more than 7 million shares of HRC stock between 1999 and 2003. He also received salary and bonus payments based on HRC's reported earnings (SEC 2003). Scrushy was eventually convicted of money laundering, extortion, obstruction of justice, racketeering, and bribery, and he spent time in a federal prison and paid hundreds of thousands of dollars in fines.

American pharmaceutical giant Pfizer Inc. agreed to pay $2.3 billion, the largest healthcare fraud settlement in the history of the US Department of Justice, to resolve criminal and civil liabilities arising from the illegal promotion of certain pharmaceuti-cal products. Bextra is an anti-inflammatory drug that Pfizer pulled from the market in 2005. Pfizer promoted the sale of Bextra for several uses and dosages that the US Food and Drug Administration specifically declined to approve due to safety concerns. The civil settlement also alleged that Pfizer paid kickbacks to healthcare providers to induce them to prescribe these, as well as other, drugs. Six whistle-blowers received payments totaling more than $102 million from the federal share of the civil recovery (DOJ 2009).

---

integrity, respect, and fairness. The *Code of Ethics* goes on to delineate the healthcare execu-tive's responsibilities to patients, the organization, employees, and the community. Like many other professional codes of ethics, it also provides clear guidance on a healthcare executive's responsibility to report the ethics violations of others.

THE ROLE OF TRANSFORMATIONAL LEADERS IN MANAGING THE STRATEGIC PLANNING PROCESS

Defining the goals of the organization is a key component of strategic planning. Organi-zational goals must meet three basic conditions with regard to organizational values and standards:

1. They must be consistent with and directly related to the values of the organization.

2. They must have specific information that explains their relation to institutional standards.

3. They must specify actions that will be taken to live up to the values and standards of the institution.

For any organization, goals that are clearly measurable and attainable and that ensure accountability are the primary prerequisite to achieving success. An organization's staff must not only understand its goals and the goals of its leaders but also embrace those goals as fundamental principles supporting change in the organization (Manion 2011). Successful transformation of any organization depends on its transformational leaders' ability to articulate these goals and get everyone in the organization motivated to achieve them.

Leaders using the transformational approach should draw on the expertise of their staff to maximize the success of the strategic planning process and chart the organization's course through difficult periods. Transformational leaders understand that their staff members are the most knowledgeable about the factors often overlooked in strategic planning and that the entire team's support is necessary to operationalize the strategic plan. Such operational support is essential to the success of new business initiatives and the long-term well-being of the organization.

Transformational leaders may successfully use the following strategies (Rubino, Esparza, and Chassiakos 2014):

1. *Uphold integrity above all else.* Dishonesty and insincerity will destroy relationships and trust, making it difficult to have followers. Being true to values and honest in interactions is critical.

2. *Get down in the trenches.* Transformational leaders do not ask people to do something they would not. Respect from followers comes from this willingness to walk in their shoes.

3. *Communicate, communicate, communicate.* Keeping open lines of communication is important. Sharing information and organizational goals and objectives increases the understanding and commitment of others.

4. *Have a meeting.* Gaining consensus on decisions is important, and more input is better. By discussing ideas—even the bad ones—with leaders, followers gain confidence and courage. This leads to employee engagement and valuable perspectives.

5. *Keep the mission of the organization in mind.* Transformational leaders are driven by the mission, vision, and values of the organization and seek to make the connection between these concepts and business decisions. This approach reinforces the importance of all employees to the mission, even the housekeeper or patient care technician.

✳ Highlight 2.3 American College of Healthcare Executives *Code of Ethics*

Preamble

The purpose of the ACHE *Code of Ethics* is to serve as a standard of conduct for members. It contains standards of ethical behavior for healthcare executives in their professional relationships. These relationships include colleagues, patients or others served; members of the healthcare executive's organization and other organizations; the community; and society as a whole.

The *Code of Ethics* also incorporates standards of ethical behavior governing individual behavior, particularly when that conduct directly relates to the role and identity of the healthcare executive.

The fundamental objectives of the healthcare management profession are to maintain or enhance the overall quality of life, dignity and well-being of every individual needing healthcare service and to create a more equitable, accessible, effective and efficient healthcare system.

Healthcare executives have an obligation to act in ways that will merit the trust, confidence, and respect of healthcare professionals and the general public. Therefore, healthcare executives should lead lives that embody an exemplary system of values and ethics.

In fulfilling their commitments and obligations to patients or others served, healthcare executives function as moral advocates and models. Since every management decision affects the health and well-being of both individuals and communities, healthcare executives must carefully evaluate the possible outcomes of their decisions. In organizations that deliver healthcare services, they must work to safeguard and foster the rights, interests and prerogatives of patients or others served.

The role of moral advocate requires that healthcare executives take actions necessary to promote such rights, interests and prerogatives.

Being a model means that decisions and actions will reflect personal integrity and ethical leadership that others will seek to emulate.

Source: Reprinted from ACHE (2011); please see ache.org for updates made since the publication of this book.

Transformational leaders need to maintain a delicate balance between using and relaxing their authority. Leaders cannot (and should not) do and be all things. Thus one of the critical activities of the transformational leader is developing a leadership team.

ESTABLISHING THE LEADERSHIP TEAM

The first step in developing a leadership team is to identify employees who think, act, and respond in a manner that supports the organization's mission, vision, and values. A team must have the attitudes and ideals that underlie a synergistic and functional leadership group.

Transformational leaders want high-performing employees on the team. However, intelligent, driven individuals can be difficult to manage because of their individuality. These nontraditional thinkers are important because they may prevent **groupthink**—a process by which groups develop monolithic thinking. Research shows that groups produce better outcomes than any individual alone. When individuals are encouraged to share their thoughts and ideas in a group, the decision-making process may be slower, but the decision is better. Greater volumes of input lead to more plausible and innovative solutions (Macleod 2011). Whereas a domineering leader can stifle the functioning of their team, a transformational leader is able to manage a highly skilled and diverse group of individuals in a manner that is most effective for the organization. A transformational leader also keeps the team focused on results (Rubino, Esparaza, and Chassiakos 2014).

Managing a team by striking a balance between leading the team itself and transforming followers into leaders is part of the fine art of transformational leadership. Transformational leaders understand that they must remain open to the input and direction of their team members and are adept at promoting effective interaction among them. Through delegation and empowerment, the transformational leader allows others to embrace the direction and operations of the organization (see Highlight 2.4 for some real-life examples).

TRANSFORMATIONAL LEADERSHIP: INTEGRAL TO MAGNET DESIGNATION

Magnet designation is awarded by the American Nurses Credentialing Center (ANCC) to hospitals or systems that have demonstrated excellence in nursing practice. It has become a high benchmark and is a key factor in the *U.S. News & World Report* Best Hospital scoring. The Magnet Model provides a framework for achieving excellence in nursing practice and serves as a road map for organizations seeking Magnet Recognition. The four components of the model are transformational leadership, structural empowerment, exemplary professional practice, and new knowledge innovations and improvements. All results are verified by empirically proven outcomes (ANCC 2015). ANCC places considerable emphasis on the chief nursing officer (CNO) as a transformational leader. It describes such a leader as one who develops a strong shared vision and philosophy, communicates expectations effectively, develops and inspires others, and leads the organization to meet strategic priorities (Clavelle et al. 2012).

The **Magnet Recognition Program**, a credentialing program that recognizes healthcare organizations for quality patient care, nursing excellence, and innovations in professional

Groupthink
Within a group, the tendency to maintain harmony by incorporating minimal input and making rapid decisions.

Magnet Recognition Program
Sponsored by the American Nurses Credentialing Center, a program recognizing healthcare organizations for quality patient care, nursing excellence, and innovations in professional nursing practice.

✳ Highlight 2.4 Transformational and Transactional Styles in the History of US Healthcare Policy

Different US presidents have developed different transformational leadership styles. John F. Kennedy inspired broad support of the civil rights movement and the space race with the Soviet Union. He was able to emotionally stir individuals from grassroots America to form networks of like-minded populations that all embraced a similar agenda. He broke down barriers of race, gender, and socioeconomic status and made people feel as though they were being personally addressed. Ronald Reagan was so successful in establishing a transformational vision of traditional, family-based values that many Americans embrace Reagan-based principles to this day.

Bill Clinton also engaged the American public with a strong message that healthcare is an inalienable right for all citizens and not an entitlement for those who can pay for it. This concept began with the advent of Medicare and Medicaid during the John F. Kennedy and Lyndon B. Johnson eras, focusing on the elderly and the poor. Before the Clinton administration, healthcare for the middle class was largely viewed as an individual responsibility. Clinton transformed the nation's views on healthcare and made reforming the healthcare system a national priority in the minds of Americans. Clinton appealed to the idea that providing care for children, the infirm, and the elderly was the "right thing to do."

Building on the growing public desire for comprehensive healthcare coverage, Barack Obama was elected in 2008 in part on a pledge to complete Clinton's vision. His election ultimately resulted in the passage of the Affordable Care Act in 2010. However, Obama was not successful in motivating Congress to pursue a shared vision and therefore relied on a transactional leadership approach to complete the process. Congress has reacted with consistent and unending criticism and attempts to repeal the law, and so without a shared vision and purpose, the legislation evolved into a fight between Democrats and Republicans.

Kennedy, Reagan, and Clinton all had an ability to unite populations of individuals behind a shared vision, though each employed different transformational techniques and skills to communicate his message. Their success in advancing agendas, swaying populations, and reorienting individual and group values is undeniable.

---

nursing practice, expects the CNO to be strategically positioned in the organization to effectively influence other executive stakeholders, including the board of directors. The CNO can and should be involved in strategic planning and is expected to have a transformational leadership style. Current research shows that such a style enhances nurse satisfaction, promotes a positive work environment, and reduces staff turnover (Clavelle et al. 2012; Merrill

2015; Rolfe 2011). The transformational leadership characteristics of the CNO are important to achieving clinical quality and positive patient care outcomes through the creation of structures and processes supporting nurse empowerment and evidence-based practice.

SUMMARY

The rapidly changing healthcare environment requires leaders who can continually reinvent strategy and successfully allocate their resources, particularly people, to perform and thrive in the marketplace. Of the different types of leadership, the transformational model seems best suited for this objective. Transformational leaders are motivators, facilitators, educators, and visionaries who focus on aligning their desires and goals with those of their followers. The transformational leadership model motivates followers through internal (i.e., values-based) rather than external (i.e., reward-based) incentives. Followers of a transformational leader are not driven by selfish aims; for them, a sense of accomplishment or community is a reward in itself. Though some aspects of transformational leadership apply to most contexts, leadership techniques that work in one culture will not necessarily work in another. In all situations, however, transformational leaders uphold strong ethics, work against groupthink, and know when structural and procedural changes need to be made to keep their organizations vital and competitive.

EXERCISES

REVIEW QUESTIONS

1. Why do organizations adopt the transformational leadership model?
2. How do organizations use transformational leadership to manage change and achieve goals?
3. In what ways are the transactional and transformational models of leadership similar? In what ways are they different?
4. How might leadership ethics apply to the healthcare field? Provide examples.

COASTAL MEDICAL CENTER EXERCISE

Does transformational leadership exist at Coastal Medical Center (CMC)?

COASTAL MEDICAL CENTER QUESTIONS

1. Does information in the case study suggest that at one time CMC embraced transformational leadership? If so, why does it no longer embrace this style?
2. Develop a plan or process by which transformational leadership might be implemented at CMC.
3. Assess the level of leadership ethics currently in place at CMC. Address any problems you see and propose potential solutions.

INDIVIDUAL AND GROUP EXERCISES: DEVELOP AN UNDERSTANDING OF EFFECTIVE LEADERSHIP TRAITS

Using the information on leadership styles in Chapter 2 as well as your knowledge and experience, complete the following exercises:

1. Individually, spend ten minutes writing down the names of five outstanding leaders in history. The leaders can be religious, political, military, and so on. Below each leader's name, write the traits that make or made this individual an outstanding leader.
2. In your group, discuss these traits and identify those leaders who exhibited transformational leadership skills. Does the issue of ethical values come up in the discussion of any of the leaders?
3. What leadership traits do you possess? What traits would you like to develop further?

REFERENCES

American College of Healthcare Executives (ACHE). 2011. "ACHE Code of Ethics." Accessed February 25, 2015. www.ache.org/abt_ache/code.cfm.

American Nurses Credentialing Center (ANCC). 2015. "Magnet Model." Accessed February 24. www.nursecredentialing.org/Magnet/ProgramOverview/New-Magnet-Model.

Baldrige Performance Excellence Program. 2015. "Baldrige Excellence Builder: Key Questions for Improving Your Organization's Performance." National Institute of Standards and Technology. Accessed August 13. www.nist.gov/baldrige/publications/upload/Baldrige_Excellence_Builder.pdf.

Bass, B. M. and R. Bass. 2008. *The Bass Handbook of Leadership: Theory, Research, and Managerial Applications*, 4th ed. New York: Free Press.

Bass, B. M., and R. E. Riggio. 2005. *Transformational Leadership*, 2nd ed. New York: Psychology Press.

Burns, J. M. 1978. *Leadership*. New York: Harper & Row.

Chartrand, G. 2010. *Unreasonable Leadership*. Ponte Vedra, FL: Unreasonable Leadership Book LLC.

Clavelle, J. T., K. Drenkard, S. Tullai-McGuinness, and J. Fitzpatrick. 2012. "Transformational Leadership Practices of Chief Nursing Officers in Magnet Organizations." *Journal of Nursing Administration* 42 (4): 195–201.

Delmatoff, J., and I. R. Lazarus. 2014. "The Most Effective Leadership Style for the New Landscape of Healthcare." *Journal of Healthcare Management* 59 (4): 245–49.

Kumar, R. 2013. "Leadership in Healthcare." *Anaesthesia and Intensive Care Medicine* 14 (1): 39–41.

Macleod, L. 2011. "Avoiding Groupthink: A Manager's Challenge." *Nursing Management* 42 (10): 44–48.

Manion, J. 2011. *From Management to Leadership: Strategies for Transforming Health Care.* San Francisco: Jossey-Bass.

McFadden, C., and E. Fieldstadt. 2015. "Recipe for Success: Calif. Eatery's Way to Give All Staff Benefits." *NBC Nightly News.* Aired February 17. www.nbcnews.com/nightly-news/recipe-success-calif-eaterys-way-give-all-staff-benefits-n292426.

Merrill, K. C. 2015. "Leadership Style and Patient Safety: Implications for Nurse Managers." *Journal of Nursing Administration* 45 (6): 319–24.

Rolfe, P. 2011. "Transformational Leadership Theory: What Every Leader Needs to Know." *Nurse Leader* 9 (2): 54–57.

Rubino, L., S. Esparza, and Y. R. Chassiakos. 2014. *New Leadership for Today's Health Care Professionals.* Burlington, MA: Jones & Bartlett Learning.

US Department of Justice (DOJ). 2009. "Justice Department Announces Largest Health Care Fraud Settlement in Its History." Published September 2. www.justice.gov/opa/pr/justice-department-announces-largest-health-care-fraud-settlement-its-history.

US Securities and Exchange Commission (SEC). 2003. "SEC Charges HealthSouth Corp., CEO Richard Scrushy with $1.4 Billion Accounting Fraud." Published March 20. www.sec.gov/litigation/litreleases/lr18044.htm.

CHAPTER 3

FUNDAMENTALS OF STRATEGIC PLANNING

Experience is a hard teacher because it gives the test first, the lesson afterwards.

—Vern Law

After you have studied this chapter, you should be able to

➤ demonstrate the ability to assess actual healthcare strategic planning problems and, using the various knowledge disciplines, develop comprehensive and practical solutions;

➤ exercise business planning techniques and demonstrate skills in professional writing and verbal communication;

➤ demonstrate a deeper understanding of the healthcare system and the management of costs, quality, and access and make sound business decisions and develop a strategy for change;

➤ successfully participate in teamwork; and

➤ use critical thinking skills and create an environment that supports innovation and entrepreneurial spirit.

KEY TERMS AND CONCEPTS

- ➤ Ambulatory surgery center
- ➤ Balanced scorecard
- ➤ Benchmarking
- ➤ Dashboard
- ➤ Efficiency frontier
- ➤ Fixed cost
- ➤ Gap analysis
- ➤ *Healthy People 2020*

- ➤ Medicare Payment Advisory Commission
- ➤ Payer mix
- ➤ Safety-net providers
- ➤ Strategic planning
- ➤ Total cost
- ➤ Variable cost

INTRODUCTION

Strategic planning brings leaders and stakeholders together to position their organization for success in an environment of uncertainty. A healthcare organization engages in strategic planning to reduce costs, improve quality and service, and ensure access to care. An innovative strategic planning process also helps an organization allocate resources more effectively to enhance the value of its services and better meet the community's healthcare needs.

The US healthcare environment is changing substantially. By 2011, healthcare employed 15.7 percent of the US workforce and reached expenditures of $2.7 trillion (Moses et al. 2013). Healthcare as a percentage of gross domestic product has doubled since 1980 to 17.9 percent in 2013. During the same period, government funding for healthcare has increased from 31 percent in 1980 to 43 percent. The rate of change in an organization's market factors or technological environment determines whether an organization's structure should be hierarchical or participatory.

In a stable environment, a hierarchical structure with centralized decision making may improve overall efficiency, provided senior leaders and managers possess sufficient knowledge and information to make informed decisions. However, in unstable environments with white-water change, the knowledge and information required for innovation must be distributed throughout multiple levels in the organization. A greater flow of information combined with decentralized decision making fosters innovation. Such participatory organizational structures may be more appropriate in the current healthcare environment.

Strategic planning
Process by which an organization determines its future direction by defining the actions that will shape it and developing objectives and techniques for measuring ongoing performance.

DEFINITION

Strategic planning is the process by which an organization determines its future overall direction and defines the actions that will shape it. Planners gather information about the internal and external environments and have in-depth discussions about the future of the organization. They also develop organizational objectives and techniques for measuring ongoing performance.

The critical components of the healthcare strategic planning model are illustrated in Exhibit 3.1 and discussed in the sections that follow.

ANALYSIS OF THE ENVIRONMENT INSIDE THE ORGANIZATION

Internal data focus on finances, personnel, key assets, and quality of care. A thorough analysis of internal data reveals an organization's strengths and weaknesses, both of which affect its ability to meet its mission.

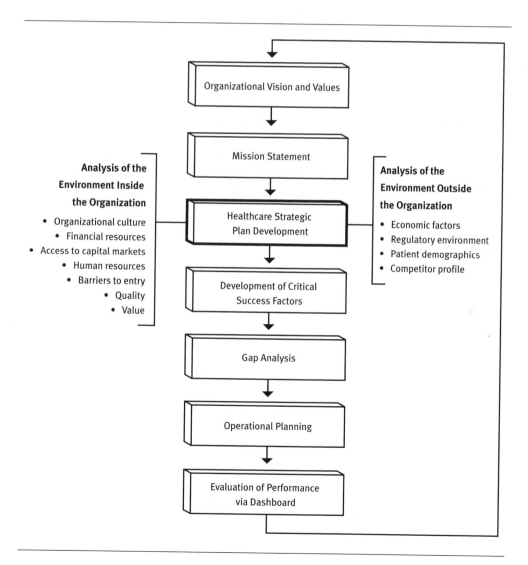

EXHIBIT 3.1
Healthcare Strategic Planning Model

Analysis of the Environment Inside the Organization

- Organizational culture
- Financial resources
- Access to capital markets
- Human resources
- Barriers to entry
- Quality
- Value

Analysis of the Environment Outside the Organization

- Economic factors
- Regulatory environment
- Patient demographics
- Competitor profile

Organizational Vision and Values

Mission Statement

Healthcare Strategic Plan Development

Development of Critical Success Factors

Gap Analysis

Operational Planning

Evaluation of Performance via Dashboard

MISSION, VISION, AND VALUES

Thomas Edison is reputed to have said that "vision without execution is hallucination." An organization's mission, vision, and values provide the foundation on which its strategic plan is built. Consistency among mission, vision, and values and clear links among all three enhance the strategic planning process and increase the chance of performance improvement. The entire workforce must also buy into the mission, vision, and values, or execution will be difficult.

CULTURE

An organizational culture is the shared values and beliefs that guide behavior in each organization (Pellegrin and Currey 2011). An organization's distinctive beliefs provide a framework for behavior. Social values in its surrounding communities shape this behavior. For example, many people believe that access to healthcare is a right, not a privilege, and patients want to be a healthcare organization's first priority. Incorporating these social values in organizational culture is important to healthcare strategic planning.

Culture also guides an organization's decisions about allocating resources and establishing priorities. For example, consumers and health professionals want access to the best technology available. An organization that emphasizes innovation and technological advancement needs to allocate its resources carefully to be able to fund this costly priority. If the organization promotes lifelong learning, it should not cut education and training budgets at the first sign of financial stress (Pellet 2013).

CRITICAL SUCCESS FACTORS

An organization's strategic plan should address improvement in five core areas:

1. Healthcare quality

2. Patient access

3. Employee retention

4. Differentiation in the market

5. Alignment of resources

Successful strategic planning in healthcare should also include a clear connection between current projects and programs, those that are regulatory directed (such as preventive services and community wellness), the strategic objectives of the organization (such as evaluation of joint ventures or participation in a health system), and the measurements being used to track success. Tracking success will reflect organizational competency and appropriate use of information technology. Implementation of the strategic plan will require collaboration between physicians and the hospital, employee training to upgrade skill levels in some instances, annual operating goals, and a plan to update every three years.

ANALYSIS OF THE ENVIRONMENT OUTSIDE THE ORGANIZATION

The healthcare strategic planning process is subject to considerable outside control and rapid change. Federal and state legislation, physician involvement, third-party payers' actions, and competitors' actions all affect operations. In addition, as healthcare organizations focus more on illness prevention and community wellness, they will need to consider educational, behavioral, and social interventions that have not been a part of the traditional, episodic system of medical treatment. In short, healthcare organizations need to focus on the external environment and future changes to the field. By gathering information from external sources, healthcare organizations increase their likelihood of achieving success.

External information describes the market position; local demographics, competitors, and payers; and the local business environment. Such data are available through online databases maintained by hospital associations, regional health-planning groups, the US Census Bureau, and the US Department of Health & Human Services.

TRENDS IN THE EXTERNAL ENVIRONMENT

Hospitals planning strategically need to be mindful of trends influencing the direction of the healthcare environment, including the advent of accountable care organizations (ACOs), expanded insurance coverage, increased hospital participation in healthcare systems, the impact of specialty hospitals, and the rise of ambulatory surgery centers.

The Advent of Accountable Care Organizations

As a part of the Affordable Care Act (ACA), the Centers for Medicare & Medicaid Services (CMS) promoted the ACO. Many ACOs create a partnership among a clinic, hospital, rehabilitation center, and nursing home. ACOs may also be a joint venture between a group of doctors or hospitals and other healthcare providers who collaborate on providing high-quality care at reduced costs. If the ACO is successful in reducing costs and improving quality at all the levels of care, the parties will share in the savings from Medicare (CMS 2015). ACOs are using strategies such as population health to manage a growing primary care base. Organizations need to consider the pros and cons of including participation in an ACO in their strategic plan. See Chapter 9 for more information about ACOs and population health.

Expanded Insurance Coverage

An estimated 10.3 million Americans became newly insured through provisions in the ACA. The greatest increase was observed among minorities and young adults. This shift will change organizational healthcare priorities to create more focus on preventive health and community well-being. Still, as of April 2014, 16.3 percent of the US population remains uninsured (Sommers et al. 2014). This uninsured segment is dependent on **safety-net providers** such as public hospitals, not-for-profit hospitals, community health centers, and local health departments. With this large number of people lining up for safety-net care, the uninsured may have long waiting periods and may therefore choose to go without.

Safety-net providers
Healthcare providers that deliver a significant amount of care to uninsured, Medicaid, and other disadvantaged patients.

Increased Participation in Healthcare Systems

Faced with lower Medicare reimbursement rates and the responsibility to provide care for the uninsured, independent hospitals are experiencing weak profit margins and a growing need for capital. As a result, they are under increasing pressure to become part of healthcare systems. Some of the benefits of system membership include lower interest rates on loans, greater negotiating power with third-party payers, and savings through group purchasing. However, in evaluating the benefits of system membership, independent hospitals should consider maintaining fiduciary control as well as local involvement in the strategic planning process to ensure that the strategic plan prioritizes and meets consumer needs in the community.

The Impact of Specialty Hospitals

Healthcare policymakers continue to debate whether physician-owned specialty hospitals that provide heart, orthopedic, and surgical services are desirable. The literature is mixed on the benefits and downsides of specialty hospitals. The potential for conflict of interest exists, but most research suggests that specialty hospitals have had little impact on general hospitals (Babu, Rosenow, and Nahed 2011).

Medicare Payment Advisory Commission (MedPAC)
Government agency composed of 17 members and established by the Balanced Budget Act of 1997 to advise Congress on issues that affect the Medicare program.

The number of specialty hospitals increased from 499 in 2000 to 956 in 2010—a 91 percent increase over the decade (Moses et al. 2013). In its 2006 report to Congress, the **Medicare Payment Advisory Commission (MedPAC)** found that physician-owned specialty hospitals did not have lower costs than competitor community hospitals did in their markets, although their patients had shorter lengths of stay. The commission also found that specialty hospitals admitted fewer severe cases and Medicaid patients than did their competitor community hospitals. Furthermore, the number of physician-owned specialty hospitals increased the most in states that have no certificate-of-need requirement (see Chapter 1, Highlight 1.13) and a growing demand for specialty services as a result of high population growth.

Other research has found that the number of people who undergo complex surgical procedures increases significantly when physician-owned specialty hospitals open. This trend stems from a greater number of physician referrals—because physicians profit from the specialty hospitals they own, they are more likely to refer their patients to them for surgery.

The Rise of Ambulatory Surgery Centers and Outpatient Surgery

In the twenty-first century, freestanding, outpatient **ambulatory surgery centers (ASCs)** were growing because they charged less than hospitals did. Most ASCs are for-profit and are located in large metropolitan areas. In 2013, 5,364 ASCs treated 3.4 million fee-for-service Medicare beneficiaries, and the Medicare program spent $3.7 billion on ASC services.

Medicare bases its payment rates on average cost of care, acuity of patients, and other factors. In addition to procedure rates, ASCs often receive professional fees for the individual physician. A high percentage of ASCs are for-profit organizations, and some argue that CMS is supporting hospital-based outpatient programs in an effort to ensure the survival of the hospitals. From 2008 through 2012, the number of Medicare-certified ASCs grew by an average annual rate of 1.7 percent, but in 2013, the number increased only by 1.1 percent. The government has shifted to higher Medicare payment rates in hospital outpatient departments (HOPDs), resulting in relatively slower growth of ASCs. In 2015, the Medicare rates were 82 percent higher for HOPDs than for ASCs. This payment difference may help explain why many hospitals have recently expanded their outpatient surgery capacity. In addition, physicians have increasingly sold their practices to hospitals, and these physicians are more likely to perform procedures at the hospitals that employ them than at freestanding ASCs (MedPAC 2015).

> **Ambulatory surgery center (ASC)**
> Facility at which outpatient surgeries (i.e., surgeries not requiring an overnight stay) are performed, often at a price that is less than that charged by hospitals.

GAP ANALYSIS

Gap analysis is a comparison of an organization's internal and external environments for the purpose of revealing, as the name suggests, gaps. *Gaps* are differences between the organization's current standing and its target performance. These gaps become the focal points that shape the strategic plan.

For example, say an organization's analysis of its internal environment reveals that its mission, vision, and values are not aligned. A primary strategic goal, then, would be to make these elements consistent with each other. Imagine that the organization finds that one of the critical success factors discussed in an earlier section is not in place—for example, its staff lacks certain skills. Organizational strategy would need to include plans for employee training to get staff up to speed.

Two of the most important gaps in organizations today are in information technology and diversity. These elements are discussed in the following sections.

> **Gap analysis**
> Comparison of an organization's current standing and its target performance.

HEALTH INFORMATION TECHNOLOGY AS A COMPETITIVE ADVANTAGE

Investments in health information technology (HIT) steadily increased over the first decade of the twenty-first century, reaching $33 billion in 2011 (Moses et al. 2013). This investment promises to increase efficiency in the healthcare system and improve quality of care through better coordination. Currently, 95 percent of US hospitals have electronic health records (EHRs) and are spending an average of 3 percent of total expenditures on HIT. Some large healthcare systems, such as the US Department of Veterans Affairs and Kaiser Permanente, are investing 4–5 percent of their revenue on HIT. Clinical information systems have the potential to improve both the inpatient and outpatient medical delivery systems. While some documentation of medical records in the United States is still paper based, EHRs offer an opportunity for the seamless exchange of clinical information. Studies examining the use of EHRs have found, in general, that EHRs have increased quality of care, reduced medication-related errors, improved follow-up on test results, and improved care coordination and communication within the care team (Nguyen, Bellucci, and Nguyen 2014).

EHRs allow the passage of real-time information to multiple users and timely feedback, both of which can foster more rapid quality improvement. In addition, users can pull information from a centralized database to supplement evidence-based research on clinical treatments. EHRs ease administrative decision making and the allocation of healthcare resources. For example, an EHR provides detailed information on patient services and current **payer mix**. This information can be linked to billing software to project reimbursement levels and measure the profitability of new business initiatives. These improvements can provide competitive advantage.

Payer mix
Percentage of revenue coming from private insurance versus government insurance versus individuals. The *mix* is important because Medicare and Medicaid often pay hospitals less than what it costs to treat patients.

To encourage the adoption of electronic information systems in the healthcare field, the Health Insurance Portability and Accountability Act (HIPAA) designated a standard electronic framework for electronic claims submission (see Highlight 3.1). Further, as part of the 2009 stimulus plan, President Obama called for a nationwide EHR system to be implemented by 2014. The program was managed through CMS and is called Meaningful Use. In 2013 the program reported that approximately 80 percent of eligible hospitals and more than 50 percent of eligible professionals have adopted EHRs and received incentive payments from Medicare or Medicaid (CMS 2013a).

As consolidation of healthcare organizations increases, more effective linkages are critical to the success of integrated delivery systems. From a risk management perspective, EHRs and supporting clinical information systems have the potential to reduce medical malpractice costs. Disjointed communication and incomplete records could become things of the past.

DIVERSITY IN THE WORKPLACE AS COMPETITIVE ADVANTAGE

Healthcare is the fastest-growing sector of the US economy and currently employs 18 million workers, 80 percent of whom are women (CDC 2015). The US hospital workforce has had an annual growth rate of 2.1 percent since 2000, when it totaled 17 million (Moses et al. 2013).

Demographic evidence shows that the US population is becoming more diverse and multicultural. In 2002, the Institute of Medicine released a report titled *Unequal Treatment:*

(✱) **HIGHLIGHT 3.1** HIPAA

HIPAA was passed in 1996 to protect the privacy and security of patient health information, particularly health information that can be used to discover a patient's identity, by

- setting national standards for the security of health information that has been stored electronically,

- permitting the confidential use of health information so that healthcare providers can analyze patient safety events and improve patient care, and

- affirming that patients own their health records and have the right to access their records.

Under HIPAA, all hospitals and healthcare providers must meet minimum information security and privacy standards. These standards allow data to be transferred between providers and other health-related entities, but the information must be coded securely and the parties doing the sharing must meet a certain list of administrative, physical, and technical safeguards and their required and addressable implementation specifications (CMS 2013b). The rules regulating information exchange are called HIPAA Transactions and Codes Sets and are based on electronic data interchange standards. The rules apply to healthcare providers, retail pharmacies, health plans, healthcare clearinghouses (organizations that do not provide care but do standardize information for providers), and covered entities (separate healthcare providers that are under one ownership). HIPAA has set rules for many types of transactions, including

- submitting claims to payers (e.g., insurance companies);

- requesting information about a patient's eligibility for certain treatments and responding to such requests;

- obtaining referrals for additional care from specialists and authorization to ensure the additional care will be covered by the payer;

- enrolling members in a health plan; and

- supplying information on patient demographics, diagnoses, or treatment plans for a healthcare services review.

Confronting Racial and Ethnic Disparities in Health Care. Since that time, healthcare organizations have made efforts to improve their cultural competence. The goal of cultural competence is to create a healthcare system and workforce that are capable of delivering the highest quality of care to every patient, regardless of race, ethnicity, culture, or language proficiency. Such a system would be equitable, of high quality, and free of disparities based on individual patient characteristics (Armada and Hubbard 2010). The American College of Healthcare Executives (2012) believes that diversity in healthcare management is both an ethical and a business imperative. Thus, to improve profitability and have a positive impact on the health status of the community, healthcare organizations should diversify their workforces. By integrating diversity into the strategic planning process, hospitals should be able to reduce health disparities in the communities they serve.

Improvement in cultural and gender diversity can be a competitive advantage for businesses. In a more diverse and inclusive workforce, individual discretionary effort improves by 12 percent, intent to stay improves by 20 percent, and team collaboration and commitment improve by about 50 percent (CEB 2012).

Greater diversity among healthcare providers can minimize language barriers and cultural differences. Improved communication between providers and patients leads to improved quality of healthcare. Under optimal conditions, the makeup of a hospital's workforce mirrors the population it serves (HRET 2011).

PLANNING AREAS

Strategic plans, at a minimum, need to address certain core areas in healthcare. These core areas include

- financial planning,
- efficiency,
- quality and value,
- management of healthcare personnel,
- current and long-term strategies,
- mix of products and services, and
- operational planning.

Each of these areas is addressed in the following sections.

FINANCIAL PLANNING

The healthcare environment has become more competitive, and healthcare leaders must improve their ability to manage resources and reduce costs. Faced with inadequate reimbursement, greater price competition, and a growing shortage of professional staff, healthcare organizations are forced to improve financial performance to gain greater access to capital and remain competitive. Hospitals are responding to these challenges by trying to provide higher volumes of care within limited financial resources. In addition, many hospitals are **benchmarking** against outstanding organizations—examining other organizations' business practices and products for purposes of comparing and improving one's own company—to improve internal operating procedures, enhance quality, maximize efficiency, and improve the value of healthcare services.

Strategic planning needs to ensure that proposed new services will attract a sufficient volume of patients to support an investment in new facilities. Before a proposal is approved, the organization should conduct a detailed study to determine whether the new service will likely generate enough revenue to justify the investment. This study should clearly define the new service line to be implemented; accurately forecast the volume of patients who will use the new service; and project construction costs, revenue, operating expenses, and overall profitability. Poor forecasting of clinical workload can lead to the approval of unnecessary and unprofitable projects.

As discussed in Chapter 1, an organization's status—for-profit or not-for-profit—affects its strategic financial planning. In general, not-for-profit hospitals have a lower return on assets, lower debt, higher occupancy rates, older facilities, and higher operating expenses per discharged patient. They also are larger and offer more clinical services. Although for-profit hospitals have higher long-term debt, they are more profitable because they use the money to invest in newer facilities. Not-for-profit hospitals have lower levels of debt because they often have difficulty borrowing money to fund facility improvements and technological advancements. Because they do a significant amount of charity care and earn lower revenues, nonprofits have difficulty paying back debt.

The strategic planning team should review key financial data as well as hospital operations data to ensure an efficient use of hospital resources, including personnel. Healthcare organizations can improve incoming cash flow by developing procedures for timely submission of correctly executed claims, rapid review of claim denials, and compliance with the organization's policy on charity care. Specifically, healthcare organizations should review their policies on charity care to ensure they are consistent with their mission and then monitor the level of charity care provided on an annual basis. In addition, healthcare organizations should perform an annual price analysis to confirm that the prices they charge for specific procedures are higher than authorized reimbursement rates so that they receive at least the maximum authorized reimbursement. This price analysis will also ensure that the reimbursement will cover the organization's **fixed cost**. Healthcare organizations should implement an audit program that reviews the accuracy of their billing and coding systems (Waugh 2014). Such a program ensures the accuracy of financial information used in the strategic planning process.

Payments from the federal Medicare program as well as from the combined state and federal Medicaid program now provide 30 percent of total hospital revenue (Harrison, Spaulding, and Mouhalis 2015). This level of government reimbursement is significant because it is set by regulation rather than market factors. As a result, much of a hospital's

Benchmarking
Examination of other organizations' business practices and products for purposes of comparing and improving one's own company.

Fixed cost
Cost incurred despite volume or use of a particular service. Examples of fixed-cost elements include buildings, equipment, and some salaried labor.

Variable cost

Cost that changes with volume or use and can be saved by the hospital if a service is not provided. Examples include medication, test reagents, and disposable supplies.

reimbursement for care does not adjust based on supply-and-demand factors. More important, in many states, Medicaid payments do not meet the **variable cost** of care or the total average cost (**total cost**) of care.

EFFICIENCY

As the population continues to age and more Americans become insured, the healthcare field is under growing pressure to improve efficiency as well as profitability. An efficient organization reduces its use of resources without worsening the outcomes of healthcare services (Harrison, Spaulding, and Mouhalis 2015). An efficiency evaluation compares organizations that share common characteristics in both clinical and administrative areas. For example, a comparison of two for-profit hospitals would be appropriate because they have similar missions. Individual hospital performance can be benchmarked against the **efficiency frontier** of "best-in-class" facilities, which model the maximal use of inputs (investment of resources) for the best possible outputs (profits and outcomes of care).

Total cost

All hospital expenditures, including facility operating costs.

Efficiency increases with greater hospital size (Harrison, Spaulding, and Mouhalis 2015). As discussed in Chapter 1, during the past ten years the number of not-for-profit hospitals with 400 or more beds has grown 15 percent and large for-profit hospitals have seen a 293 percent increase. Efficiency combined with improved quality represents greater value for healthcare services—an important consideration in the healthcare field as reimbursement for hospital services moves from a volume-based model to a value-based model as a result of the ACA.

Efficiency frontier

The best investment of resources for the best possible profits and outcomes of care.

QUALITY AND VALUE

Strategic planning in healthcare is often conducted by administrators focused on the business components and clinicians focused on patient care and quality. Striking a balance is important. Ongoing tension is often present in healthcare organizations between the value-driven approach and the volume-driven approach to service delivery. In times of economic strain, the temptation to decrease resources dedicated to quality is great; however, now, more than ever, quality and safety cannot be ignored in the strategic plan. The importance of publicly reported quality measures and patient experience scores will continue to increase and will be tied to reimbursement (Knight 2014).

The challenge in the planning process is finding a differentiating factor related to quality. Everyone is striving to be "the best," but doing so will require more than developing a quality scorecard. Thoughtful exercises in brainstorming what clients need or want is a part of considering quality and value. Some areas for consideration are improving access and patient flow, using Lean processes to improve efficiencies in care processes, leveraging technology, aligning with providers, managing population health, and creating a positive patient experience (Knight 2014).

One definition of value is that for which the customer would willingly and knowingly pay. The consumer decides on the timeliness as well as the quality level of the product or service she is purchasing. The government even calls this value-based purchasing (see Chapter 12). Although consumers would prefer to purchase healthcare of the best quality, resource limitations tend to redirect their focus on cost. This is where the consumer starts to look hard at the best value for her time and money.

MANAGEMENT OF HEALTHCARE PERSONNEL

Healthcare organizations should continually monitor personnel costs and productivity against industry benchmarks. In particular, they should routinely perform salary surveys to compare their salary rates with those of local and state peers.

Hospitals require adequate numbers of well-trained and highly credentialed healthcare professionals. Research has shown there is a strong relationship between adequate nurse-to-patient ratios and safe patient outcomes (ANA 2014). Ensuring adequate staffing levels has been shown to reduce medical and medication errors, decrease patient complications, decrease mortality, and improve patient satisfaction. Yet 54 percent of nurses report excessive workload. One in three nurses report inadequate staffing levels. Two in five units are short-staffed (ANA 2015).

High-quality healthcare is provided by teams of physicians, nurses, and allied health professionals trained in more than 50 different medical specialties. Good communication and close collaboration are required to ensure that the 200 or more professional interactions that occur during an average hospital admission result in high-quality care (Nancarrow et al. 2013). Research has shown that healthcare organizations with well-coordinated teams report lower long-term illness and mortality. Patient satisfaction also improves when healthcare professionals communicate clearly, express empathy, and demonstrate good listening skills. Good communication skills can be taught, and healthcare organizations must foster an environment in which good provider–patient communication is a priority.

CURRENT AND LONG-TERM STRATEGIES

Excellent strategic planning is a key for healthcare organizations that have proved profitable in the long term. Strategic planning provides a framework for integrating marketing, efficiency, personnel management, and outstanding clinical quality while ensuring financial performance. The development of process improvement teams is vital, and so is the use of real-time data to monitor performance on key metrics. Accurate data on community demographics, market share, payer mix, costs, and medical staff performance allow executives to make sound decisions.

By comparing these internal data with competitor and industrywide benchmarks, leaders can develop sound strategic plans and financial targets. Good data enable them to accurately forecast future demand over the next five to ten years. Short-term performance also must be monitored to make sure it is consistent with the organization's long-term vision. Once new business initiatives become fully operational (typically 24 months after start-up), the organization should evaluate them to ensure that they are fulfilling the objectives of the strategic plan. (Performance measurement and evaluation will be covered in greater detail later in the chapter.) In addition to performance measurement, creativity and a focus on community needs are important to long-range strategic planning.

MIX OF PRODUCTS AND SERVICES

Hospitals' reimbursement rates have been decreased as a result of federal government spending cuts, and insurance payers are following government strategies. Patients are reconsidering healthcare spending because of the economic downturn and growing insurance deductibles. The impact of these trends on a hospital's bottom line can be significant. One response is significant cost reductions, but cutting costs can often restrict a hospital's ability to increase revenue, creating a downward spiral for the facility. Healthcare leaders should find ways to redirect current resources to create more effective growth strategies. Growth is paramount in this very tumultuous time (Clark and Lindsey 2013).

Many hospitals located in growing communities are expanding their inpatient and outpatient capacities. While many services are profitable, these organizations need to operate unprofitable services such as obstetrics, pediatrics, and emergency services. As a result, many of these hospitals are participating in joint ventures with physicians to improve clinical quality and develop a more varied product mix. Healthcare organizations should routinely monitor their medical staff network to maximize clinical services while ensuring a profitable mix. Such an assessment should take into consideration changing community demographics and needs and the product mixes that competitors offer. Healthcare organizations can gather information on changing community needs from community leaders, board members, hospital employees, and physicians on the medical staff.

Joint ventures enable organizations to preserve capital, expand services, and better meet community healthcare needs. A healthcare organization seeking a joint venture should identify potential partners that demonstrate ethical, cultural, and quality-of-care factors that are consistent with its strategic plan. Once these model partners have been identified, the strategic planning process can pinpoint clinical areas in which joint ventures may be most appropriate. Such areas could be new service lines, the development of facilities that are more convenient or easier for patients to access, or high-level services that enhance the hospital's reputation. Any new service should be financially profitable and provide long-term value to the organization. Value may take the form of increased clinical volume, greater market share, or limited competition from other hospitals.

OPERATIONAL PLANNING

Operational plans set strategic plans in motion and carry out the tasks they prescribe. Each operational plan should be assigned to a senior leader and linked to specific activities with deadlines. Responsibilities should be assigned to individual leaders who are held accountable for performance. By pushing operational goals down the ranks of the organization, the strategic plan becomes a reality for all staff and creates a unified endeavor. The strategic plan should prioritize operational goals according to the resources available to the organization at any given point in time.

EVALUATION OF PERFORMANCE

Once strategic plans are in operation, organizations must evaluate the results of strategic actions. To align behaviors, clear goals must be linked with the measurement of outcomes. Organizations that are able to create such an alignment are more likely to be successful, but they should monitor their performance on a routine basis. For example, performance data could be collected monthly and then evaluated over time.

One useful tool for linking strategic goals to annual operating performance is called a **dashboard**. Like the gas gauge, speedometer, and temperature gauge on a car dashboard, an organizational dashboard contains numerous indicators of performance. Just as the indicators on a car dashboard must all reflect good performance for the car to reach its destination, an organization's strategic success depends on the collective performance shown by the indicators on its dashboard. An example of a hospital dashboard is shown in Exhibit 3.2.

Dashboard
Tool that links strategic goals to operating performance.

Dashboard measures might include quality of care (nosocomial infection rates[1] and 30-day readmission rates[2]), patient satisfaction, market penetration, operating efficiency (by emergency wait time, average length of stay, or cost per procedure), and financial performance (net operating income and cash on hand). The dashboard should include visual cues, such as green representing favorable performance, yellow representing areas of growing concern, and red representing areas of poor performance.

On the basis of these indicators, the organization can modify its strategy to improve areas of poor performance. For example, say a hospital wants to build a particular service line, but its dashboard shows that it does not have enough staff to do so. The hospital would then need to focus on recruiting and training additional staff while ensuring that it can afford to compensate the new staff and will still make a profit.

As shown in Exhibit 3.1, evaluation of performance ends the strategic planning cycle, but not the strategic planning process. Strategic planning is a continuous activity. In healthcare, change occurs rapidly, both internally and externally. Once a strategy has been implemented and evaluated, the cycle begins again. An organization modifies its strategy as needed, reimplements it, and evaluates it again, and new strategies are developed in response to the changing environment.

EXHIBIT 3.2
Sample Hospital
Dashboard

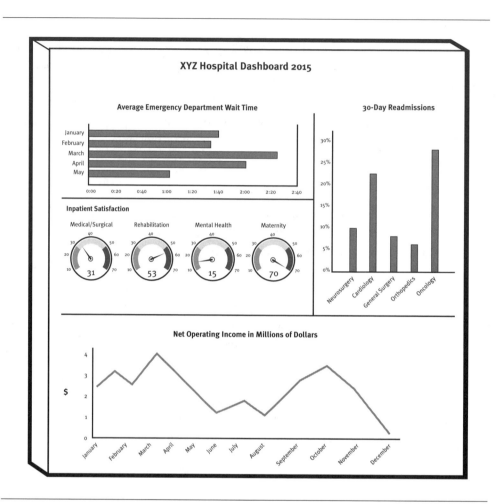

*Balanced scorecard
(BSC)*
Tool that allows
organizations to
assess their missions
by evaluating specific
objectives and metrics
across multiple
domains.

Another tool is the **balanced scorecard (BSC)**, which allows a corporation to view its performance. The BSC is a strategy and management system that focuses an organization on several areas of performance measurement. Prior to the introduction of the BSC, in most cases, performance was measured on the basis of financial achievements alone.

The BSC shows, at a glance, an organization's goals and how it aims to achieve them. The BSC is divided into several areas that the organization considers important to achieving its mission—for example, human resources, patient satisfaction, financial position, quality and safety outcomes, or employee professional development. For each area, the organization states objectives and identifies specific measurements that will demonstrate how it is progressing in that area. Target results are also listed to indicate what an organization hopes or expects to achieve. For example, the human resources section of the BSC might measure and list targets for employee turnover that include the turnover rate, cost per hire, length of employment, and so forth. The BSC allows everyone in the organization to see easily what the organization's priorities are and which areas need improvement.

Specific metrics should meet the following criteria: (1) importance to organization and staff, (2) measurability, (3) data validity, and (4) actionability. The BSC is balanced because it meets four goals. First, it provides a broad view of performance; second, it creates transparency and accountability; third, it communicates goals and engages staff; and last, it ensures the use of data in the strategic planning process.

PLANNING AT THE LOCAL, REGIONAL, AND NATIONAL LEVELS

Organizational planning at the local level is different from regional and national healthcare planning. As a result of the growth in health systems, many healthcare organizations are doing more regional and national planning.

LOCAL PLANNING

In general, healthcare in the United States is a local commodity produced to meet local demand. For this reason, much of an organization's strategic plan is developed using local data. A good understanding of community needs is necessary for local healthcare planning. More important, local governmental entities and other organizations in the community can provide additional funding and thus significantly influence the allocation of healthcare resources.

Measuring the availability of physicians, allied healthcare providers, hospital beds, and long-term care resources in the local geographic area is a responsibility of the local health-planning council. State government also assesses the effect of its communities' economic status on the availability of healthcare services in the area. Economic factors affect individuals' ability to pay for healthcare services, the number of uninsured, and, ultimately, the community's overall health. Common economic factors affecting local planning include per capita income and the percentage of unemployed in the community.

REGIONAL PLANNING

As healthcare complexity increases in the United States, a case can be made for allocating healthcare resources at the regional (e.g., state) level. Such an approach could reduce costs through improved efficiency and ensure a consistently high level of healthcare quality.

Regional planning at the state level includes an analysis of population demographics and the development of mathematical models designed to determine the need for health services in local communities. These activities address a variety of questions associated with regional health planning, such as the location of hospitals; the number of hospital beds, hospitals with open-heart surgery units, ASCs, imaging centers, and nursing homes;

and the availability of hospice programs. Typically, academic medical centers generate the strongest presence on a regional level, followed by larger tertiary community hospitals. Some hospitals have differentiated themselves by affiliating with academic medical centers or health systems (Beckham 2014).

The ACA broadened Medicaid's role, making it the foundation of coverage for nearly all with incomes up to 138 percent of the federal poverty level. However, the 2012 US Supreme Court ruling on *National Federation of Independent Businesses v. Sebelius* made the decision to implement the Medicaid expansion optional for states. For those that expand, the federal government will pay 100 percent of Medicaid costs of those newly eligible for Medicaid from 2014 to 2016. The federal share will phase down gradually to 90 percent in 2020, where it remains well above traditional federal medical-assistance percentage rates. As of March 2015, 29 states (including the District of Columbia) had adopted the Medicaid expansion, though debate continues in other states (Dorn et al. 2015). The low-income population and its increased access to medical care should be considered in the planning process depending on the state's position on Medicaid.

NATIONAL PLANNING

A framework for healthcare strategic planning at the national level is important. The passage of the ACA provided the foundation of a national strategic healthcare plan that integrates the priorities of key stakeholders, including patients, employers, plans, healthcare providers, and medical suppliers. The strategic plan was developed by the federal government and then implemented by governmental authorities at the local and regional levels.

Healthy People 2020
A comprehensive analysis of the US population's healthcare needs and a statement of goals and measures by the US Department of Health & Human Services, around which local and regional planning can take place. Also the name of a ten-year effort to achieve the goals it outlines.

The United States experienced significant improvement in the health status of its population between 2005 and 2015. However, research demonstrates that minorities suffer disproportionately from many diseases. The federal and state governments are working to reduce these disparities through such projects as the ***Healthy People 2020*** report—a statement of healthcare objectives, around which local and regional planning can take place, produced by the US Department of Health & Human Services. Also the name of a ten-year effort to promote the goals it outlines, this comprehensive analysis of the US population's healthcare needs specifies healthcare improvement goals and measures by which progress toward those goals can be monitored.

Healthy People 2020 contains 42 topic areas with more than 1,200 objectives. The *Healthy People 2020* objectives, called Leading Health Indicators, were selected to communicate high-priority health issues and actions that can be taken to address them. Great strides have been made over the past decade: Life expectancy at birth has increased; rates of death from coronary heart disease and stroke have decreased. Nonetheless, public health challenges remain, and significant health disparities persist.

The *Healthy People 2020* Leading Health Indicators place renewed emphasis on overcoming these challenges as we track progress up to the year 2020. The indicators will be used to assess the health of the nation, facilitate collaboration across sectors, and motivate action at the national, state, and community levels to improve the health of the US population (HHS 2015).

Many believe local communities have the greatest understanding of healthcare needs and therefore should have significant influence over healthcare planning decisions. As such, local communities should be included in the strategic planning process and in any national healthcare reform initiative.

ENDNOTES

1. *Nosocomial infections* are infections that are not caused by a patient's condition but are acquired in hospitals and other healthcare facilities.

2. A *30-day readmission rate* is the percentage of patients who were treated for a particular condition and discharged from the hospital but who had to be readmitted to the same or another hospital within 30 days of the initial discharge.

SUMMARY

Strategic planning is a process by which healthcare organizations determine their future direction. An important part of strategic planning is the allocation of resources to maximize the delivery of healthcare services. Research suggests that good strategic planning leads to lower healthcare costs, improved quality of care, and greater patient satisfaction.

Healthcare strategic planning is grounded in an organization's mission, vision, and values. Building on this foundation, the organization develops a strategic plan based on analyses of the internal environment of the organization and the external environment in which it operates.

As part of the process, organizations identify factors necessary to achieving outstanding performance and then complete a gap analysis designed to identify where improvement is needed. At the operational level, developing programs and services that support the overall strategic plan and turn plan objectives into action is important for healthcare organizations.

An effective tool for linking the strategic plan to operating performance is a dashboard analysis. Measurement of performance via a dashboard is part of an ongoing feedback process that drives future strategic planning. Programs are implemented, performance is measured, and any remaining performance gaps prompt the cycle to begin again.

EXERCISES

REVIEW QUESTIONS

1. What roles do boards of directors, senior leaders, physicians, employees, and community organizations play in a healthcare organization's strategic planning process?

2. Do you agree that healthcare organizations should monitor key business metrics throughout the year? Evaluate this idea and provide an example from the chapter that illustrates the monitoring of organizational performance.

3. Should a healthcare organization do a community health assessment as part of its strategic planning? Why or why not?

4. Does the diversity of a healthcare organization's staff have any impact on organizational performance?

COASTAL MEDICAL CENTER EXERCISES

According to Chapter 3 and the Coast Medical Center (CMC) case study, does CMC have the organizational capabilities for future success?

Richard Reynolds, the newly hired CEO, has been actively investigating the declining performance of CMC. During the hiring process, the board of directors assigned him the responsibility of getting the organization back on track. Help Mr. Reynolds develop a strategic planning process that will place CMC on a new road to success by considering five new business initiatives, creating a dashboard, and evaluating CMC based on these metrics. Outline a strategic planning process appropriate for CMC.

COASTAL MEDICAL CENTER QUESTIONS

1. Many stakeholders described the past CEO of CMC, Don Wilson, as a visionary who helped the organization grow and prosper for more than 20 years. His successor, Ron Henderson, took the organization from profitability to significant financial losses within two years and was fired as a result. Name five areas in which Mr. Henderson's performance was weak.

2. Of the five areas of new business initiatives to improve performance, which one should be the first priority?

3. How is CMC positioned relative to its competitors?

4. How should CMC create new and innovative approaches to community needs?

5. What do you see as the future of strategic planning at CMC?

REFERENCES

American College of Healthcare Executives. 2012. "Statement on Diversity." Revised March. www.ache.org/policy/diversity.cfm.

American Nurses Association (ANA). 2015. "Nurse Staffing." Accessed August 12. www. nursingworld.org/nursestaffing.

————. 2014. "Safe Staffing Literature Review." Published August. www.nursingworld.org/ MainMenuCategories/ThePracticeofProfessionalNursing/NurseStaffing/2014-Nurse-Staffing-Updated-Literature-Review.pdf.

Armada, A. A., and M. F. Hubbard. 2010. "Diversity in Healthcare: Time to Get REAL!" *Frontiers of Health Services Management* 26 (3): 3–17.

Babu, M. A., J. M. Rosenow, and B. V. Nahed. 2011. "Physician-Owned Hospitals, Neurosurgeons, and Disclosure: Lessons from Law and the Literature." *Neurosurgery* 68 (6): 1724–32.

Beckham, D. 2014. "Differentiating Physicians for Competitive Advantage." *H&HN Daily*. Published June 17. www.hhnmag.com/Daily/2014/Jun/061714-beckham-physician-differentiation.

Centers for Disease Control and Prevention (CDC). 2015. "Healthcare Workers." Accessed April 14. www.cdc.gov/niosh/topics/healthcare/default.html.

Centers for Medicare & Medicaid Services (CMS). 2015. "Accountable Care Organizations (ACO)." Last modified January 6. www.cms.gov/Medicare/Medicare-Fee-for-Service-Payment/ACO/index.html.

————. 2013a. "Data Show Electronic Health Records Empower Patients and Equip Doctors." Published July 17. www.cms.gov/Newsroom/MediaReleaseDatabase/Press-Releases/2013-Press-Releases-Items/2013-07-17.html.

————. 2013b. "Privacy and Security Standards." Last modified April 2. www.cms.gov/ Regulations-and-Guidance/HIPAA-Administrative-Simplification/HIPAAGenInfo/Privacy andSecurityStandards.html.

Clark, B., and S. Lindsey. 2013. "Growth Is the Answer: 3 Ways to Grow Your Hospital Business." *Becker's Hospital Review*. Published May 30. www.beckershospitalreview.com/hospital-management-administration/growth-is-the-answer-3-ways-to-grow-your-hospital-business.html.

Corporate Executive Board (CEB). 2012. "Creating Competitive Advantage Through Workforce Diversity: Seven Imperatives and Inventive Ideas for Companies That Want to Get It Right." Accessed August 12, 2015. http://img.en25.com/Web/CEB/diversity-whitepaper.pdf.

Dorn, S., N. Francis, L. Snyder, and R. Rudowitz. 2015. "The Effects of the Medicaid Expansion on State Budgets: An Early Look in Select States." Kaiser Family Foundation. Published March 11. http://kff.org/medicaid/issue-brief/the-effects-of-the-medicaid-expansion-on-state-budgets-an-early-look-in-select-states/.

Harrison, J., A. Spaulding, and P. Mouhalis. 2015. "The Efficiency Frontier of For-Profit Hospitals." *Journal of Health Care Finance* 41 (4): 1–23.

Health Research & Educational Trust (HRET). 2011. *Building a Culturally Competent Organization: The Quest for Equity in Health Care*. Published June. www.hret.org/quality/projects/resources/cultural-competency.pdf.

Institute of Medicine. 2002. *Unequal Treatment: Confronting Racial and Ethnic Disparities in Health Care*. Washington, DC: National Academies Press.

Knight, E. 2014. *Strategic Planning for Hospitals and Healthcare Systems*. Coker Group. Published October. www.cokergroup.com/2012-09-26-20-46-16/white-papers?...29.

Medicare Payment Advisory Commission (MedPAC). 2015. "Report to the Congress: Medicare Payment Policy March 2015." Accessed August 12. www.medpac.gov/documents/reports/mar2015_entirereport_revised.pdf.

Moses, H., D. Matheson, E. R. Dorsey, B. George, D. Sadoff, and S. Yoshimura. 2013. "The Anatomy of Health Care in the United States." *Journal of the American Medical Association* 310 (18): 1947–64.

Nancarrow, S. A., A. Booth, S. Ariss, T. Smith, P. Enderby, and A. Roots. 2013. "Ten Principles of Good Interdisciplinary Team Work." *Human Resources for Health* 11 (19): 2–11.

Nguyen, L., E. Bellucci, and L. T. Nguyen. 2014. "Electronic Health Records Implementation: An Evaluation of Information System Impact and Contingency Factors." *International Journal of Medical Informatics* 83 (11): 779–96.

Pellegrin, K . L., and H. S. Currey. 2011. "Demystifying and Improving Organizational Culture in Health-Care." In *Organization Development in Healthcare: Conversations on Research and Strategies*, edited by J. A. Wolf, H. Hanson, M. J. Moir, L. Friedman, and G. T. Savage, 3–23. Volume 10 of *Advances in Health Care Management*. Bingley, UK: Emerald Group Publishing.

Pellet, L. 2013. "Organizational Culture Is Created by What Leaders Allocate Attention and Resources To." *Talent Space* (blog). Published November 8. www.halogensoftware. com/blog/organizational-culture-is-created-by-what-leaders-allocate-attention-and-resources-to.

Sommers, B., T. Musco, K. Finegold, M. Gunja, A. Burke, and A. McDowell. 2014. "Health Reform and Changes in Health Insurance Coverage in 2014." *New England Journal of Medicine* 371 (9): 867–74.

US Department of Health & Human Services (HHS). 2015. "Leading Health Indicators." Healthy People 2020. Accessed April 3. www.healthypeople.gov/2020/Leading-Health-Indicators.

Waugh, J. L. 2014. "Education in Medical Billing Benefits Both Neurology Trainees and Academic Departments." *Neurology* 83 (20): 1856–61.

CHAPTER 4

STRATEGIC PLANNING AND SWOT ANALYSIS

I skate where the puck is going to be, not where it has been.

—Wayne Gretzky

LEARNING OBJECTIVES

After you have studied this chapter, you should be able to

➤ demonstrate the ability to integrate the various disciplines into a comprehensive framework to assess healthcare strategic planning problems;

➤ exercise strong individual managerial problem-solving skills through the use of SWOT analysis;

➤ formulate strategy and implement change through the use of gap analysis and force field analysis; and

➤ discuss multidisciplinary teamwork required within organizations that allows leaders and individual team members to efficiently implement change.

KEY TERMS AND CONCEPTS

➤ Bundled payment

➤ Churn rate

➤ Downstream value

➤ Force field analysis

➤ Opportunities

➤ Strengths

➤ SWOT analysis

➤ Threats

➤ Weaknesses

INTRODUCTION

Healthcare organizations must continually make adjustments to maintain optimal function. The high rate of change in healthcare is shortening the strategic planning window for healthcare organizations that are adapting to healthcare reform (Zuckerman 2014). Leading organizations believe strategic planning is more important than ever and focus on allocating resources for the short and long term, integrating geographically separated organizations, and developing a team that can focus on a clear strategy. As a result, strategic planning is evolving into a more continuous and integrated process. A number of different techniques can be used to determine where adjustments need to be made. One essential technique involves a discussion of an organization's strengths, weaknesses, opportunities, and threats, commonly called **SWOT analysis**. SWOT analysis has been used extensively in other industries but has not yet been widely used in healthcare (Makos 2014).

Prior to strategic planning, a panel of experts who can assess the organization from a critical perspective perform a SWOT analysis. This panel could comprise senior leaders, board members, employees, medical staff, patients, community leaders, and technical experts. Panel members base their assessment on utilization rates, outcome measures, patient satisfaction statistics, organizational performance measures, and financial status. While based on data and facts, the conclusions drawn from SWOT analysis are the expert opinion of the panel.

The annual strategic planning process should incorporate strategic planning, action planning, and operational oversight into an ongoing cycle (Zuckerman 2014). Many of the elements discussed in SWOT analysis are a part of this process, including environmental factors, organizational structure, capital financing, operational planning, and measurement of financial performance.

SWOT analysis
Examination of an organization's internal strengths and weaknesses, its opportunities for growth and improvement, and the threats the external environment presents to its survival.

DEFINITION

SWOT analysis is an examination of an organization's internal strengths and weaknesses, its opportunities for growth and improvement, and the threats the external environment presents to its survival. Originally designed for use in other industries, it is gaining increased use in healthcare.

Steps in SWOT Analysis

The primary aim of strategic planning is to bring an organization into balance with the external environment and to maintain that balance over time. Organizations accomplish this balance by evaluating new programs and services with the intent of maximizing organizational performance. SWOT analysis is a preliminary decision-making tool that sets the stage for this work.

Step 1 of SWOT analysis involves the collection and evaluation of key data. Depending on the organization, these data might include population demographics, community health status, sources of healthcare funding, and the current status of medical technology in the organization. Once the data have been collected and analyzed, the organization assesses its capabilities in these areas.

After the data on the organization are collected, in step 2 it is sorted into four categories: strengths, weaknesses, opportunities, and threats. Strengths and weaknesses generally stem from factors in the organization, whereas opportunities and threats usually arise from external factors. Organizational surveys are an effective means of gathering some of this information, such as data on an organization's finances, operations, and processes (Makos 2014). Exhibit 4.1 illustrates step 2 of SWOT analysis in a hypothetical example

Exhibit 4.1
Sample SWOT
Matrix

	Helpful to Objective	Harmful to Objective
Internal Origin	**Strengths** • Worldwide reputation • Focus on patient care • Focus on quality and value • Experience in medical imaging • Location of hospital • High-tech facility and equipment • No capital expenditures	**Weaknesses** • Some increase in staffing • Some dissatisfaction by employees working on Saturdays • Increased workload for radiologists already working at peak performance
External Origin	**Opportunities** • Local community targeted marketing • Improvements in payer mix • Improvements in integrated care	**Threats** • Local competitors offering Saturday MRIs • Loss of potential market share and revenue to competitors • Unknown implications of healthcare reform

of an outpatient clinic considering the value of adding Saturday MRI (magnetic resonance imaging) appointments in response to increasing demand.

Step 3 involves the development of a SWOT matrix for each business alternative under consideration. For example, say a hospital is evaluating the development of an ambulatory surgery center (ASC). It is looking at two options: The first is a wholly owned ASC, and the second is a joint venture with local physicians. The hospital's expert panel would complete a separate SWOT matrix for each alternative.

Step 4 involves incorporating the SWOT analysis into the decision-making process to determine which business alternative best meets the organization's overall strategic plan.

STRENGTHS

Traditional SWOT analysis views **strengths** as current factors that have prompted outstanding organizational performance. Examples include the use of state-of-the-art medical equipment, investments in healthcare informatics, and a focus on community healthcare improvement projects.

Strengths
Current factors that have prompted outstanding organizational performance.

To draw an example from real life, Mayo Clinic is a nonprofit, integrated, multispecialty medical practice with more than 60,000 employees. Mayo is an outstanding organization because it integrates the provision of healthcare through teamwork, the use of real-time patient healthcare information, and the application of advanced technology to provide high-quality care to the patient at an affordable cost (Berry and Beckham 2014). For example, treatment at an academic medical center during the last two years of life for a patient with at least one of nine chronic conditions might cost $93,000, while similar treatment at Mayo would cost $53,000 (Wennberg et al. 2008). Mayo's strengths also include investing in structural tools such as comprehensive electronic health records, which connect individual clinicians with the latest clinical information available for treating the patient.

Patients at Mayo frequently have complex medical conditions that benefit from the pooling of knowledge inside the organization and among the integrated healthcare team. Mayo fosters a culture that considers teamwork essential to delivering patient-centered care. This attitude translates to a unified focus on shared values to achieve a high level of collaboration across the team. This teamwork enhances learning, inspires confidence, and promotes camaraderie among the clinical team. Research suggests that top-tier organizations nurture teamwork and recruit individuals who are likely to be team players (Beckham 2013).

For other healthcare organizations, potential organizational strengths might include highly competent personnel, a clear understanding among employees of the organization's goals, and a focus on quality improvement. Future strengths include growth through mergers and acquisitions as healthcare organizations consolidate into larger organizations with annual revenues in excess of $2 billion (Zuckerman 2014). These larger organizations have the ability to reach economies of scale and reduce costs in the future by 3–5 percent annually. This reduction in costs combined with improved quality results in greater value for the patient.

WEAKNESSES

Weaknesses are organizational factors that increase healthcare costs or reduce healthcare quality. Under healthcare reform, it is increasingly clear that hospitals that seek to "go it alone" will find it difficult to acquire the financial and human resources necessary to build the infrastructure required for coordinated care.

The fundamental Affordable Care Act (ACA) model for integrated care shifts the healthcare system from volume-driven fee-for-service care provision to chronic disease management and value-driven episodes of care (see Highlight 4.1). The shift is occurring piecemeal, one payer and one contract at a time—forcing hospitals to operate in both the volume- and value-driven models at the same time. As a result, hospital mergers have increased in order to find strategic partners that can manage the transition from a volume-driven to a value-driven marketplace. In 2000, 52 percent of hospitals were part of multihospital systems, whereas by the end of 2013, 62 percent of hospitals had joined multihospital systems (AHA 2014). As organizations now position themselves for value-based reimbursement with shared savings and **bundled payments** (single payments made to providers or healthcare facilities for all services rendered to treat a given condition or provide a given treatment), freestanding hospitals will increasingly be unable to provide integrated healthcare (Lineen 2014).

Other hospital weaknesses include aging facilities and a lack of continuity in clinical processes, which can lead to duplication of efforts. Weaknesses can be broken down further to identify underlying causes. For example, disruption in the continuity of care often results from poor communication. This fragmentation leads to inefficiencies in the entire system—weaknesses also breed other weaknesses. Thus, poor communication disrupts the continuity of care. Inefficiencies, in turn, deplete financial and other resources.

The growth in integrated delivery systems allows greater efficiency across the continuum of healthcare. As a result, hospitals will need to develop ambulatory care networks and enhance their relationship with multispecialty physician groups. Failing to market ambulatory services in the face of increasing competition could prove to be a fatal weakness as patient referrals migrate to larger health systems.

Other common weaknesses include poor use of healthcare informatics, insufficient management training, lack of financial resources, and an organizational structure that limits collaboration with other healthcare organizations. A payer mix that includes large numbers of uninsured patients or Medicaid patients can also negatively affect an organization's financial performance, and lack of relevant and timely patient data can increase costs and lower the quality of patient care.

OPPORTUNITIES

Traditional SWOT analysis views **opportunities** as significant new business initiatives available to a healthcare organization. For example, healthcare organizations could collaborate through the development of healthcare delivery networks, pursue increased funding for

> (✳) **HIGHLIGHT 4.1** Value-Driven Episodes of Care
>
> The US Department of Health & Human Services (HHS) is testing and expanding new healthcare payment models that can improve healthcare quality and reduce its cost. HHS has adopted a framework that categorizes healthcare payment according to how providers receive payment to provide care:
>
> - Category 1—Fee-for-service with no link of payment to quality
>
> - Category 2—Fee-for-service with a link of payment to quality
>
> - Category 3—Alternative payment models built on fee-for-service architecture
>
> - Category 4—Population-based payment
>
> Value-based purchasing includes payments made in categories 2–4. Moving from category 1 to category 4 involves two shifts: (1) increasing accountability for both quality and total cost of care and (2) a greater focus on population health management as opposed to payment for specific services.
>
> Prior to 2011, many Medicare payments to providers were tied only to volume, rewarding providers based on, for example, how many tests they ran, how many patients they saw, or how many procedures they did, regardless of whether these services helped (or harmed) the patient. But under the ACA and because of other changes, by 2014, an estimated 20 percent of Medicare reimbursements had shifted to categories 3 and 4, directly linking providers' reimbursement to the health and well-being of their patients (CMS 2015).

healthcare informatics, partner with communities to develop new healthcare programs, or introduce clinical protocols to improve quality and efficiency. Additional opportunities include obtaining increased reimbursement; instituting value-based purchasing; increasing patient satisfaction; providing new clinical services aligned with population health needs; and delivering integrated, patient-focused care. Healthcare organizations might also improve patient satisfaction by increasing public involvement and ensuring patient representation on boards and committees.

Organizations that are successful at using data to improve clinical processes have lower costs and higher-quality patient care. For example, healthcare organizations with Centers for Medicaid & Medicare Services (CMS) Hospital Compare quality scores above the 90th national percentile are eligible for CMS pay-for-performance incentives (see Chapter 6 for information on CMS Hospital Compare). Pay-for-performance incentive programs vary payment among providers on the basis of quality and efficiency measures so that desired outcomes occur through changed behavior. The greater the number of organizations achieving such scores, the greater patients' access to quality healthcare. Such scores also enhance an organization's reputation in the community. While there will always be a certain number of hospitals at the 90th percentile, the bar continues to keep getting higher. Even the best have to continue to improve.

THREATS

Threats
Factors that could negatively affect organizational performance.

Churn rate
Ratio indicating the quantity of new patients relative to existing patients.

Threats are factors that could negatively affect organizational performance. Examples include political or economic instability, increasing demand by patients and physicians for expensive medical technology that is not cost-effective, increasing state and federal budget deficits, and increasing pressure to reduce healthcare costs. Additional threats include healthcare funding cuts, the increasing cost of technology, and the potential for reduced access to capital.

One of the basic threats to a healthcare organization's survival is **churn rate**, the quantity of new patients relative to existing patients. Hospital churn rates can vary, but a good target is 15 percent new patients annually. This rate replaces lost business while maintaining significant growth. A high churn rate can be good news. A low churn rate suggests that an organization is losing potential new patients to its competitors and poses a significant threat if the number of existing patients also declines. Such a decrease in the number of existing patients can come from many sources; patients may move out of the area, die, or age into a cohort requiring a different type of provider. Referral patterns among primary physicians may also change. Low churn rates clearly reflect an organization's inability to attract new patients, possibly driven by low patient satisfaction.

SWOT ANALYSIS: INTERNAL AND EXTERNAL PERSPECTIVE

As shown in Exhibit 4.1, SWOT has an internal as well as an external focus. Strengths and weaknesses are primarily internal in origin. Examples of these internal factors include patient satisfaction, cost per procedure, and level of quality. Conversely, opportunities and threats are primarily external in origin. These could include the level of competition in the market, the availability of integrated care, and the economy of scale as measured by an organization's market share. Strengths and opportunities are helpful to the objective; weaknesses and threats are harmful to the objective.

FORCE FIELD ANALYSIS

Healthcare organizations' responsibility to implement change that is beneficial to the patient, staff, and organization is increasing. The primary drivers of change in healthcare are the push for quality improvement, the need for customer satisfaction, the desire to improve working conditions, and the diversification of the healthcare workforce.

Force field analysis (see Exhibit 4.2) takes SWOT analysis a step further by identifying the forces driving or hindering change—in other words, the forces driving an organization's strengths, weaknesses, opportunities, and threats. Kurt Lewin's (1951) force field analysis and force field diagrams are the founding theory for this exercise. Forces that propel an organization toward goal achievement are called *helping forces*, while those that block progress toward a goal are called *hindering forces*. After identifying these positive and negative forces, an organization can develop strategies to strengthen the positives and minimize the negatives. For an organization to achieve success, the helping forces must outweigh the hindering forces. When this state is reached, an organization is able to move from its current reality to a preferred future.

Effective force field analysis considers not only organizational values but also the needs, goals, ideals, and concerns of individual stakeholders. Individuals who promote change are

Force field analysis
Examination of the forces helping or hindering organizational change.

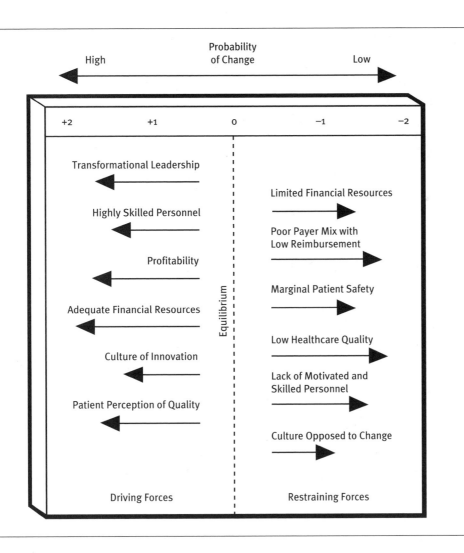

EXHIBIT 4.2
Healthcare Model for Force Field Analysis

helping forces, whereas those who resist change are hindering forces. As a result, understanding individuals, their attitudes, and the culture of the organization is important. A group performing force field analysis should also identify the key stakeholders in an issue and develop a plan to gain their support. Counteracting organizational inertia (the hindering forces) and creating an environment that proactively supports future change (the helping forces) is vital. Such change is accomplished by modifying current attitudes ("unfreezing" an organization's perspective on a particular issue), emphasizing the positive aspects of change, and then incorporating the new attitudes in the organization's processes ("refreezing" the new attitudes so that they and their associated behavior patterns become entrenched in the institution).

A participative management style that solicits input from inside the organization is important in implementing change. This approach also fosters the development of consensus within work groups, which helps to refreeze the new behaviors in the organization.

GAP ANALYSIS

To further refine planning decisions, SWOT analysis can be supplemented by gap analysis, which reveals differences between the organization's current standing and its target performance. Knowing where to focus efforts improves the efficiency of interventions. Obtaining data that can be used for local benchmarking and improvement is a key step in raising awareness and driving quality improvement. Research shows that while we have seen improvement, there are still gaps of quality care in healthcare practice. For example, in 2010, 287,000 women died worldwide from causes related to pregnancy and childbirth. Also, during the same year, 3.1 million babies died in their first month of life (Dean et al. 2014). These mortality rates clearly show that improvement is needed in the continuum of care for these patients. *Preconception care* is a solution that would improve the continuum of care by ensuring ongoing health surveillance and early intervention so that women begin pregnancy in the best possible health. Some potential tools include community-based studies to identify need and availability of resources, education programs, women's support groups, and counseling on topics such as smoking, obesity, nutrition, diabetes, hypertension, and depression. By closing the gap through preconception care, health professionals can enhance the community's health status and improve clinical outcomes for women, mothers, and infants.

Implementing a gap analysis framework to improve quality of care for patients requires an organization to ask and answer a series of tough questions (Dick, Gaudreault, and Shakir 2010; see Exhibit 4.3).

Gaps also exist between people's expectations of high-quality care and situations in which they receive low-quality healthcare. Low-quality healthcare may be the result of providers' lack of responsiveness, marginal competence, unreliability, weak communication skills, and breaches of confidentiality. Performance variations also result from trade-offs in the allocation of healthcare resources (Kasti 2013). For example, some healthcare organizations

What to Ask	How to Answer
What are we trying to accomplish?	Identify the target population and improvement goal.
	Pinpoint gaps and who falls through them.
What changes can we make that will result in improvement?	Identify the causes and barrier behind the gap.
	Determine what changes would improve care or close the gap.
	Plan and implement change.
	Monitor results.
How will we know if a change is an improvement?	Collect data.
	Plot or display the data for analysis.

EXHIBIT 4.3
Performing a Gap Analysis

may lack the financial resources to purchase new equipment or hire additional staff when experiencing increased demand because they have allocated their resources for another purpose; as a result, patients experience excessive waiting times.

DOWNSTREAM REVENUE

Understanding **downstream value**—the revenue captured by the services a patient uses after his initial visit—can provide a hospital with a better foundation for strategic planning and resource allocation. Although hospitals tend to think in terms of transactions, in the rapidly changing healthcare environment, hospitals must increasingly look beyond the dollars spent on the initial transaction and incorporate downstream revenue. Patients generate two to ten times the value of the initial transaction in the two years following that encounter from sources such as subsequent testing or return visits (Sturm 2009).

Downstream value
Revenue captured by the services a patient uses after his initial visit, such as subsequent testing or return visits.

A full-time physician brings in an average of $1.45 million in net revenue every year to the hospital with which she is affiliated, and some specialties bring in almost double that amount. In 2013, primary care physicians brought in more revenue to their hospitals than specialists did. Primary care physicians generated $1.57 million in downstream revenue for their hospitals, compared to $1.42 million from specialists. This figure did not include indirect revenue they may have created from patient referrals to specialists (Herman 2013).

Downstream revenue can provide a strong foundation of resources for future strategic planning. Moreover, as changes in reimbursement drive transactional revenue down, positive patient relationships that produce an ongoing revenue stream from repeated and clinically appropriate visits are critical.

SUMMARY

SWOT analysis is performed prior to the strategic planning process. Ideally, SWOT analysis includes a comprehensive review of the healthcare literature, in-depth data analysis, and input from a panel of SWOT analysis experts. Findings from the analysis are sorted into four categories: strengths, weaknesses, opportunities, and threats. Force field analysis supplements SWOT analysis by identifying the forces driving the strengths, weaknesses, opportunities, and threats. To refine these analyses even further, gap analysis may be performed to determine where deficiencies exist in an organization's delivery of care. Such analyses promote (1) a better understanding of barriers to change, innovation, and the transfer of knowledge to practice; (2) improved outcomes; and (3) more efficient allocation of healthcare resources.

A review of service lines allows organizations to identify new promotable products. These promotable products should have a high profit margin and downstream revenue opportunity and should allow for low-cost ease of entry as a reasonable payback period. Other signs of market potential are leading indicators in the geographic area such as housing starts, employment rates, and per capita income, which can be harbingers of future activity in a healthcare service line.

EXERCISES

REVIEW QUESTIONS

1. How does SWOT analysis set the stage for strategic planning?
2. Discuss the use of force field analysis in promoting change in a healthcare organization.
3. Provide examples of how gap analysis can be used to improve the quality of healthcare services.
4. Provide an example of how a hospital's strategic plan can affect downstream revenue.

COASTAL MEDICAL CENTER EXERCISES: SWOT ANALYSIS AND HOSPITAL EMERGENCY DEPARTMENT EXPANSION

Using the four steps of SWOT analysis discussed in Chapter 4, create a panel of experts and perform a SWOT analysis for Coastal Medical Center (CMC). Use SWOT analysis to identify factors that are key to getting CMC back on track and moving forward on a new road to success.

CMC CEO Richard Reynolds has met with Dr. John Warren, the chief medical officer, and Dr. Debra Jones, the director of the CMC emergency department (ED). They discussed the quality-level data included in the following report. They also discussed a workload report of the ED service volume for the past year. The data show a high level of ED utilization. The average charge for a hospital ED visit is $1,000 plus $500 in ancillary charges such as laboratory, radiology, and pharmacy. However, the data also suggest that a percentage of the ED patients are leaving without being seen. Mr. Henderson, Dr. Warren, and Dr. Jones are concerned about lost revenue because hospital data show that, in addition to the ED charges, if admitted to the hospital, patients generate an average of $100 in profit per inpatient day.

COASTAL MEDICAL CENTER QUESTIONS

Use the following report to answer these questions:

1. Based on your evaluation of the ED data, do you see any current problems?
2. Based on the data provided, calculate the potential lost revenue for ED visits over the past year.
3. Based on the data provided, calculate the potential lost downstream hospital revenue from ED admissions who walked out over the past year.
4. Make a recommendation to Mr. Henderson, Dr. Warren, and Dr. Jones for how to deal with the ED problem.

CMC Hospital Data	
Annual discharges	40,720
Average length of stay (days)	5.1
Average daily census	423
Inpatient surgeries	13,000
Outpatient surgeries	14,900
Births	2,400
Outpatient visits	245,000
Emergency department (not admitted)	36,400
Emergency department (admitted)	24,700
Total emergency department patients	61,100

ED Quality-Level Comparison

Measure	Score		
	CMC	State Average	National Average
Average (median) time patients spent in ED before admission	340 minutes	282 minutes	272 minutes
Average (median) time patients spent between decision to admit and departing for inpatient room	130 minutes	108 minutes	97 minutes
Average time patients spent in ED before being sent home	150 minutes	143 minutes	133 minutes
Average time patients spent in ED before being seen by a healthcare professional	36 minutes	23 minutes	24 minutes
Average time patients with broken bones waited for pain medication	70 minutes	56 minutes	55 minutes
Percentage of patients who left ED before being seen	4%	2%	2%
Percentage of patients who came to ED with stroke symptoms and received brain scan results within 45 minutes	55%	67%	61%

REFERENCES

American Hospital Association (AHA). 2014. "Fast Facts on US Hospitals." Updated January 2015. www.aha.org/research/rc/stat-studies/fast-facts.shtml.

Beckham, D. 2013. "Building a Team of Teams." *Hospitals & Health Networks*. Published February 19. www.hhnmag.com/Daily/2013/Feb/beckham021913-4960002469.

Berry, L. L., and D. Beckham. 2014. "Team-Based Care at Mayo Clinic: A Model for ACOs." *Journal of Healthcare Management* 59 (1): 9–13.

Centers for Medicare & Medicaid Services (CMS). 2015. "Better Care. Smarter Spending. Healthier People: Paying Providers for Value, Not Volume." Published January 26.

www.cms.gov/Newsroom/MediaReleaseDatabase/Fact-sheets/2015-Fact-sheets-items/2015-01-26-3.html.

Dean, S., Z. Lassi, A. Imam, and Z. Bhutta. 2014. "Preconception Care: Closing the Gap in the Continuum of Care to Accelerate Improvements in Maternal, Newborn and Child Health." *Reproductive Health* 11 (Suppl. 3): S1.

Dick, S., S. Gaudreault, and F. Shakir. 2010. "Implementing a Gap Analysis Framework to Improve Quality of Care for Your Patients." US Agency for International Development. Accessed August 15, 2015. www.usaidassist.org/sites/assist/files/hci.ghc_gap_framework_workbook.14jun10_1.pdf.

Herman, B. 2013. "Which Physicians Generate the Most Revenue for Hospitals?" *Becker's Hospital Review.* Published May 8. www.beckershospitalreview.com/hospital-physician-relationships/which-physicians-generate-the-most-revenue-for-hospitals.html.

Kasti, M. 2013. "Model for Healthcare Performance: GAP #1—The Strategy Gap." *Mo Kasti.com* (blog). Published November 9. www.mokasti.com/model-for-healthcare-performance-gap-1-the-strategy-gap/.

Lewin, K. 1951. *Field Theory in Social Science: Selected Theoretical Articles.* Edited by D. Cartwright. New York: Harper & Row.

Lineen, J. 2014. "Hospital Consolidation: 'Safety in Numbers' Strategy Prevails in Preparation for a Value-Based Marketplace." *Journal of Healthcare Management* 59 (5): 315–17.

Makos, J. 2014. "How to Conduct SWOT Analysis in Healthcare Organizations." Pestle Analysis. Published October 28. http://pestleanalysis.com/swot-analysis-in-healthcare.

Sturm, A. 2009. "Five New Ways to Look at Generating Revenue." *Healthcare Financial Management* 63 (11): 68–74.

Wennberg, J. E., E. S. Fisher, D. C. Goodman, and J. S. Skinner. 2008. *Tracking the Care of Patients with Severe Chronic Illness: The Dartmouth Atlas of Health Care 2008.* Dartmouth Institute for Health Policy and Clinical Practice Center for Health Policy Research. www.dartmouthatlas.org/downloads/atlases/2008_Chronic_Care_Atlas.pdf.

Zuckerman, A. 2014. "Successful Strategic Planning for a Reformed Delivery System." *Journal of Healthcare Management* 59 (3): 168–72.

CHAPTER 5

HEALTHCARE MARKETING

Art Layne and Jeffrey P. Harrison

Look before, or you'll find yourself behind.

—Benjamin Franklin

After you have studied this chapter, you should be able to

➤ apply basic principles of marketing to healthcare products and services;

➤ identify social, environmental, and fiscal factors affecting healthcare marketing;

➤ assess current market trends in the healthcare marketplace;

➤ evaluate criteria for implementing marketing strategies;

➤ describe the theories and concepts foundational to marketing; and

➤ provide examples of how marketing theory is applied in health management.

KEY TERMS AND CONCEPTS

➤ Community health needs
   assessment

➤ Digital media

➤ Five Ps of healthcare marketing

➤ Indirect marketing

➤ Marketing plan

➤ Medical tourism

➤ Print media

➤ Radio and television media

➤ Social media

INTRODUCTION

Healthcare spending in the United States accounted for 17.9 percent of gross domestic product in 2013 and is projected to reach 19.6 percent by 2021 (Spaulding, Zhao, and Haley 2014). From a marketing perspective, this increase creates significant opportunities for healthcare organizations that want to get a share of the growing business opportunity. Those organizations with the greatest marketing ability can anticipate taking away market share from their local competitors. Conversely, organizations without an effective marketing plan can anticipate a loss of market share, making them a likelier candidate for acquisition.

No one working in the field today can deny that the business of healthcare has become part of a growing "eHealth" landscape. Patients and other consumers, clinicians, and the field in general have embraced emerging forms of digital technology (e.g., the Internet, social media, mobile health applications) that can influence healthcare information, including consumption and delivery. A 2015 survey showed that 72 percent of US adults looked for health information online during the past year, and 52 percent of smartphone users used their devices to search for health information (Mackey and Liang 2015).

Many believe that the provision of healthcare services is a local phenomenon that requires a marketing strategy specific to the local community (Kent 2015). However, such an approach runs counter to the current growth in the regional healthcare systems expanding across the United States. Regional healthcare systems must engage in strategic marketing to ensure their activities are appropriate for local markets. This chapter introduces the key concepts of healthcare marketing and proposes a process for marketing across the spectrum of healthcare services. This marketing can be accomplished through a strategic process that supports an innovative approach to the use of tools that reflect improved service to the local, regional, and even international community.

From a management perspective, excellent strategic marketing provides a path to profitability and can lead to greater market share. Marketing can have a positive impact on healthcare organizations. Its design should involve the board of directors, leaders, and physicians as well as community stakeholders. An outstanding marketing plan is a way to improve operations and transform the organization.

DEFINITION

A **marketing plan** is a written document that guides marketing activities by considering the competitive marketplace, the healthcare organization's capabilities, and the service lines with the greatest economic potential. The marketing plan can include the development of websites, social media, educational seminars, radio or television advertising, printed brochures, and other materials and activities to promote a new business initiative. This process helps an organization shape its overall direction in future years. Marketing can help ensure that available healthcare services are well known in targeted communities. As a result, the marketing plan should include information about the internal and external environment and focus on service lines that community leaders believe are important for future growth.

STRATEGIC HEALTHCARE MARKETING

Marketing can help improve operations—but to do so, organizations should create a strategic marketing plan with input from key stakeholders.

Strategic management theory emphasizes the importance of positioning the healthcare organization relative to its environment to achieve its objectives and ensure its survival. This theory is important to the marketing process because it allows the organization to develop a strategy appropriate for the targeted market. A good marketing plan will enhance the managerial decisions made throughout the organization. In addition, marketing provides a solid foundation for meeting the need for essential healthcare services efficiently. Hospital executives have the ability and the responsibility to choose a marketing strategy that will maximize their organization's position in the healthcare market and enhance its performance.

According to strategic adaptation theory, an organization's actions can shape its environment and improve its performance. Among these actions are marketing decisions, which can improve financial performance and enhance profitability. The four primary components of a marketing plan are growth and financial outlook, service-line strategy, care quality, and clinical innovation. With more publicly reported quality measures available, citing positive quality outcomes can be a major strategy and also an internal motivator for continued improvement.

Working from a strategic management perspective, marketing is vital for maximizing the allocation of scarce healthcare resources and ensuring the success of new healthcare services. Most important, because healthcare organizations operate in a dynamic environment, a sound marketing plan can lead to organizational growth and increased effectiveness.

THE FIVE PS OF HEALTHCARE MARKETING

The five Ps are fundamental marketing elements designed to assess a business strategically. Building a brand for a healthcare business in a consistent way is important. Using the five Ps can help healthcare leaders think about products that can add value and offer a service that is different from those of competitors. Using the five Ps can also identify areas for improvement or change needed to meet the needs of your target market.

The **five Ps of healthcare marketing** are shown in Exhibit 5.1. They include

1. *people*—patient demographics, along with the physicians and healthcare workers required to deliver a quality service line in the local market;

2. *product*—the mission-driven type of healthcare services offered and the data or quality outcomes measured;

3. *price*—the fee schedule or rate of reimbursement for the service, adjusted for payer mix;

4. *place*—the location of the service, including the facility, parking, signage, and access to major highways; and

5. *promotion*—the method of advertising to be used to appeal to physicians, patients, health plans, and local businesses. This method could include focus groups, corporate branding, or indirect marketing and an evaluation of the competitor's marketing strategies.

Five Ps of healthcare marketing
Key marketing elements that are used to ensure a complete assessment of needs. In healthcare, they include people, product, price, place, and promotion.

An analysis of patient demographics is important because the demand for new healthcare business initiatives is often a function of age, gender, culture, and economic status. When forecasting the profitability of a new initiative, evaluating payer mix and the level of charity care the new business is expected to generate is also important. The marketing plan should ensure an appropriate payer mix to maximize profitability. A high percentage of patients with commercial insurance will increase the level of profitability for a new business initiative, whereas a high percentage of patients who are dependent on Medicaid reimbursement or who have no way to pay will reduce profitability.

While the Internet is driving much of marketing today, promotion should also consider traditional methods such as local radio, cable television, and billboards, especially for organizations with larger marketing budgets. Sponsorship of local and regional events can be a cost-effective way to show consumers how you and your business are associated with the community. Direct mail and some print advertising, including appointment-reminder postcards, continue to be affordable traditional options and can be beneficial (Lavinsky 2013). Two keys to success are as follows:

Exhibit 5.1
Five Ps of
Healthcare
Marketing

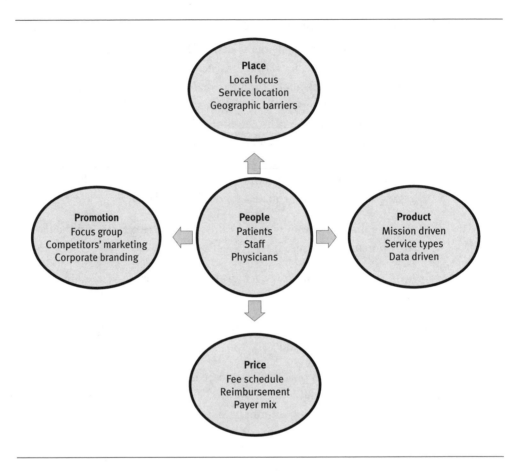

1. *Know who your customers are and target them.* The best marketing message in the world delivered to the wrong consumer is a waste of money. You would likely not, for instance, advertise cataract surgery on ESPN.

2. *Develop a compelling, unique selling proposition that makes you stand out.* Are you better, faster, or less expensive than your competitors? Why would patients come to you instead of your competitor? What can you offer them? Consider what would persuade them to take action (Lavinsky 2013).

MARKETING MEDIA IN THE CURRENT ENVIRONMENT

The healthcare strategic planning process is subject to considerable outside control and rapid change. Federal and state legislation, physician involvement, and the actions of third-party payers and competitors all affect an organization's operations. As a result, healthcare organizations need to focus on the external environment and future changes to the industry. By gathering information from external sources, healthcare organizations increase their likelihood of achieving success.

External information includes market position; data on local demographics, competitors, and payers; and information on the business environment. Such data are available through online databases maintained by hospital associations, regional health-planning groups, the US Census Bureau, and the US Department of Health & Human Services. Major healthcare trends include growth in managed care and accountable care organizations, new population health initiatives, participation in healthcare systems, and the expansion of ambulatory healthcare services. These innovations are all potential selling points.

TRENDS IN PRINT MEDIA

One of the more traditional modes of advertisement and marketing for hospitals has been the use of **print media** such as newspapers, magazines, brochures, and billboards. These methods are often combined with patient education materials by including healthcare organization logos and contact information. Outdoor advertising such as billboards and ads displayed on public transit continue to be a method used by larger hospitals and institutions. Magazine ads have seen a consistent decline in dollars spent, dropping by about 20 percent between 2008 and 2013. Newspaper ads have become cost prohibitive. In 2013, a color healthcare ad in a Sunday *New York Times* cost $28,900 for less than half a page and $41,200 for a half a page to a full page (Landen 2013).

> **Print media**
> Newspapers, magazines, brochures, and billboards.

Advertisements for healthcare often use emotional appeal and usually avoid cost information. Of 102 cancer centers that placed 409 unique clinical advertisements in top media markets in 2012, the majority (88 percent) of advertisements promoted treatments, and less than 5 percent mentioned insurance coverage or costs, risks, or benefits. Emotional appeals were frequent (85 percent), evoking hope for survival. Nearly half included patient testimonials, which were usually focused on survival rather than what a typical patient may expect (Vater et al. 2014). More research is needed to determine how these advertisements influence patient understanding and expectations.

TRENDS IN RADIO AND TELEVISION MEDIA

Healthcare organizations can purchase a span of programming on **radio** or **television media**, typically using it to market a product or service. These segments are produced and paid for by the organizations themselves.

> **Radio and television media**
> Programming distributed via television or radio.

Between 2008 and 2009, while Internet marketing increased, television marketing fell 7 percent from $395.3 million to $369.3 million. Yet spending on television marketing was 6.5 times larger than on digital media. In 2010, while television advertising rose 10 percent to $407.9 million, Internet ad spending more than tripled to $202.1 million, half of the television total. In 2011, the average national 30-second television spot cost $354,000 (Landen 2013). The cost-effectiveness of digital media makes it accessible to all organizations, while television is restricted to larger healthcare organizations. Radio can be used to target a specific audience.

Direct-to-consumer advertising (DTCA) is a form of marketing promotion that is aimed toward the end users—the patients—rather than healthcare professionals. For example, pharmaceutical companies frequently use television ads for this purpose and research indicates that it raises prescription rates. Physicians report filling DTCA-prompted patient requests for interventions that they considered inappropriate 70 percent of the time; prescribing rates for antidepressants were 22 percent higher when patients made brand-specific requests that they heard about through advertisements (Wang and Kesselheim 2013).

TRENDS IN DIGITAL MEDIA

Digital technology has become mobile. People are constantly connected via smartphones and tablets. As of January 2014, 90 percent of US adults owned a cell phone and 58 percent of US adults owned a smartphone (Pew Research Center 2015). They have come to expect the same at a hospital, and they research hospitals on the Internet. Technology trends suggest that patients will soon be able to check into the hospital with their portable devices, using the devices to select their preferences for television shows and dinner options before they are even assigned a room (White 2014). Digital marketing media have the potential to improve the efficiency of the healthcare delivery system and to increase market share. Accordingly, Internet marketing by hospitals, clinics, and medical centers rose about 20 percent from $47.5 million to $57.2 million between 2008 and 2009 (Landen 2013). While the majority of healthcare marketing in the United States is done via print, radio, and television, digital marketing provides important opportunities to exchange information about an organization's services and its use of evidence-based treatment. Such digital marketing can provide a competitive advantage by furnishing multiple consumers with up-to-date information and creating an opportunity for online consumer response. During 2012, 72 percent of Internet users looked online for health information (Pew Research Center 2015).

Digital marketing can also allow for the telling of patient stories, a technique that is very effective in healthcare. Appealing to emotions can be more effective than touting quality or specialty care (Landen 2013). Digital marketing information can be updated from a centralized database and provides efficient allocation of scarce marketing resources. This use of digital marketing can improve efficiency and quality in marketing healthcare services.

As consolidation in the healthcare field increases, the need for more effective digital marketing is critical to the success of integrated delivery systems. Four types of **digital media**—web-based methods of making contact with consumers, including organizational websites, social media, patient portals, and digital bulletin boards located in patient waiting areas—are discussed here in detail:

Digital media
Web-based methods of making contact with consumers.

1. *Organizational websites.* Hospital websites should be evaluated on five dimensions: (1) accessibility, (2) content, (3) marketing, (4) technology, and (5) usability. Up-to-date content is a positive indicator to consumers that

the organization is engaged in state-of-the-art activities. Routinely adding and changing content to remain current and explicitly documenting the dates that webpages are updated should be standard practice. Search engine optimization is also an important aspect of marketing and should be tested for specific clinical topics or points of interest for the public. Huerta and colleagues (2014) examined 2,407 unique web domains covering 2,785 hospital facilities and scored their websites in these five dimensions. They scored each dimension on a scale of 0–10 and gave the hospital an average score. They determined the top 100 hospitals by ranking each dimension and calculating an average ranking. The best site overall in their evaluation was jaxhealth.com, the website for St. Vincent's Healthcare in Jacksonville, Florida, with a score of 29.6. It ranked fifteenth in accessibility, sixty-first in content, fifty-second in marketing, fourteenth in technology, and sixth in usability.

2. *Social media.* **Social media** encompass websites and applications that enable users to create and share content or participate in social networking sites on Facebook and LinkedIn, blogs, content-hosting sites (e.g., WebMD), and virtual communities. In a recent report called *Engaging Patients Through Social Media*, the IMS Institute for Healthcare Informatics states that the use of social media among US adults has grown from 8 percent in 2005 to 72 percent in 2013 (Collier 2014). Other research has found that the adoption of social media varies across hospitals, with 94 percent having a Facebook page and 50 percent having a Twitter account (Griffis et al. 2014). A majority of hospitals have a Yelp page, and almost all hospitals have comments on Foursquare. The social media pages of large, urban, not-for-profit, and teaching hospitals are more likely to be visited. A strong social media presence can help increase market share by supporting a hospital's reputation and ability to attract patients. For example, patients may perceive hospitals with a social media presence to be more likely to offer advanced technologies in the course of evidence-based treatments. Some institutions now include experts in social media as part of their public relations team.

Social media
Websites and applications that enable users to create and share content or to participate in social networking sites, collaborative services, blogs, content hosting sites, and virtual communities.

3. *Patient portals.* Patient portals are web-based applications that enable patients to interact and communicate with their healthcare providers. The adoption and active use of patient portals continues to increase across the United States, driven by Stage 2 meaningful use (MU) requirements. These federally mandated changes began in October 2013 for hospitals and in January 2014 for physicians. Stage 2 MU requires providers to adopt and use technology that allows patients to view, download, and transmit copies of their own health records electronically (Tulu et al. 2015). Patient portals are the key

technologies that will help providers meet these requirements. In addition, providers that adopt patient portals will enjoy a competitive advantage, as patients increasingly demand convenient, 24/7 access to their financial and clinical data (Frost and Sullivan 2013). While accessing data is the first step, the future of the patient portal is to look for more advanced solutions for patient engagement that can motivate patient compliance and sustain behavioral change.

4. *Digital bulletin boards located in patient waiting areas.* Larsson (2015) conducted a study to evaluate the effectiveness of a digital bulletin board in an emergency department in Montana. She was trying to promote the home testing of radon levels, a health risk in that area of the country. The bulletin board encouraged viewers in the waiting room to participate in the radon program. The message addressed price only in terms of the convenience of mailing completed tests from home in a postage-paid envelope. No information about the research study, the dollar cost of the radon test kits, or participant incentives was included in the message. The intent was for people to be persuaded to action by only the information provided, which is the preferred outcome of a social-marketing approach. Larsson found that participation in the radon program increased by more than 50 percent at the intervention site without requiring providers to present the information. This increase occurred during a time that participation in the program declined at two control sites.

Digital media cannot be ignored in a marketing plan, but setting up a system to ensure the accuracy and currency of the information is important. Dealing with the prolific flow of health information on the Internet and the crucial need for better governance to enable evidence-based sources are both vital factors in good execution. Healthcare leaders need to ensure that the health domains on the Internet are safe, regulated spaces for health marketing (Mackey et al. 2014).

INDIRECT MARKETING

Indirect marketing is not targeted directly to consumers but rather consists of leveraging brand recognition and awareness of a provider in the community. Healthcare organizations are well positioned for indirect marketing because they focus on community need and wellness. For example, hospitals will sponsor charity events, host speakers for the community, conduct free health clinics and health fairs, or provide healthcare services for athletic teams. Hospital and facility signage is one of the cheapest and most effective marketing tools available to healthcare organizations. Because healthcare is a local commodity, signage placed in a prominent place on the building and sized in a way consistent with the maximum

Indirect marketing
Advertising that does not directly communicate with consumers, but rather leverages brand recognition and consumer awareness of an organization's presence in the marketplace.

authorized by local ordinance is appropriate. This signage should be lighted after dark and remain lighted until dawn, regardless of the operating hours of the facility.

Word-of-mouth advertising by patients, physicians, and staff is the most powerful indirect marketing tool influencing decision making for prospective patients. A satisfied consumer will return and might even bring two or three family members as consumers. On the other hand, an unhappy patient can be expected to discuss her bad experience with the community at large over an extended period of time, frequently reaching hundreds of potential consumers.

HEALTHCARE MARKETING AT THE LOCAL AND REGIONAL LEVELS

The vast majority of healthcare services are provided within ten miles of an individual's home. In this context, geographic barriers such as rivers, bridges, and interstate highway networks affect healthcare marketing. As a result, local healthcare marketing is essential for organizational survival and is the foundation for creating a strong patient referral network.

LOCAL MARKETING

By many accounts, healthcare in the United States is a local commodity produced to meet local demand. For this reason, much of an organization's marketing plan is developed using local data. A good understanding of community needs is necessary to develop a local marketing plan.

The Affordable Care Act, enacted March 23, 2010, added new requirements that hospital organizations must satisfy to be considered not-for-profit or charitable. One of the requirements is to conduct a **community health needs assessment (CHNA)** at least once every three years to identify key health needs and issues through systematic, comprehensive data collection and analysis. This information can help develop a community health improvement plan by justifying how and where resources should be allocated to best meet community needs. A CHNA can also serve as another method for indirect marketing by improving organizational and community coordination and collaboration. Such local marketing efforts should stress the availability of physicians, the quality of hospital infrastructure, and the use of advanced technology.

Community health needs assessment (CHNA)
State, tribal, local, or territorial health assessment that identifies key health needs and issues through systematic, comprehensive data collection and analysis.

REGIONAL MARKETING

As healthcare complexity increases and health systems in the United States gain market share, healthcare systems will increasingly market at the regional level. Such an approach can help integrate highly complex healthcare services and reduce costs through greater purchasing power with media vendors.

Medical tourism
Traveling outside one's local area for higher-value or unique healthcare services; also called medical travel, health tourism, or global healthcare.

The European concept of **medical tourism** is gaining favor in the United States. Mayo Clinic, for instance, is promoting itself as a *destination medical center*—a healthcare organization that draws patients from outside the local area because it offers higher-value or unique services. Such medical centers must provide a service that moves patients to drive past their local providers on their way to an alternate healthcare organization.

As air travel has become cheaper and exchange rates more stable, medical tourism is becoming more viable. More than 50 countries have identified medical tourism as a national industry, often for highly specialized treatments that may be unavailable in home countries for cancer, reconstructive surgery, cardiovascular disease, or organ transplant. Other services include eye surgery, joint replacement, dental surgery, cosmetic surgery, and bariatric surgery. Providers and customers usually find each other via the Internet. Developed countries such as the United Kingdom, Germany, and the United States are prominent medical tourism destinations (Connell 2015).

Medical tourism is a relatively new industry that is becoming increasingly competitive and consumer oriented. When marketing specific procedures for medical tourism, marketing departments should consider highlighting quality metrics that exceed established US standards of care. With access to quality and cost data, healthcare consumers are better able to assess the value of services among regional and international healthcare organizations. However, medical tourism can create an ethical dilemma because it raises concerns about the need to provide quality care to local, as opposed to international, patients (Connell 2015). In some ways, medical tourism represents a dynamic restructuring of healthcare from an industry once assumed to be local to one that is international in scope. This globalization of healthcare will require new and innovative approaches to marketing.

SUMMARY

Healthcare marketing is a method of educating consumers on the attributes of a healthcare organization's services. A marketing plan should focus on outstanding clinical services that lead to improved quality and greater customer satisfaction. Many organizations use a multiplatform, multichannel approach—television, outdoor and digital advertising, radio, print, giveaways, and public relations. When appropriate, healthcare marketing can also address low costs and increased efficiency. High-quality, low-cost care enhances the value of healthcare. An outstanding marketing plan that stresses customer satisfaction will result in higher profits and reduced costs.

EXERCISES

REVIEW QUESTIONS

1. Evaluate the idea that healthcare marketing is an annual process done by senior leadership with limited involvement from key stakeholders.

2. Provide an example from your own personal or work experience that illustrates a marketing initiative that had a positive influence on an organization's reputation.
3. Does the diversity of a healthcare organization's staff have any impact on the success of a healthcare marketing plan?

COASTAL MEDICAL CENTER EXERCISE

According to Chapter 5 and the case study, does Coastal Medical Center (CMC) have the organizational capabilities to develop a marketing plan?

After investigating the declining performance of CMC, the new CEO believes that a new marketing plan is necessary to gain market share. Based on your research, use the following questions to help the CEO develop a marketing plan that will place CMC on a new road to success.

COASTAL MEDICAL CENTER QUESTIONS

1. Outline a general healthcare marketing plan that is appropriate for CMC.
2. CMC is experiencing declining inpatient and outpatient volumes. Develop a list of five marketing initiatives to improve clinical workload.
3. Who should be involved in developing the CMC marketing plan, and at what point in the planning process should you consult them?
4. How will you know your healthcare marketing plan is a success?

REFERENCES

Collier, R. 2014. "Patient Engagement or Social Media Marketing?" *Canadian Medical Association Journal* 186 (8): E237–E238.

Connell, J. 2015. "From Medical Tourism to Transnational Health Care? An Epilogue for the Future." *Social Science in Medicine* 124 (January): 398–401.

Frost and Sullivan. 2013. "Market Disruption Imminent as Hospitals and Physicians Aggressively Adopt Patient Portal Technology." Published September 26. www.frost.com/prod/servlet/press-release-print.pag?docid=285477570.

Griffis, H. M., A. S. Kilaru, R. M. Werner, D. A. Asch, J. C. Hershey, S. Hill, Y. P. Ha, A. Sellers, K. Mahoney, and R. M. Merchant. 2014. "Use of Social Media Across US Hospitals: Descriptive Analysis of Adoption and Utilization." *Journal of Medical Internet Research* 16 (11): e264. doi:10.2196/jmir.3758.

Huerta, T. R., J. L. Hefner, E. W. Ford, A. S. McAlearney, and N. Menachemi. 2014. "Hospital Effective Consumer Engagement." *Journal of Medical Internet Research* 16 (2): e64. doi:10.2196/jmir.3054.

Kent, M. 2015. "Six Ways for Healthcare Marketers to Win at Local Advertising." *Rise Interactive*. Published April 27. www.riseinteractive.com/blog/post/six-ways-for-healthcare-marketers-to-win-at-local-advertising.

Landen, R. 2013. "Telling Their Stories: Healthcare Marketing, Advertising Emphasize the Personal Approach as Providers Find New Ways to Connect with Patients." *Modern Healthcare*. Published August 3. www.modernhealthcare.com/article/20130803/MAGAZINE/308039952.

Larsson, L. S. 2015. "The Montana Radon Study: Social Marketing via Digital Signage Technology for Reaching Families in the Waiting Room." *American Journal of Public Health* 105 (4): 779–85.

Lavinsky, D. 2013. "Is Traditional Marketing Still Alive?" *Forbes*. Published March 8. www.forbes.com/sites/davelavinsky/2013/03/08/is-traditional-marketing-still-alive/.

Mackey, T. K., and B. A. Liang. 2015. "It's Time to Shine the Light on Direct-to-Consumer Advertising." *Annals of Family Medicine* 13 (1): 82–85.

Mackey, T. K., B. A. Liang, J. C. Kohler, and A. Attaran. 2014. "Health Domains for Sale: The Need for Global Health Internet Governance." *Journal of Medical Internet Research* 16 (3): e62. doi:10.2196/jmir.3276.

Pew Research Center. 2015. "Health Fact Sheet." Accessed June 21. www.pewinternet.org/fact-sheets/health-fact-sheet/.

Spaulding, A., M. Zhao, and D. R. Haley. 2014. "Value-Based Purchasing and Hospital Acquired Conditions: Are We Seeing Improvement?" *Health Policy* 118 (3): 413–21.

Tulu, B., J. Trudel, D. M. Strong, S. A. Johnson, D. Sundaresan, and L. Garber. 2015. "Patient Portals: An Underutilized Resource for Improving Patient Engagement." *Chest*. Published June 11. doi:10.1378/chest.14-2559.

Vater, L. B., J. M. Donohue, R. Arnold, D. B. White, E. Chu, and Y. Schenker. 2014. "What Are Cancer Centers Advertising to the Public? A Content Analysis." *Annals of Internal Medicine* 160 (12): 813–20.

Wang, B., and A. S. Kesselheim. 2013. "The Role of Direct-to-Consumer Pharmaceutical Advertising in Patient Consumerism." *American Medical Association Journal of Ethics* 15 (11): 960–65.

White, J. 2014. "Technology Trends: 3 Reasons Hospitals Should Expand IT Networks." *Healthcare Business and Technology*. Published July 31. www.healthcarebusinesstech.com/hospital-technology-trends/.

CHAPTER 6

STRATEGIC PLANNING AND HEALTH INFORMATION TECHNOLOGY

The difference between what we do and what we are capable of doing would suffice to solve most of the world's problems.

—Gandhi

LEARNING OBJECTIVES

After you have studied this chapter, you should be able to

➤ understand the concept of healthcare information, including how it is collected, stored, accessed, and utilized;

➤ communicate technical health information system concepts in a language that can be understood by healthcare staff;

➤ articulate an understanding of the role of health information system development and integration;

➤ demonstrate the use of healthcare information in management and organizational decision making;

➤ critically analyze current issues surrounding health information systems within the healthcare environment; and

➤ identify the strategic impact of health information systems.

KEY TERMS AND CONCEPTS

➤ Big data

➤ Clinical information systems

➤ Critical access hospital

➤ Direct-to-consumer telehealth

➤ E-health

➤ Healthcare data analysts

➤ Healthcare data warehouse

➤ Meaningful use

➤ Patient portal

➤ Telehealth

➤ Value-based purchasing

INTRODUCTION

As healthcare organizations face increased competition and changing reimbursement rates, the future of strategic planning in healthcare will require developing data-use strategies that incorporate quality and efficiency. Organizations will need to manage population health as they shift from fee-for-service reimbursement to bundled payment and **value-based purchasing** (an initiative that rewards acute care hospitals with incentive payments for the quality of care they provide to people with Medicare). This transition will require the use of electronic health records (EHRs) to develop integrated systems between healthcare organizations that foster provider collaboration across the continuum of care. In addition, healthcare organizations will need to enhance their analytical capabilities to mine quality and safety data as they move forward. Simply having a data repository in the EHR is not enough. We must be able to interpret and manage the data through data analytics to obtain information that is useful in improving patient outcomes.

Data management is a major challenge and will require access to and exchange of healthcare data. In addition, as healthcare organizations move data between local, regional, and national geographic areas, they will need to address system architecture requirements. This chapter discusses the use of **health information technology (HIT)**—the comprehensive management of health information across computerized systems and its secure exchange among consumers, providers, government and quality entities, and insurers—in strategic decision making and in delivering quality patient care in the digital environment. It discusses a wide range of databases currently available as resources for strategic planning. It also discusses the technologies, governmental policies, and data management strategies necessary to position an organization for future success.

Value-based purchasing
Centers for Medicare & Medicaid Services initiative that rewards acute care hospitals with incentive payments for the quality of care they provide to people with Medicare.

Changing organizational culture remains a significant obstacle as healthcare organizations are forced to transform the way they use and analyze data. This transformation becomes more important as they move to integrated delivery systems and personalized care. Such a change in culture requires hospital executives, medical group leaders, and integrated health systems to work together to develop new organizational entities such as accountable care organizations (ACOs). The situation is further complicated by the recent growth of clinics staffed by physicians and other healthcare providers at retail locations such as Walmart, Walgreens, and CVS. These organizations are new healthcare competitors with the ability to fill prescriptions and make referrals for other diagnostic and therapeutic services. To effect change, the leaders of healthcare organizations will be forced to overcome cultural inertia through the use of transformational leadership.

In 2013, 78 percent of physician outpatient practices used EHRs, up from only 18 percent in 2001 (Hsiao and Hing 2014). This trend makes available a significant amount of patient data for the improvement of clinical practice and enhancement of healthcare quality. EHRs have created an increasing need for physicians and other healthcare providers to integrate mobile devices into their routine clinical practices.

Clinical information systems are technology applied at the point of care and designed to support the acquisition of information and storage and processing capabilities. They provide information on patient outcomes and practitioner performance and include clinical alerts, reminder systems for disease management, and medication administration systems. These systems are important because they use HIT to standardize clinical practice. By integrating multiple systems, they improve decision making and communication among an organization's healthcare staff.

Given the dynamic nature of the healthcare environment, healthcare executives, clinical providers, and HIT executives are facing significant challenges, including reimbursement increasingly based on value; the systemwide tracking of quality metrics such as complication rates, hospital-acquired infections, and patient costs; and bundled payments. These challenges require the use of new HIT systems and the recruitment of individuals with HIT analytical skills. Investment in these technologies and individuals will require an ongoing commitment of HIT resources. While attempting to maximize the use of these data in real-time clinical practice, healthcare also faces Health Insurance Portability and Accountability Act (HIPAA) requirements that protect individual health information.

There is also a growing need to manage **big data**—data sets of such massive size that they are difficult to process using traditional computation tools—through the use of advanced analytics that improve both individual care and the population health of the local community. The use of big data will allow healthcare professionals to use millions of cases to improve the standard of care, participate in population health by defining the needs of subpopulations, and identify and intervene on behalf of groups at risk for poor outcomes (Riskin 2012). If the healthcare industry could use big data effectively and creatively to improve quality and safety, it could add $300 billion in value by reducing

Clinical information system
Technology applied at the point of care and designed to support the acquisition of information as well as provide storage and processing capabilities.

Big data
Data sets of such massive size that they are difficult to process using traditional computation tools.

expenses (Manyika et al. 2011). As a result, healthcare organizations need to expand their HIT budgets to allow the acquisition of new software and to invest further in skilled data analysts and clinical-information experts.

The Nebraska Health Information Initiative is a statewide health information exchange launched in 2009. It conducted a survey of healthcare providers in 2013. Of those responding, 63 percent indicated satisfaction with HIT. Improvement in patient care (56 percent) and ease of sending (40 percent) and receiving (48 percent) information within the referral network were among the most common reasons for adoption. The most important feature identified was a comprehensive medication list. Major barriers included cost (38 percent) and loss of productivity (36 percent) (Cochran et al. 2015).

MEANINGFUL USE

Meaningful use is the common term for a program of the Centers for Medicare & Medicaid Services (CMS) that imposes a standard for using certified EHR technology to improve the overall quality of healthcare by providing financial incentives. The program uses certified EHR technology designed to result in better clinical outcomes, improved population health outcomes, increased transparency and efficiency, and more robust research data. Eligible professionals and hospitals must achieve specific objectives to qualify for CMS financial incentive programs. This change has put the need to incorporate HIT in strategic planning into high gear.

> *Meaningful use*
> CMS-sponsored
> program imposing
> a standard for
> using certified EHR
> technology to improve
> the overall quality of
> healthcare by providing
> financial incentives.

Meaningful use is being implemented in three stages. Stage 1, enacted 2011–2012, was devoted to data capture and sharing. Stage 2, in 2014, focused on advancing clinical processes such as implementation of computerized provider order entry and medication reconciliation; Stage 3, to begin in 2017, will deal with improved outcomes (HHS 2015b). As of 2014, 91 percent have received incentive payments for Stage 1, indicating they met the requirements. Only eight hospitals have submitted validation for Stage 2 out of 75 eligible hospitals; hospitals are eligible for Stage 2 after demonstrating validation or attesting for two years at Stage 1 (Pennic 2014).

The Office of the National Coordinator for Health Information Technology (ONC) will be focusing on Stage 3 of meaningful use, which also includes the interoperability of EHRs. In healthcare, the Healthcare Information and Management Systems Society (HIMSS) defines interoperability as the ability of different information technology systems and software applications to communicate, exchange data, and use the information that has been exchanged. Data exchange and standards should allow data to be shared among clinician, lab, hospital, pharmacy, and patient regardless of the application or application vendor. The ONC sets HIT standards and creates a coordinated system architecture. It will set guidelines on sharing data and determining who has access to the data. These guidelines will probably include a federated system in which individual organizations maintain their own data, which are coordinated and distributed as appropriate. This approach will ensure a high level of interoperability between the EHRs of different systems.

E-Health

E-health
Broad range of data
processing and
computer networking
applications (including
use of the Internet) in
healthcare.

Information technology introduces a new language and set of terms into healthcare that are often unfamiliar to practitioners—including different terms used for similar concepts, which makes comprehension even more difficult. For instance, the terms *telemedicine*, *telehealth*, and *e-health* are often used interchangeably by both healthcare providers and consumers. *Telemedicine* was originally used to describe medical service provision across a distance. As telemedicine became a broader possibility with more applications, the term *telehealth* was introduced to reflect a broader scope of health-related functions. Since that time, **e-health**, used to cover a broad range of data processing and computer networking applications (including the Internet) in healthcare, has emerged. The newer themes of telehealth and e-health are broader and expand on the original term of telemedicine (Fatehi and Wootton 2012). To clarify terms used in this chapter, definitions for frequently used terms are introduced in the following sections.

As healthcare organizations respond to the Affordable Care Act (ACA), they will increasingly use digital health data to reduce costs and improve accountability. In addition, the transition from fee-for-service payment to pay-for-performance payment is forcing providers to deliver quality care at a reduced cost. The growth of health systems and ACOs requires analyzing and sharing patient data securely across the continuum of care. This requirement has led to the emergence of wireless technologies and mobile devices. Strategic planners in healthcare should pay attention to this shift—as of January 2014, 58 percent of American consumers reported having a smartphone and 42 percent have a tablet computer (HIMSS Analytics 2014b).

Telehealth
Use of telecommunica-
tions to deliver health
services.

Telehealth is the use of telecommunications between patient and provider to deliver health services and information that support patient care, administrative activities, and health education. Telehealth has evolved from simply using digital systems to support patient care and administrative activities to new **direct-to-consumer telehealth** services—online medical services that market directly to individual patients (Perna 2015). This change was driven in great part by search engines such as Google, which created an infrastructure that allows individuals to search for health information and then connect with a doctor from a healthcare organization. Marketing telehealth services directly to the consumer is a growing trend. Such a system builds a link between patients and physicians in their medical practices and provides access to specialty care at larger hospitals.

*Direct-to-consumer
telehealth*
Online medical services
that market directly to
individual patients.

Direct-to-consumer telehealth services improve access and convenience and reduce cost. For example, a telehealth system allows an individual to communicate with her physician, obtain a treatment plan, and have a prescription sent to the pharmacy without a face-to-face appointment and therefore with no work time lost (Perna 2015). This type of convenience is driven by significant advancements in telehealth technological capabilities. For example, Mayo Clinic has kiosks available to patients who need to connect with remote physicians. These kiosks have video capabilities and stethoscopes, scales, and other examination equipment. This innovation is only the beginning; there is a growing number of direct-to-consumer telehealth applications for iPhones. As of 2015, some commercial health plans were reimbursing direct-to-consumer telehealth services at $49 per healthcare encounter (Perna 2015).

Telehealth comprises numerous technologies. Telehealth innovations are particularly valuable in rural communities where access to healthcare is limited. This type of care can also play an important role in the management of chronically ill patients because it establishes and maintains an ongoing connection with the clinical care team. It also helps to coordinate care among primary care and specialty physicians and prevent unnecessary office and emergency room visits and costly hospitalization.

There were 5 billion mobile phones in use in 2010 (Manyika et al. 2011). Thirty-six percent of clinical providers believe the use of smartphone and tablet computers will improve the efficiency and quality of healthcare and provide for better coordination. Mobile devices optimize the use of clinicians' time, and 50 percent of clinicians report that using smart phones and computer tablets has improved their job satisfaction. In 2014, more than half of US hospitals reported the use of smart phones and tablet computers at their facilities. In addition, 59 percent of hospitals reported that they used these devices to access clinical information. However, only 33 percent of hospitals stated that all clinical data could be accessed via these devices (HIMSS Analytics 2014a).

Complex medical problems involve the management of chronic disease and the monitoring of critical health indicators. Mobile devices help patients and health providers to address medical conditions proactively through real-time monitoring and treatment regardless of the location of the patient or health provider. The use of mobile devices for healthcare will save money, improve access, and provide higher-quality care. Mobile devices also provide access to the growing body of knowledge on evidence-based medicine, patient genetics, pharmaceutical products, and clinical practice (West 2013).

A **patient portal** is a website that gives patients 24-hour access to personal health information. Using a secure username and password, patients can view health information such as medical records, medications, immunization histories, allergies, and lab and radiology results.

Patient portal
Secure website that gives patients 24-hour access to personal health information.

In 2014, 62 percent of US hospitals had a patient portal. However, only 23 percent of those portals allowed patients to access their EHR and diagnostic results (HIMSS Analytics 2014b). The patient portal supports patient engagement and will be a foundation of future healthcare systems. If only 23 percent of healthcare organizations are maximizing the use of their patient portals by allowing individual patients to access their patient records, opportunities for improvement exist.

Advanced patient portals allow patients to

◆   communicate via secure e-mail with their healthcare teams,

◆   request prescription refills,

- ◆ schedule appointments,

- ◆ check insurance coverage,

- ◆ update personal information,

- ◆ make payments,

- ◆ download and complete forms, and

- ◆ view educational materials.

The advantages of patient portal implementation include enhanced patient–provider communication, empowered patients, the provision of support care between clinical visits, and improved patient outcomes (HealthIT.gov 2015).

Healthcare data warehouse
Database that integrates multiple types of data, such as patient demographic information, comprehensive clinical information, and resource utilization data.

All these new data require storage. **Healthcare data warehouses** are databases that integrate multiple types of data, such as patient demographic information, comprehensive clinical information, and resource utilization, to provide a foundation for decision making. This use of big data represents the next frontier in innovation and will be a key to productivity, competitiveness, and future growth (Manyika et al. 2011). These databases are large and require special software for storage, management, and analysis. As of 2015, these databases can be measured in terabytes (thousands of gigabytes); however, as technology advances, they will increase in size. Healthcare data warehouses also provide common linkable identifiers so that analysis can be performed. This new technology furnishes an opportunity to improve the global economy and enhance US healthcare by fostering an environment of innovation. For example, clinical data from all Veterans Health Administration (VHA) sites are maintained in Austin, Texas. Because the data that data warehouses contain are comprehensive and voluminous, they allow researchers and strategic planners to efficiently collect and evaluate data on large patient populations.

STRATEGIC HEALTH INFORMATION TECHNOLOGY INITIATIVES
E-HEALTH INITIATIVES

Numerous new e-health tools help healthcare researchers and physicians improve the health of the population (DeGaspari 2015). These tools include the EHR, which allows the capture of more data in a more timely manner. The data can then be used to improve the public health status of the local population. Many organizations, including the Centers for Disease Control and Prevention, are using analytical tools to monitor these online databases and identify public health trends at the local, state, and national levels. This use of data can improve clinical practice and track changes in disease incidence rates. By analyzing big data we can create partnerships between clinical providers and public health systems. These partnerships and the use of real-time data can identify potential epidemics before they become community crises and provide key metrics for a community's health status.

Under the ACA, hospitals and other providers face growing pressure to improve efficiency and enhance the movement of patients through the continuum of care. The creation of health information networks and the use of standardized data systems improve communication, which leads to better integration of healthcare providers and improved quality of care for patients. E-health can link ambulatory care, hospital care, skilled nursing care, and home care through regional data exchanges and telehealth.

CLINICAL INFORMATION SYSTEMS INITIATIVES

At the time of this writing in 2015, worldwide IT spending was on pace to total $3.5 trillion (Lovelock et al. 2015). HIT will represent a $10 billion market by 2020 (Manyika et al. 2011). As a result, healthcare organizations need to implement a data-driven big data strategy to create value and improve healthcare efficiency.

Health information systems improve coordination of care, and better coordination of care leads to improved medical outcomes. HIMSS's Electronic Medical Record (or EMR, another term for EHR) Adoption Model measures the level of clinical information systems adoption in US hospitals (see Exhibit 6.1). It rates hospitals' level of adoption using a seven-stage scale, where Stage 0 indicates the lowest level of adoption and Stage 7 indicates the highest level of adoption. The first stage is adding laboratory, radiology, and pharmacy services to electronic formats. The stages end with a complete EHR; the ability to share data across applications; data warehousing; and a single record shared between inpatient, emergency department, and outpatient services. Only 3.3 percent of hospitals have not started their EHR journey (HIMSS Analytics 2015).

As of February 2015, more than nine out of ten hospitals eligible for the Medicare and Medicaid EHR Incentive Program had achieved meaningful use of certified HIT. Exhibit 6.1 describes the stages and percentages of hospitals meeting those stages as of second quarter 2015.

By July 2015, more than 1,300 hospitals had achieved Stage 6 adoption and 205 had achieved Stage 7, the highest level of EMR adoption (HIMSS Analytics 2015). This change represents a significant increase in the use of clinical information systems.

ELECTRONIC HEALTH RECORD INITIATIVES

Approximately 5,400 US hospitals are tracking their use of EHRs using the HIMSS EMR Adoption Model. At Stage 7, hospitals no longer use paper charts, have created a data warehouse, and readily share clinical information in the organization across the healthcare continuum (HIMSS Analytics 2014a). In addition, they have developed mechanisms for the exchange of health information with other nonassociated organizations via a data-sharing agreement. This highest level of EHR adoption requires a clear strategic vision and provides the opportunity for increased efficiency and future advancements in clinical care.

Stage	Cumulative Capabilities	2015 Q1	2015 Q2
Stage 7	Complete EMR, CCD transactions to share data, Data warehousing, Data continuity with ED, ambulatory with ED, OP	3.7%	3.7%
Stage 6	Physician documentation (structured templates), full CDSS (variance and compliance), full R-PACS	22.2%	23.6%
Stage 5	Closed loop medication administration	30.8%	32.3%
Stage 4	CPOE, Clinical Decision Support (clinical protocols)	13.6%	13.2%
Stage 3	Nursing/clinical documentation (flow sheets), CDSS (error checking), PACS available outside Radiology	19.7%	18.2%
Stage 2	CDR, Controlled Medical Vocabulary, CDS may have Document Imaging, HIE capable	4.3%	3.6%
Stage 1	Ancillaries-Lab, Rad, Pharmacy-All installed	2.2%	1.9%
Stage 0	All Three ancillaries not installed	3.5%	3.3%

Source: Reprinted from HIMSS Analytics. Used with permission.

CCD: Continuity-of-care document (electronic document-exchange standard for sharing patient summary information between all applications or web browsers and EHRs)

CDR: Call detail record or file type

CDS: CERN document server (a type of software used to organize categories of data)

CDSS: Clinical decision support system (system designed to assist physicians and other health professionals with clinical decision-making tools)

CPOE: Computerized provider order entry

ED: Emergency department

HIE: Health information exchange (method of electronically moving patient data)

OP: Outpatient

PACS: Picture-archiving and communications system

R-PACS: Radiology picture-archiving and communications system

The VHA is a good example of the implementation of one system of EHR. The VHA has grown from operating 54 hospitals in 1930 to operating 152 medical centers, in addition to approximately 1,400 community-based outpatient clinics, community living centers, and veterans centers in 2015. Together, these healthcare facilities provide care to more than 8.3 million veterans each year (VA 2015). The VHA had developed its own EHR system, called the Veterans Health Information Systems and Technology Architecture (VistA). Within VistA, the Computerized Patient Record System is an integrated, comprehensive suite of clinical applications that work together to create a display of a veteran's EHR over time.

The federal government has made the computer source code for VistA available as free operating software. As a result, some rural Medicare-certified **critical access hospitals** (rural hospitals able to charge a fee-for-service rate in return for providing the community with emergency department and basic hospital services), Indian Health Service hospitals, and nursing homes have implemented it. For healthcare organizations with limited financial resources, the adoption of open-source EHR software is a viable alternative to expensive software packages.

In July 2015, the US Department of Defense (DoD) awarded an up to $11 billion, ten-year contract to a team led by Leidos and Cerner to develop a new EHR system called the Defense Healthcare Management System Modernization initiative. DoD's new health record promotes greater interoperability with the VHA's VistA health record. The exchange of health information among the DoD, the VHA, and private-sector businesses using EHRs is critical for providing seamless care delivery. The VHA will work with the DoD to meet the interoperabilty challenge (Walker 2015).

Critical access hospital
Rural hospital certified to charge a fee-for-service rate in return for providing community access to emergency department and basic hospital services.

EVIDENCE-BASED MEDICINE INITIATIVES

Personalized medicine is driving continuous change in evidence-based medicine (Raths 2015). President Obama's 2016 budget includes $215 million to provide clinicians with new tools, knowledge, and therapies that will work best for individual patients. For example, personalized medicine can involve genetic mapping to identify which medications will have the maximum effect on a specific cancer. In the future, healthcare organizations might build a genetic database that includes those medications and therapies that can best treat genetic mutations in cancer. A physician portal that allows clinicians to access the research and clinical analytics necessary to identify the highest-quality treatment for their individual patients is also a possible innovation. The beginning of such a personalized medicine portal was the creation of the Global Alliance for Genomics and Health, formed in 2013 to create a standard framework for the secure sharing of genomic and clinical data. To date, membership includes large, research-oriented medical centers, but in the future it could also include hospitals and physician practices. The concept of personalized medicine informatics is a major advancement in evidence-based care because it offers a real-time tool for decision making that is structured to benefit each individual patient.

STRATEGIC PLANNING FOR HEALTH INFORMATION TECHNOLOGY

The future of HIT is exciting. It involves further enhancements in healthcare applications such as EHRs, e-health, and a wide range of clinical tools. It also provides opportunities for great efficiency through the measurement of dashboard performance metrics and the collaboration of clinicians across the continuum of healthcare.

Exhibit 6.2 is an example of an HIT checklist that healthcare organizations can use to evaluate their progress in HIT planning and benchmark against other organizations.

Exhibit 6.2

Health Information
Technology
Checklist

HEALTH INFORMATION DASHBOARD

	Yes	No
Shared IT vision	☐	☐
Multidisciplinary IT planning committee	☐	☐
Integration of IT systems	☐	☐
Data warehouse	☐	☐
Electronic linkage between patients and physicians	☐	☐
Evidence-based medicine	☐	☐
Computerized provider order entry (>50% of orders)	☐	☐
High-quality IT staff and technology	☐	☐
Sufficient capital investment in IT (≥3%)	☐	☐
Community IT health initiatives	☐	☐

DATA SECURITY

Ensuring data security and compliance with all HIPAA requirements is critical to any strategic HIT initiative. Use of firewalls and password protection should be a part of the IT infrastructure. Some larger organizations are moving toward a two-factor identification that might include, for instance, a password and a fingerprint. Hackers from other countries and within the United States have targeted medical records as a way to obtain personal information, including Social Security numbers. Black market sales of medical records have become profitable. Identity thieves have discovered that medical records can sell for 20 times the price of a stolen credit card number (Pettypiece 2015).

There are several examples of huge data breaches in recent years. In 2013, Target announced that data from 40 million credit and debit cards were stolen. Sony Pictures Entertainment was hacked in 2014, and hackers obtained e-mails, pictures, executive salary information, and more. Even the government is not exempt, as evidenced by the hacking of the US Office of Personnel Management in 2015 when 4 million current and former federal employees had personal information exposed (OPM 2015). Of hospitals and physician groups, 90 percent have reported a cyber attack. Protection against these incidents is estimated to cost the US healthcare system $6 billion per year (Pettypiece 2015).

In addition, system backup and recovery are a necessary part of any disaster plan. As hospitals become more dependent on electronic documentation, disasters such as electricity failure or network failure can be devastating. Planning for these unexpected or unplanned outages is important.

THE GROWING HIT WORKFORCE

The healthcare field is experiencing a growing need for expert data analysts and clinical informatics specialists to lead it into the age of big data. As of 2011, the United States had a 50–60 percent shortage in expert **healthcare data analysts**—individuals hired by healthcare organizations to compile, validate, and analyze crucial medical data. By 2018, there will be between 140,000 and 190,000 unfilled expert healthcare data analyst positions and a shortage of 1.5 million data managers who understand the use of big data (Manyika et al. 2011).

Healthcare data analysts
Individuals hired by healthcare organizations to compile, validate, and analyze crucial medical data.

Healthcare data analysts use cutting-edge tools in advanced analytics to help interpret data, discover new information, and evaluate data quality. These analytical reports provide important information to senior leadership that is used in the strategic planning process to evaluate potential new service lines. The information is also used by operating managers to track the performance of ongoing projects via the organizational dashboard. Healthcare data analysts need a unique mix of healthcare knowledge, business acumen, understanding of applied mathematics, and expertise in computer science. These experts use analytic tools to work on projects such as

- ◆ optimization of operating room schedules to maximize productivity and utilization rates,

- ◆ optimization of appointment scheduling to meet patient demand,

- ◆ simulation for capacity operation in the emergency department during seasonal peaks,

- ◆ analysis of service-line volume to identify potential new markets,

- ◆ forecasting workload and revenue by departments, and

- ◆ forecasting changes in key performance metrics in the dashboard.

Much time can be spent on gathering data, validating methods of data acquisition, reformatting, and so on. But to make the most of healthcare analysts, healthcare administrators should ensure these professionals are doing more than just collecting data. Transforming raw data into meaningful analytics can be broken down into three stages—data capture, data provisioning (moving data into readable forms for healthcare practitioners), and data analysis (Staheli 2015).

Given that US healthcare can use databases to improve efficiency and quality, the shortage of HIT professionals is damaging. The optimal use of big data could save $300 billion annually and reduce national healthcare expenditures by 8 percent. Among for-profit hospitals big data has the potential to increase operating margins by 60 percent (Manyika et al. 2011).

HEALTHCARE INFORMATION RESOURCES

The Internet offers a wide variety of informational resources useful to healthcare strategic planners. This section outlines some of the most important for decision making and strategic planning.

INTERNATIONAL DATA
NationMaster

Using NationMaster (www.nationmaster.com), healthcare professionals can research and compare nations. A massive statistical database compiled from such sources as the Central Intelligence Agency's *World Factbook*, the United Nations, and the Organisation for Economic Co-operation and Development, NationMaster provides

- information on disasters, such as the extent of their devastation and the losses incurred by affected countries;

- economic information, such as gross domestic product, aid received, per capita income, debt, inflation, trade balance, foreign investment, and government spending; and

- health statistics from countries around the world, including birth weights; smoking rates; incidences of HIV infection, cancer, and circulatory and other diseases; infant and maternal mortality rates; life expectancies; suicide rates; teenage pregnancies; and health expenditures.

NATIONAL DATA
Centers for Medicare & Medicaid Services

CMS is part of the US Department of Health & Human Services (HHS). CMS is a federal agency whose primary responsibility is to administer Medicare, Medicaid, the Children's Health Insurance Program, and parts of the ACA. As part of this responsibility, CMS maintains extensive data on annual Medicare and Medicaid expenditures and national healthcare expenditures (available online at www.cms.gov).

Healthy People Project

The Healthy People 2020 program outlines opportunities to avoid preventable diseases, disability, injury, and premature death. HIT is an integral part of the implementation and success of the program. Efforts include building the public HIT infrastructure for interventions, health literacy, and health communication. The program maintains a database called DATA2020 that can be used to search for data related to four measures of health. They are (1) general health status, including life expectancy, chronic disease prevalance, and years of potential life lost; (2) health-related quality of life and well-being; (3) determinants of health such as biology, genetics, the environment, and access to health services; and (4) disparities and inequities, including those based in race or ethnicity, gender, physical and mental abilities, and geography (HHS 2015a). The *Healthy People 2020* report integrates input from public health experts; federal, state, and local government officials; more than 2,000 organizations; and the public.

The project's associated website (www.healthypeople.gov) provides innovative approaches to helping communities track their progress as they develop an agenda for health improvement. The site allows users to tailor information to their needs and explore evidence-based resources for implementation.

FedStats

FedStats (http://fedstats.sites.usa.gov) provides a full range of official statistical information produced by the federal government. The site provides links to more than 100 agencies that provide data and trend information on such topics as the economy, population trends, crime, education, healthcare, aviation safety, energy use, and farm production.

US Census Bureau

The US Census Bureau (www.census.gov) provides extensive information from the American Community Survey (ACS). The statistics are broken down to the zip code level. Instead of collecting census data every ten years, as the decennial census does, the ACS collects population and housing data on an annual basis. The current information provided by the ACS helps communities determine where to locate services and allocate resources.

National Center for Health Statistics

The National Center for Health Statistics (NCHS; www.cdc.gov/nchs), the nation's principal health statistics agency, compiles statistical information, mainly through surveys (e.g., the

National Ambulatory Medical Care Survey), to guide health policy and improve the health of the population. The NCHS's statistics document the health status of the population; disparities in health status by race and ethnicity, socioeconomic status, and region; and trends in healthcare delivery.

STATE DATA
StateMaster

StateMaster (www.statemaster.com) is a statistical database that provides a multitude of data on US states. Healthcare data available through StateMaster include state health status (in terms of such indicators as life expectancy and obesity levels) and comparisons of the health of residents by region. Its primary sources of data are the US Census Bureau, the Federal Bureau of Investigation, and the National Center for Educational Statistics. In addition to numerical data, StateMaster displays data in visual formats, such as pie charts, maps, graphs, and scatterplots.

State Health Facts

State Health Facts (http://kff.org/statedata/) is a statistical database sponsored by the Kaiser Family Foundation. It contains extensive state-level demographic healthcare information, data on residents' income and employment, and other, similar content.

California HealthCare Foundation

California has the largest population in the United States. Its more than 36 million residents represent 12 percent of the total US population. In partnership with the University of California at San Francisco Philip R. Lee Institute for Health Policy Studies and the California Hospitals Assessment and Reporting Taskforce, the California HealthCare Foundation developed calqualitycare.org (www.calqualitycare.org), a source of current data on quality in California hospitals. The 218 hospitals rated on this site account for 82 percent of hospital admissions in California, and the rated procedures (for heart attack, heart failure, heart bypass surgery, pneumonia, and maternity) are the five most common conditions requiring admission to a hospital. The site also provides measures pertaining to surgery patients and patients admitted to intensive care units. Hospitals on this site are rated on quality and timeliness of care, overall patient experience, and adherence to recommended patient safety practices.

Florida Department of Health

Florida is one of the most populous states in the United States. Its 17.7 million residents represent more than 6 percent of the total US population. The Florida Department of Health (www.floridahealth.gov) provides a wide range of healthcare data on the state's providers and residents through its databases, including annual vital health statistics data, public health data, information on hurricanes, practitioner profiles, and professional licensure listings.

HOSPITAL DATA

Agency for Healthcare Research and Quality

The Agency for Healthcare Research and Quality (AHRQ) is the health services research arm of the HHS. AHRQ funds research in the following areas:

- ◆ Quality improvement and patient safety

- ◆ Outcomes and effectiveness of care

- ◆ Clinical practice and technology assessment

- ◆ Healthcare delivery systems

- ◆ Primary care and preventive services

- ◆ Healthcare costs and financing

AHRQ's website (www.ahrq.gov) provides links to research data, survey reports, and tools, including AHRQ's Healthcare Cost and Utilization Project (www.ahrq.gov/data/hcup).

GuideStar

GuideStar (www.guidestar.org) is a publisher of financial and other data on not-for-profit organizations that are IRS-recognized tax-exempt organizations. Visitors to the site can view an organization's past three years of tax returns or find out more about its mission, programs, and finances. Thanks to generous funding from a number of foundations, GuideStar's basic service is available at no charge.

Hospital Compare

Hospital Compare (www.hospitalcompare.hhs.gov) is a collaborative effort of CMS, the Hospital Quality Alliance, and the nation's hospitals to create and publicly report hospital quality information. The hospital quality measures show recommended care for some of the most common and costly conditions. The measures are based on scientific evidence about treatments known to produce the best results. Healthcare experts and researchers are constantly evaluating the evidence to make sure that the guidelines and measures continue to reflect the most up-to-date information.

NURSING HOME DATA

Nursing Home Compare

CMS's Nursing Home Compare tool (www.medicare.gov/nursinghomecompare/search.html) evaluates nursing homes at the local, state, and national levels. CMS's Online Survey, Certification, and Reporting (OSCAR) database and Long-Term Care Minimum Data Set (MDS) repository supply the information found on the site. OSCAR itself is populated with information documented from state nursing home inspections, which assess such factors as resident care, staffing levels, and living environment. The MDS repository is populated with data on every resident in a Medicare- or Medicaid-certified nursing home. CMS collects information on residents' health, physical functioning, mental status, and general well-being and compares it with MDS quality standards.

SUMMARY

HIT is a dynamic environment and is facing growing volumes of patient data. As a result, creating an IT infrastructure that is flexible, allows collaboration among clinicians, incorporates mobile devices, and ensures access to patient data in real time is essential for healthcare organizations. Clinicians must also have access to information supporting the latest evidence-based approach to clinical care or the ability to provide real-time access to personalized medicine that is specifically designed for the individual patient.

HIT has important strategic value in the competitive healthcare environment. By implementing technology and processes that will improve patient care, healthcare providers can increase efficiency and profitability, enhance quality, and better coordinate care across the continuum of health services. As consolidation in the healthcare field increases, HIT provides linkages necessary for the successful integration of healthcare delivery systems. From a risk management perspective, EHRs and supporting clinical information systems have the potential to reduce medical malpractice costs.

E-health initiatives such as telehealth have the potential to improve the health status of patients at the local, regional, and national levels, particularly those in rural communities. E-health also promotes more efficient use of medical resources and helps reduce administrative costs.

In the strategic planning process, healthcare leaders' support of healthcare informatics is essential. Leadership support of IT steering committees and leadership involvement in the development of IT disaster recovery plans are particularly important. Most vital, future advances in personalized medicine provide opportunities for improved clinical outcomes for individual patients.

EXERCISES

REVIEW QUESTIONS

1. What role does information play in strategic planning in healthcare?
2. How can HIT help healthcare providers adapt to the rapidly changing healthcare environment? Provide examples of several HIT systems experiencing significant growth.
3. Health information websites are an important source of information for patients and providers. Identify three websites that provide healthcare data, and describe the type of information they contain.

COASTAL MEDICAL CENTER EXERCISE

Based on the data in the Coastal Medical Center (CMC) case, how can the information contained in the multiple databases discussed in Chapter 6 be used to improve CMC's performance?

COASTAL MEDICAL CENTER QUESTIONS

1. CMC failed to plan for investment in HIT. Develop a list of three types of HIT it should consider implementing and the impact they could have on the organization.
2. Develop an IT strategic plan for CMC.
3. Who should be involved in IT strategic planning, and at what point should you involve them?
4. How would you determine whether the IT strategic plan was successful?

INDIVIDUAL EXERCISE: DEVELOPING A DATA-USE PLAN FOR A CENTER OF EXCELLENCE IN WOMEN'S HEALTHCARE

A center of excellence is a team, a shared facility, or an entity that models leadership, best practices, research, support, and training for a particular area of medical expertise. You have been chosen to lead an initiative to evaluate the creation of a new center of excellence in women's healthcare at your organization. Using the information in the book presented thus far and the databases discussed in this chapter, answer the following questions.

1. Based on our discussion of leadership and your knowledge of hospital staffing patterns, identify five hypothetical individuals, by specialty role or category, whom you would like to include on your planning team.

2. Using the databases introduced in this chapter, list which ones would be most useful in the strategic planning process you would use in developing the new center of excellence in women's healthcare.
3. Identify the type of data provided by each website, and explain its use in the planning process.

REFERENCES

Cochran, G. L., L. Lander, M. Morien, D. E. Lomelin, H. Sayles, and D. G. Klepser. 2015. "Health Care Provider Perceptions of a Query-Based Health Information Exchange: Barriers and Benefits." *Journal of Innovation in Health Informatics* 22 (2): 302–8.

DeGaspari, J. 2015. "Making Sense of an Onslaught of Data in Public Health." *Healthcare Informatics*. Published January 21. www.healthcare-informatics.com/article/top-ten-tech-trend-making-sense-onslaught-data-public-health.

Fatehi, F., and R. J. Wootton. 2012. "Telemedicine, Telehealth or E-health? A Bibliometric Analysis of the Trends in the Use of These Terms." *Journal of Telemedicine and Telecare* 18 (8): 460–64.

HealthIT.gov. 2015. "What Is a Patient Portal?" Accessed August 13. www.healthit.gov/providers-professionals/faqs/what-patient-portal.

HIMSS Analytics. 2015. "Validated Stage 6 & 7 Providers List." Accessed August 27. www.himssanalytics.org/stage7.

———. 2014a. "Essentials Brief: Mobile Devices Study." Published December 9. www.himssanalytics.org/research/essentials-brief-mobile-devices-study.

———. 2014b. "Essentials Brief: Patient Engagement Series: Patient Portal Study." Published October 28. www.himssanalytics.org/research/essentials-brief-patient-engagement-series-patient-portal-study.

Hsiao, C., and E. Hing. 2014. "Use and Characteristics of Electronic Health Record Systems Among Office-Based Physician Practices: United States, 2001–2013." National Center for Health Statistics Data Brief 143. Published January. www.cdc.gov/nchs/data/databriefs/db143.pdf.

Lovelock, J.-D., K. Hale, A. O'Connell, W. L. Haden, R. Atwal, and C. Graham. 2015. "Forecast Alert: IT Spending, Worldwide, 2Q15 Update." Gartner. Published June 29. www.gartner.com/doc/3084417.

Manyika, J., M. Chui, B. Brown, J. Bughin, R. Dobbs, C. Roxburgh, and A. H. Byers. 2011. "Big Data: The Next Frontier for Innovation, Competition, and Productivity." McKinsey & Company. Published May. www.mckinsey.com/insights/business_technology/big_data_the_next_frontier_for_innovation.

Pennic, J. 2014. "Only 8 Hospitals Have Attested for Meaningful Use Stage 2." HIT Consultant. Published June 17. http://hitconsultant.net/2014/06/17/only-8-hospitals-have-attested-for-meaningful-use-stage-2/.

Perna, G. 2015. "Direct-to-Consumer: Alternative Methods of Telehealth Take Hold." *Healthcare Informatics*. Published January 21. www.healthcare-informatics.com/article/top-ten-tech-trends-direct-consumer-alternative-methods-telehealth-take-hold.

Pettypiece, S. 2015. "Rising Cyber Attacks Costing Health System $6 Billion Annually." *Bloomberg Business*. Published May 7. www.bloomberg.com/news/articles/2015-05-07/rising-cyber-attacks-costing-health-system-6-billion-annually.

Raths, D. 2015. "Setting the Roadmap for FHIR." *Healthcare Informatics*. Published January 21. www.healthcare-informatics.com/article/top-ten-tech-trends-setting-roadmap-fhir.

Riskin, D. 2012. "Big Data: Opportunity and Challenge." *Healthcare IT News*. Published June 12. www.healthcareitnews.com/news/big-data-opportunity-and-challenge.

Staheli, R. 2015. "4 Ways Healthcare Data Analysts Can Provide Their Full Value." Health Catalyst. Accessed August 29. www.healthcatalyst.com/healthcare-analytics-best-practices.

US Department of Health & Human Services (HHS). 2015a. "Framework." Accessed August 29. www.healthypeople.gov/sites/default/files/HP2020Framework.pdf.

————. 2015b. "Meaningful Use Definition and Objectives." Accessed January 29. www.healthit.gov/providers-professionals/meaningful-use-definition-objectives.

US Department of Veterans Affairs (VA). 2015. "Where Do I Get the Care I Need?" Accessed August 29. www.va.gov/health/FindCare.asp.

US Office of Personnel Management (OPM). 2015. "OPM Announces Steps to Protect Federal Workers and Others from Cyber Threats." Published July 9. www.opm.gov/news/releases/2015/07/opm-announces-steps-to-protect-federal-workers-and-others-from-cyber-threats/.

Walker, M. B. 2015. "Leidos, Cerner Win 'DHMSM,' DoD's $11B Electronic Health Record Contract." *FierceGovHealthIT*. Published July 29. www.fiercegovhealthit.com/story/breaking-leidos-cerner-win-dhmsm-dods-11b-electronic-health-record-contract/2015-07-29.

West, D. M. 2013. "Improving Health Care Through Mobile Medical Devices and Sensors." Brookings Institution. Published October 22. www.brookings.edu/research/papers/2013/10/22-improving-health-care-mobile-medical-devices-apps-sensors-west.

CHAPTER 7

STRATEGIC PLANNING AND THE HEALTHCARE BUSINESS PLAN

The way to get started is to quit talking and begin doing.

—Walt Disney

Think ahead. Don't let day-to-day operations drive out planning.

—Donald Rumsfeld

LEARNING OBJECTIVES

After you have studied this chapter, you should be able to

➤ analyze and address challenges in strategic planning for healthcare organizations through the use of financial information;

➤ create a business plan for a new service line in a healthcare organization;

➤ assess the appropriate organizational structure for a new business initiative, including corporate structure and scope of leadership;

➤ understand the management of costs, quality, and access; and

➤ demonstrate the ability to make financial decisions and develop a strategy for change.

KEY TERMS AND CONCEPTS

➤ Cost of capital

➤ Financial plan

➤ Healthcare business plan

➤ Horizontal integration

➤ Income statement

➤ Internal rate of return

➤ Net present value

➤ Payback period

➤ Pro forma financial statement

➤ Regression analysis

➤ Vertical integration

INTRODUCTION

As healthcare moves into an age of reform, accountable care, and bundling, the question of how to align physicians with the goals and priorities of the hospital is even more important. The healthcare business plan serves an important role in successfully aligning hospitals and physicians through financial integration and by incorporating joint incentives for profitability, quality, and clinical productivity (Levin and Gustave 2013).

Effective business planning is a formal, measurable process that evaluates resource allocation, performance, and the current business environment and forecasts potential demand for new services. Business planning will become increasingly important as traditional federal healthcare policies change and move toward bundled payments and population health–based outcomes as a reimbursement strategy. Consistent with the overall strategic plan, the completion of a comprehensive business plan will evaluate new business initiatives and ensure the initiatives meet a demonstrated community need and are the most appropriate use of the organization's scarce resources.

DEFINITION

Healthcare business plan
Method by which a healthcare organization evaluates future investment in a new business initiative.

A **healthcare business plan** is a method by which a healthcare organization evaluates future investment in a new business initiative. To create a comprehensive business plan, the organization must gather a wide range of information and forecast future demand. A sample business plan outline appears in Exhibit 7.1. The website of the US Small Business Administration offers a number of additional resources, including

◆ an outline for writing a business plan (www.sba.gov/writing-business-plan);

◆ an electronic form for creating a written business plan (www.sba.gov/sites/default/files/SBA%201010C.pdf); and

◆ the SBA Business Planner, with a wide range of information and data sources useful in the business planning process (www.sba.gov/sites/default/files/ SBA%20Export%20Business%20Planner.pdf).

HEALTHCARE BUSINESS PLAN

An organization's healthcare business plan should be consistent with its overall mission and vision and should consider the competitive market. While the business plan is a written document, it is subject to change. Factors such as a shift in community demographics or competitors' actions will require an organization to revisit its plan and revise it as necessary.

The typical business plan includes a detailed discussion of the proposed healthcare service, the identification of target markets, and financial projections. After the new service has been implemented, planners evaluate it over a multiyear period, usually three years. The initiative's development can be monitored by setting targets and seeing whether those targets are met in that three-year time frame. Periodic evaluation over multiple years will return a fair, realistic assessment of the initiative's progress.

HEALTHCARE BUSINESS PLANNING WORKFLOW

While the business plan outline provides the components of the company's workflow, Exhibit 7.2 illustrates how data are gathered for the plan. The following sections provide additional explanations for these steps in the process.

EXHIBIT 7.1
Sample Business Plan Outline

I. Executive Summary	IV. Financial Data
II. Statement of Purpose	A. Pro forma financial statement
III. Description of the Business	1. Income statement
A. Competition/market	2. Balance sheet
B. Operating procedures	B. Capital funding
C. Personnel	C. Break-even analysis
D. Facilities	D. Three-year summary
E. Strategic capital allocation	E. Internal rate of return
	V. Alternatives
	VI. Recommendation

Exhibit 7.2
Healthcare
Business Planning
Workflow

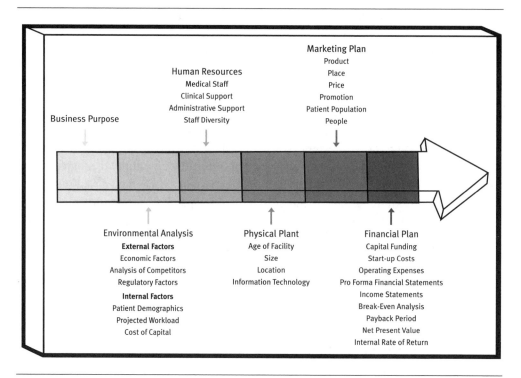

Horizontal integration
Expansion along current lines of business into new geographic areas, often through mergers with other organizations, for purposes of increasing market share.

Vertical integration
Expansion to a new line of business located somewhere along the continuum of care (e.g., a hospital that normally provides acute care opening a primary care clinic or acquiring a skilled nursing facility).

Business Purpose

The statement of purpose should define the company's core goals and purpose and form the basis for the company brand and promises to consumers. A statement of purpose focuses primarily on the short message that will guide the company in formulating its business practices and strategy. It should also contain consumer needs and attainable goals (Lister 2015). A corporate strategy that includes business expansion should be grounded in a business plan. For example, organizations can expand their current lines of business into new geographic areas through mergers with other organizations (a strategy of **horizontal integration**), or they can choose to expand into new lines of business somewhere along the continuum of care—such as outpatient clinics, ambulatory surgery centers, or skilled nursing facilities—or to acquire and integrate physician group practices (a strategy of **vertical integration**). Vertically integrated businesses leverage mass-production principles of efficiency and dominated the corporate world until the later part of the twentieth century. However, in the 1990s, businesses started to consider why they needed to own the whole process and how to collaborate with others for some of the components and processes needed to create, produce, distribute, sell, and support their product. By 2012, both strategies were being used, depending on the model that yielded the best product, experience, availability, price, service, and support for consumers (Taylor 2012).

Environmental Analysis

Historically, healthcare has been less affected by economic factors than other industries have been. However, sound business decision making is necessary in the healthcare field to ensure future success because the business climate is changing. External factors to consider in the course of writing a business plan include the current economy, regulatory law, and the results of competitor analysis. The federal government is extending its influence on healthcare through legislation on healthcare delivery processes and reimbursement for care. In addition, the Medicare and Medicaid programs continue to focus on healthcare compliance, evidence-based clinical care, and Health Insurance Portability and Accountability Act privacy statutes in support of the patient population. As healthcare providers struggle to meet these requirements, hospital–physician partnerships can be mutually beneficial in providing patient care in adherence to current healthcare policy legislation (Kauk, Hill, and Althausen 2014).

Healthcare is delivered in local communities and is affected by market competition, making an evaluation of current and potential competitors essential to the business planning process. A highly competitive market increases the vulnerability of a healthcare organization's strategic position by lowering profit margins and reducing operating capital. As market competition increases, healthcare organizations often consider mergers, acquisitions, or joint ventures in an attempt to reduce costs, share risks, and enhance reputations. Research suggests that consolidation can create economies of scale, help organizations maximize their use of resources in the local market, reduce administrative overhead costs, and lower the **cost of capital**—the opportunity cost of making a specific investment, or alternately stated, the rate of return an organization must achieve to make a capital investment worthwhile (see Highlight 7.1). The cost of capital reflects what could have been earned by putting the same money into a different investment with equal risk. However, if successful, the increased market share from a new initiative may also reduce operating costs and improve patients' awareness of the services an organization offers. Cost of capital is one of the internal factors to consider during strategic planning, along with patient demographics and projected workload.

Cost of capital
Opportunity cost of making a specific investment; that is, the rate of return an organization must achieve to make a capital investment worthwhile.

An analysis of a for-profit, publicly traded healthcare competitor can be completed online using the competitor's name or stock symbol. On Yahoo! Finance (http://finance.yahoo.com), for example, analysts can enter the company's name or stock symbol and then select "profile" for a description of that company. Selection of other subheadings on the company's page will reveal stock price fluctuations based on corporate performance and other useful information.

Regulatory Factors

When exploring new business initiatives, organizations must be mindful of government regulations pertaining to healthcare development, including the Stark laws, which regulate

---

⊛ **HIGHLIGHT 7.1** Cost of Capital

When an organization has two investment opportunities of equal risk and must choose one, it hopes that the one it chooses will yield a greater rate of return. Say Hospital X can either open a new outpatient clinic or build a new parking lot. The hospital forecasts that it will earn a 7 percent return if it invests in a clinic and a 5 percent return if it invests in a parking lot, so it chooses to invest in a clinic. The 5 percent return the hospital "gave up" by choosing to invest in the clinic instead of the parking lot is part of the cost of capital.

The interest on the funds used to make the investment also figures into the cost of capital. When an organization borrows money, it must pay back that money plus interest. Interest is a consideration even for organizations wealthy enough not to have to borrow money. The money that organization has in the bank is earning interest—for example, Hospital X's savings earn 3 percent. If it withdraws that money to make an investment, the hospital will stop earning that 3 percent interest. In both cases, the interest is part of the cost of capital, and the organization hopes that the return it will make on its investment will be greater than the interest it is paying (in the case of the organization that has to borrow money) or not earning (in the case of the wealthy organization that is withdrawing money from its bank account).

---

hospital partnerships with physicians (see Highlight 7.2). Some states are subject to certificate-of-need regulations, which require health services planners to obtain approval from state officials to build a new healthcare facility (see Chapter 1, Highlight 1.13). The intent of these regulations is to limit the duplication of services in a geographic area.

Human Resources

Human resources are a critical factor in healthcare business planning and may determine the success of new business initiatives. Because of the increasing complexity of healthcare services, the inclusion of clinicians on teams working to develop business plans is important, including physicians, nurses, and allied health professionals. Effective planning aligns human resources with organizational strategy and measures the status of human resources as part of the organization's balanced scorecard (see Chapter 3). For example, human resources could be measured according to the number and specialties of physicians and medical staff members, the level of certification held by clinical support personnel, and the overall diversity of the organization's staff.

HIGHLIGHT 7.2 Stark Laws

The original Stark legislation—the Ethics in Patient Referral Act—took effect in 1992. The intent of this federal legislation was to reduce conflicts of interest regarding physician referrals and to limit overutilization of healthcare services. The statute was expanded in 1995 under Stark II to prohibit physicians or their family members from referring Medicare patients to healthcare organizations in which they have a financial interest, including clinical laboratories and organizations that provide physical therapy, occupational therapy, radiology services, radiation therapy, durable medical equipment, home health services, and hospital services.

Stark III regulations went into effect on December 4, 2007, to institute exceptions to Stark II. These exceptions, called *safe harbors*, were designed to provide clear guidance in support of governmental healthcare policy. Under this revised legislation, for example, these safe harbors allow for ownership, investment, and compensation for intrafamily referrals in rural areas. This safe harbor was designed to protect the healthcare infrastructure of rural communities and to encourage healthcare providers to practice in rural areas. Stark III also allows employed physicians to refer to other providers in their healthcare system. This modification helps bond independent physicians in the community to the healthcare system, which, theoretically, should promote better continuity of care.

Violations of the Stark statutes are punishable by a $15,000 civil penalty, and any claim paid as the result of an improper referral is considered an overpayment, which the provider must pay back. Organized schemes to evade the statutes can be punished by a $100,000 civil penalty (Stark Law 2015).

In one important human resources trend, physicians are being hired by hospitals or joining group practices. In 2000, 53 percent of physicians were independent from their hospitals; in 2012, that number dropped to 23 percent. With the advent of accountable care organizations (ACOs) and the expansion of Medicare, health systems have sought greater efficiency through integration of care. These changes have shifted the market from single physicians or group practices to healthcare institutions (Moses et al. 2013).

Because of this changing healthcare environment, effective leaders who wish to maximize organizational performance focus their efforts on recruiting the best individuals available. Organizations start by identifying individuals who have a track record of success and who reflect the changing demographics of the population they serve. Once these individuals are on board and have demonstrated their knowledge and outstanding performance, they should be rewarded with appropriate financial compensation and other organizational recognition. Such recognition helps retain those who will lead the organization to future success.

A management style that values employee contributions and supports team decision making will result in lower employee turnover. Organizations that exhibit an organizational culture of trust, respect, and employee recognition have the lowest turnover rates (Levin and Gustave 2013).

Physical Plant

Many health systems are deferring routine maintenance and other capital expenditures on aging facilities (Wong-Hammond and Damon 2013). Unfortunately, these capital expenditures cannot be delayed indefinitely. As a result, health systems should develop a capital allocation plan that aligns funding sources with mission-driven growth initiatives. In this context, many health systems face operating environments of declining demand for inpatient services and limited growth in inpatient revenue. Further declines in hospital operating margins are possible because of the shift away from hospital inpatient care toward ambulatory care provided in outpatient settings.

Communities' evolving healthcare needs require investments in new facilities. Successful organizations develop a facility master plan that incorporates high-performance work processes and the latest technology. Development of new processes is even more critical for organizations with old facilities because their existing processes may be inappropriate for new facilities. Organizations planning for replacement facilities should consult process improvement experts to maximize organizational efficiency.

Under certain capital market conditions, highly rated health systems can take advantage of lower interest rates. For example, in 2013, an investment-grade not-for-profit health system was able to issue $300 million in new 30-year tax-exempt bonds at 4.5 percent interest, a low rate for that period. This advantage provides a low-cost source of capital that many strong health systems can use in their business planning process (Wong-Hammond and Damon 2013).

The first step in facility planning is a community needs assessment to identify current and future healthcare needs. Using this information, hospital leaders can create a plan that adds facilities as they are required by the community. Many hospitals create master campus plans, which include facilities inside and outside the main hospital. The plans also sometimes incorporate smaller new initiatives, such as expanded outpatient services, that do not require major facility expenditures. A master facility plan can improve patient care, enhance community health status, and have a positive impact on overall profitability.

Historically, many health systems' business plans were oriented toward the acquisition of physical assets (e.g., real estate, property, equipment, hospital facilities). As of 2015, with health systems facing a more complex operating environment, organizations are more heavily focused on acquiring physicians, investing in clinical health information technology

(HIT), and improving their ambulatory care capacity to better meet the changing healthcare delivery models (Wong-Hammond and Damon 2013).

New investments in HIT provide a synergistic effect for any new hospital construction. By combining high-performance work processes and investments in new facilities with state-of-the-art technology, healthcare organizations can streamline clinical processes, improve patient care, and enhance the organization's profitability. The cumulative effect of new processes, investments in technology, and hospital construction sets the stage for increased quality and profitability.

Marketing Plan

As discussed in Chapter 5, a strong marketing plan is important to ensuring the success of new business initiatives. As a result, the development of a formal marketing plan is an important part of the process of developing a business plan. The marketing plan considers the demographic characteristics of the population in the service community. It also takes into account the competitive marketplace, the healthcare organization's capabilities, and the areas with the greatest economic potential. Separate parts of the marketing plan should be designed to attract the attention of physicians; patients; and major employers, which can be a source for contracts and employee health services.

An analysis of patient demographics—part of the first P in the five Ps of a marketing plan (Chapter 5)—is important because the demand for new healthcare business initiatives is often a function of age, sex, culture, and economic status. In addition, a high percentage of patients with commercial insurance will increase the level of profitability for a new business initiative, whereas a high percentage of patients who are dependent on Medicaid reimbursement or who have no way to pay will reduce profitability.

Financial Plan

While the intent of this book is not to teach a full finance course, it is necessary for healthcare administrators to understand some financial terms and concepts in order to complete a business plan. The following sections discuss these ideas as part of the financial plan component.

Organizations compose **financial plans**—documents analyzing financial information on potential performance—to model the future of a new business initiative. Capital funding is most often needed to obtain buildings, land, and equipment that cost more than a certain dollar amount. Other expenses can come from operating revenue. A capital acquisition strategy is key to any healthcare business plan and should consider the following (Wong-Hammond and Damon 2013):

Financial plan
Document that analyzes financial information to demonstrate potential performance of a new business initiative.

◆ How to access external debt such as bank loans or bond financing; additionally, for-profit hospitals have the ability to use equity capital, which is the sale of common stock

◆ The use of business plans to set targets, create objectives, and reprioritize

◆ Multiple finance options, such as lease strategies versus buy strategies

◆ Levels of risk associated with an initiative in order to calculate the needed financial returns

Pro forma financial statement
Statement prepared before a business initiative is undertaken to model the anticipated financial results of the initiative.

A financial plan will also include start-up costs and operating expenses for any new business initiative. As part of this process, planners summarize the anticipated financial results of an initiative in **pro forma financial statements**. The accurate forecasting of clinical workload is key to these statements. Because accurate forecasts are often difficult to make, healthcare organizations frequently develop pro forma statements reflecting different workload scenarios. These statements reflect the potential revenue stream of the proposed initiative several years into the future because an ongoing cash flow is necessary to pay back debt and meet operating expenses.

Income Statement

Income statement
Summary of an organization's revenue and expenses over a certain period.

An **income statement** is a summary of an organization's revenue and expenses over a defined period. A *statement of operations* is similar to an income statement, except it is used by not-for-profit organizations and reflects the fact that they do not generate profits. A pro forma income statement for a new physical therapy clinic is shown in Exhibit 7.3.

Payback Period

Payback period
Length of time it takes a new business initiative to recoup the cost of the original investment.

A **payback period** is the length of time a new business initiative will take to recoup an organization's original investment. The shorter the payback period, the more rapidly an organization is able to recover its original capital investment and redeploy its resources to new projects. When prioritizing new business initiatives, organizations often pick projects that will have the shortest payback period.

Exhibit 7.4 shows a payback period for the proposed physical therapy clinic featured in Exhibit 7.3. Note that it considers three scenarios, as do the pro forma financial statements discussed earlier in the financial plan section. These scenarios could differ based on volume or model of care. In the case of this clinic, the scenarios are based on projected workload or volume. The graph in Exhibit 7.4 is a summary of the information provided in Exhibit 7.5.

Net Present Value

Net present value (NPV)
Figure calculated on the basis of discounted cash flow to evaluate the financial worth of a business initiative; the amount of money a business initiative is projected to earn minus the amount of money originally invested in it.

Net present value (NPV) is a figure investors calculate to determine whether a capital project will be worth the investment. In basic terms, it is the amount of money a business initiative is projected to earn minus the amount of money invested in it. If NPV is greater than zero, the initiative is probably worth the investment; it will generate more money than the organization's original investment in it. If NPV is less than zero, the initiative is probably not worth the investment; it will not generate enough money to repay the investment in

Cost Center	Projected Revenue and Expenses
REVENUE	
1010 PHYSICAL THERAPY REVENUE	$384,155
EXPENSES	
100 SALARIES—GENERAL	−85,000
1585 FRINGE BENEFITS	−9,750
3500 MED/SURG SUPPLIES	−1,435
3800 MARKETING	−5,000
4600 OFFICE SUPPLIES	−175
4640 POSTAGE/SHIPPING	−134
4800 MINOR EQUIPMENT	−1,314
5550 SUPPLIES AND MATERIALS	−1,306
5630 LINEN EXPENSE	−1,232
5640 REPAIRS AND MAINTENANCE	−366
7030 BUILDING DEPRECIATION	−24,000
7060 EQUIPMENT DEPRECIATION	−1,612
7600 LEASE/RENT—EQUIPMENT	−2,336
9100 PROFESSIONAL DUES	−495
TOTAL EXPENSES	−134,155
NET INCOME	$250,000

EXHIBIT 7.3
Pro Forma Physical Therapy Clinic Annual Income Statement

it. NPV uses *discounted cash flow* (see Highlight 7.3), which takes into account the cost of the capital invested in the project and the fact that money loses value over time because of inflation. The value of the project is obtained by discounting expected cash flows (the residual cash flows after all operating expenses), but prior to debt payments, at the weighted average cost of capital (the cost of the different components of financing used by the company,

EXHIBIT 7.4
Projected Physical
Therapy Clinic
Payback Period

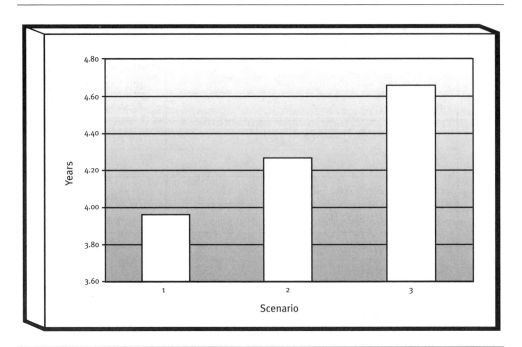

weighted by their market value proportions). A 12 percent cost of capital is used in the NPV calculations for the projected physical therapy clinic's payback analysis in Exhibit 7.5, showing different scenarios of projected workload (100 percent, 90 percent, and 80 percent). The rate is determined by the individual organization to reflect the cost associated with borrowing money for a project. Note that Year 0 in all three scenarios includes the same building costs and net cash flows (and the resulting cumulative cash flows)—essentially, the

---

⊛ HIGHLIGHT 7.3 Discounted Cash Flow

Discounted cash flow is used to determine the value of an amount of money over time. It revolves around the principle that a dollar today is worth more than a dollar tomorrow and uses a discount rate (also called a *weighted average cost of capital*) to calculate worth. The discount rate accounts for changes in value because of factors such as inflation as well as the return that could have been earned by investing the money.

The principle of discounted cash flow implies that an investment today is worth whatever amount it will earn for the investor in the future. For example, if you invest $1,000 today and expect it to earn another $100 in five years, the value of that money is actually $1,100. Put another way, the $1,100 that you have in five years is worth $1,000 today.

Exhibit 7.5
Projected Physical
Therapy Clinic
Payback Analysis

Physical Therapy Clinic Payback Period Scenarios (Cost of Capital 12%)

Payback Period, 100% of Projected Workload

	Sq. Ft.	Year 0	Year 1	Year 2	Year 3	Year 4	Year 5	Totals
Building costs		($750,000)	$ –	$ –	$ –	$ –	$ –	($750,000)
Net income		$ –	$250,000	$255,000	$260,100	$265,302	$270,608	$1,301,010
Net cash flows		($750,000)	$250,000	$255,000	$260,100	$265,302	$270,608	$551,010
Cumulative payback		$ –	$ 250,000	$505,000	$765,100	$1,030,402	$1,031,010	
Cumulative cash flows		($750,000)	($500,000)	($245,000)	$15,100	$280,402	$551,010	

Payback period (years) = 3.96   NPV = $183,787   IRR = 21.3%

Payback Period, 90% of Projected Workload

	Sq. Ft.	Year 0	Year 1	Year 2	Year 3	Year 4	Year 5	Totals
Building costs		($750,000)	$ –	$ –	$ –	$ –	$ –	($750,000)
Net income		$ –	$225,000	$229,500	$234,090	$238,772	$243,547	$1,170,909
Net cash flows		($750,000)	$225,000	$229,500	$234,090	$238,772	$243,547	$420,909
Cumulative payback		$ –	$ 225,000	$454,500	$688,590	$927,362	$1,170,909	
Cumulative cash flows		($750,000)	($525,000)	($295,500)	($61,410)	$177,362	$420,909	

Payback period (years) = 4.27   NPV = $90,409   IRR = 16.7%

Payback Period, 80% of Projected Workload

	Sq. Ft.	Year 0	Year 1	Year 2	Year 3	Year 4	Year 5	Totals
Building costs		($750,000)	$ –	$ –	$ –	$ –	$ –	($750,000)
Net income		$ –	$200,000	$204,000	$208,080	$212,242	$216,486	$1,040,808
Net cash flows		($750,000)	$200,000	$204,000	$208,080	$212,242	$216,486	$290,808
Cumulative payback		$ –	$ 200,000	$404,000	$612,080	$824,322	$1,040,808	
Cumulative cash flows		($750,000)	($550,000)	($346,000)	($137,920)	$74,322	$290,808	

Payback period (years) = 4.66   NPV = ($2,970)   IRR = 11.8%

cost of the building. In the first year, the net income is different depending on the volume, or the number of appointments the clinic has filled. Then each year, the net income uses a 2 percent market share increase. In the first scenario of 100 percent projected workload, the net income accumulated for 3.96 years results in the payback of the building cost and expenses over time. From that point on, the revenue stream has covered the fixed costs and is generating significant net income.

Internal Rate of Return

Internal rate of return (IRR) is a term used in capital budgeting to measure and compare the profitability of investments. It is the interest rate at which the NPV of all the cash flows (both positive and negative) from a project or an investment equal zero. In the same way that payback period may be used to prioritize projects (as discussed earlier in the chapter), an organization could choose the project with the highest IRR from a list of potential projects, thereby maximizing overall profitability. The IRR for the first scenario of the

Internal rate of return (IRR)
Interest rate at which the NPV of all the cash flows (both positive and negative) from a project or an investment equal zero. The term is used in capital budgeting to measure and compare the profitability of investments.

potential physical therapy clinic, at 100 percent of projected workload (i.e., the amount of work expected to be completed by the clinic), is shown in Exhibit 7.5.

PLANNING TOOLS

BUSINESS PLANNING SOFTWARE

A variety of software is available to assist business plan development. Business planning software helps the business leader define the proposed product or service, identify the specific market or markets for that product or service, conduct market research, analyze the competition, determine the market position of competitors' products and services, and describe the clinical care process. It also helps analyze financial performance, develop a staffing plan, and determine the legal structure (e.g., wholly owned, for-profit or not-for-profit subsidiary corporation; joint venture corporation owned partly by a healthcare organization; physician group).

FINANCIAL ANALYSIS TOOLS

Microsoft offers a suite of financial planning tools in Excel that can be used for healthcare business planning. These tools—which can be accessed by clicking on "fx Insert Function" under the Formulas tab—can calculate IRR, payback period, NPV, and other values. Additional information on these capabilities can be found at Matt H. Evans's website (www. exinfm.com/excel%20files/npv_irr.xls).

FORECASTING TOOLS

Developing accurate workload projections is another important part of healthcare business planning. Future demand for a new service can be estimated by looking at patient demographics in the market area. Age, sex, cultural diversity, per capita income, unemployment rate, and payer mix are all factors to consider in assessing the potential profit of a new business initiative. Consideration of referral information from physicians, health plans, and other healthcare organizations in combination with demographic data increases the accuracy of this estimate.

Regression analysis
Mathematical method of determining the relationships between variables, usually the effect of one variable on another, such as the effect of a price increase on demand.

Regression analysis (see Highlight 7.4) is a useful tool for forecasting changes in healthcare workload over multiyear periods. This method provides an accurate estimate of future workload and can be adjusted to reflect seasonal fluctuations in the demand for health services. For example, healthcare organizations experience increased demand for services during flu season, which normally runs from October through February. While forecasting, taking into account both long-term trends and short-term variations in the healthcare business planning process is important. Examples of long-term trends in

HIGHLIGHT 7.4 Regression Analysis

Regression analysis is a mathematical method of determining the relationship of one variable to another—for example, determining whether the number of patient visits to the emergency department (ED) is related to the day of the month. To discover whether there is a relationship between these two variables, the analyst would gather data about both (the number of patient visits to the ED and the calendar day) and graph the results. If she finds a relationship, a formula can be constructed that will allow a healthcare provider to predict traffic to the ED on any given day.

Multiple regression analysis is the same as "basic" regression analysis, except a greater number of variables are tested. For example, to further analyze the patient flow in the ED, you might include time of day and length of time spent waiting in the emergency department in addition to the number of visits on specific days.

healthcare include a shorter length of stay for hospital inpatient care and the increased use of outpatient services. Several types of regression analysis can be performed in Excel, including linear regression, exponential regression, and multiple regression.

SUMMARY

Quality and efficiency are becoming increasingly important to the success of hospitals in the new, value-based environment of healthcare reimbursement. In addition, physicians must increasingly become accountable for cost-effective care. Opportunities also exist to take advantage of payment incentives through the Centers for Medicare & Medicaid Services for hospitals and physicians as they participate in ACO models and other approaches to bundling healthcare reimbursement. By controlling costs, health systems have an opportunity to manage to Medicare reimbursement for treatments and procedures, which in the aggregate will allow them to become low-cost providers and succeed in the healthcare market of the future (Levin and Gustave 2013).

Effective business planning enables integrated healthcare systems to allocate healthcare personnel, facilities, and information technology efficiently and deliver healthcare services to the local community in an organized fashion. To maintain a competitive position in the market, healthcare organizations must pursue new business initiatives. Successful business planning and accurate forecasts for these new initiatives depend on the collection and analysis of historical data, input from clinical providers, patient demographic data, physician referral patterns, and competitors' market share. The use of forecasting tools such as regression analysis increases the accuracy of forecasts by accounting for seasonal fluctuations in the demand for health services, short-term variations, and long-term industry trends.

The healthcare planning methods discussed in this chapter provide a framework on which to base the process of developing a business plan. Part of this framework is the marketing plan, which is a written document that guides marketing activities. Preparation of the marketing plan requires a clear understanding of the competitive marketplace in which an organization operates as well as the organization's capabilities. When evaluating potential new healthcare services, the organization should focus on areas with the greatest economic potential. A plan for growth is also not complete without the numbers to back it up. The financial section of a business plan looks forward, providing a projection of what numbers are anticipated based on the analysis. Planners use tools and reports such as payback period, IRR, and NPV to make these predictions. A plan is not an accounting report or a tax return, but rather an educated guess (Wasserman 2010). Ending with clear alternatives and recommendations so that the decision makers can draw conclusions needed is important. Using pie charts, graphs, and other visuals will further aid in selling the plan. The business plan is one of the major components of strategic planning overall.

EXERCISES

REVIEW QUESTIONS

1. What is a healthcare business plan? What key sections are included in a healthcare business plan?
2. What are horizontal integration and vertical integration? How does vertical integration reflect a change of strategic direction for an organization?
3. Discuss the importance of financial planning in healthcare organizations. Describe several of the techniques used in the financial planning process.

COASTAL MEDICAL CENTER EXERCISE

On the basis of the information provided in the Coastal Medical Center (CMC) case and what you learned in Chapter 7, develop a healthcare business plan for CMC's possible new physical therapy clinic. Exhibits 7.3, 7.4, and 7.5 may be used as CMC's data. Make sure to consider the following questions.

COASTAL MEDICAL CENTER QUESTIONS

1. Who should be involved in developing the healthcare business plan?
2. How will you know if the healthcare business plan is a success?
3. What do you see as the value of the healthcare business plan for CMC's future success?

INDIVIDUAL EXERCISE: PLANNING FOR POPULATION HEALTH ON THE ISLAND OF HISPANIOLA

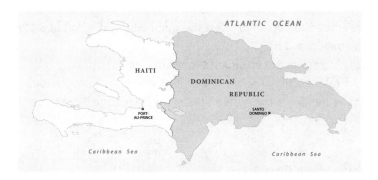

Hispaniola is an island in the Caribbean that is divided into two nations, Haiti and the Dominican Republic. Complete the following table using the NationMaster website (www. nationmaster.com).

	United States	Dominican Republic	Haiti
Population[1]			
Population growth[2]			
Education[3]			
Murder rate[4]			
Drinkable water[5]			
Gross domestic product per capita			
Infant mortality[6]			
Life expectancy[7]			
Physicians per capita[8]			

1 Total population of nation

2 Average annual percentage change in population

3 Average years of schooling received

4 Homicide rate per year per 100,000 inhabitants

5 Percentage of population with access to clean water sources

6 Annual number of infant deaths (aged less than one year) per 1,000 live births

7 Number of years a newborn infant would live if prevailing patterns of mortality at the time of his birth stay the same throughout his life

8 Number of graduates of any facility or school of medicine who are working in the country in any medical field (practice, teaching, research)

GROUP EXERCISE: PLANNING FOR POPULATION HEALTH ON THE ISLAND OF HISPANIOLA

1. Are the health and well-being of a population important?
2. How does education appear to affect the well-being of the United States, the Dominican Republic, and Haiti?
3. What is the importance of economics to healthcare?
4. What is the relationship of public health infrastructure to population health status?
5. Would you rather live in the United States, the Dominican Republic, or Haiti?
6. What is the cause of the difference between the three countries?

Additional Hispaniola Resources

- www.nytimes.com/2014/11/30/travel/driving-the-seam-of-hispaniola.html
- www.nytimes.com/2012/01/09/opinion/haiti-can-be-rich-again.html
- www.dw.com/en/haiti-and-the-dominican-republic-one-island-two-worlds/a-16593022

REFERENCES

Kauk, J., A. Hill, and P. Althausen. 2014. "Healthcare Fundamentals." *Journal of Orthopedic Trauma* 28 (Suppl. 1): S25–S41.

Levin, L. S., and L. Gustave. 2013. "Aligning Incentives in Health Care: Physician Practice and Health System Partnership." *Clinical Orthopaedics and Related Research* 471 (6): 1824–31.

Lister, J. 2015. "Statements of Purpose for Businesses." *Houston Chronicle*. Accessed September 4. http://smallbusiness.chron.com/statements-purpose-businesses-26026.html.

Moses, H., D. M. Matheson, E. R. Dorsey, B. P. George, D. Sadoff, and S. Yoshimura. 2013. "The Anatomy of Health Care in the United States." *Journal of the American Medical Association* 310 (18): 1947–63.

Stark Law. 2015. "Stark Law FAQ's." Accessed September 4. http://starklaw.org/stark-law-faq.htm.

Taylor, T. 2012. "Vertical vs. Horizontal Integration: Which Is a Better Operations Strategy?" *OPS Rules* (blog). Published November 9. www.opsrules.com/supply-chain-optimization-blog/bid/241648/Vertical-vs-Horizontal-Integration-Which-is-a-Better-Operations-Strategy.

Wasserman, E. 2010. "How to Write the Financial Section of a Business Plan." Inc.com. Published February 1. www.inc.com/guides/business-plan-financial-section.html.

Wong-Hammond, L., and L. Damon. 2013. "Financing Strategic Plans for Not-for-Profits." *Healthcare Financial Management* 67 (7): 70–76.

CHAPTER 8

COMMUNICATING THE STRATEGIC PLAN

Communication is the real work of leadership.

—Nitin Nohria

You see things; and you say, "Why?" But I dream things that never were; and I say, "Why not?"

—George Bernard Shaw

LEARNING OBJECTIVES

After you have studied this chapter, you should be able to

➤ exercise an understanding of basic communication theory and the appropriate use of communication technology;

➤ analyze healthcare situations and choose the most effective way to communicate with the audience;

➤ demonstrate strong communication skills when conducting research, writing, and verbally presenting healthcare strategic plans;

➤ develop effective interpersonal communication skills;

➤ apply basic principles of critical thinking, problem solving, and communication in the development of healthcare business plans; and

➤ apply skills in written, visual, and oral communication.

KEY TERMS AND CONCEPTS

➤ Electronic whiteboard

➤ Intranet

➤ Motivation

➤ Stage charisma

➤ Webcast

INTRODUCTION

The ability to communicate the strategic plan is a critical factor for successfully implementing change (Kash et al. 2014). Previous chapters of this book discussed the technical aspects of developing a strategic plan. To ensure the plan is implemented, the next step is to communicate it to the healthcare organization's stakeholders, both in writing and verbally. These stakeholders include the board of directors, the leadership team, the medical staff, the nursing staff, administrative personnel, and key community leaders. A leader's ability to persuasively communicate the strategic plan can help an organization motivate staff, disseminate accurate information, and align its culture and communications efforts with the strategic planning process.

PRESENTATION OF THE STRATEGIC PLAN

Communications pertaining to strategy can take many forms. Presentation of an organization's strategic plan to community groups, routine reporting of operational results following implementation of new healthcare services, and community education on accessing new healthcare services are just a few examples. The advent of the Affordable Care Act (ACA) and the way it was marketed to the public provide an interesting healthcare communications case study as well (see Highlight 8.1).

The strategic plan must be communicated both in writing and verbally. This chapter outlines strategies for persuading groups using both methods.

WRITTEN COMMUNICATION

Effective internal communication can be used to inform staff of the strategic plan, enabling the board of directors, medical staff, nursing staff, and administrative personnel to become

Highlight 8.1 Healthcare Communication and the Affordable Care Act

In October 2013, the ACA implemented a communication plan designed to market insurance for sale on the federal exchanges. The government found that when communicating complex mathematical issues to the public, using widely recognized visual cues is important. For example, Medicare chose to market the ACA plans as bronze, silver, gold, and platinum. These visual cues represent a spectrum from low cost–low benefit (bronze) to high cost–high benefit (platinum). Medicare found that individuals who were below the mean in mathematical ability were able to make informed choices among the plans.

Medicare also found that options listed at the top of the website menu had a higher likelihood of selection. Government marketing staff also deemphasized complicated financial information about premiums, copayments, deductibles, out-of-pocket costs, and so on because it may overwhelm potential enrollees. Seven million people purchased insurance in the new federal market, suggesting the wisdom of this approach. The second round of enrollment showed similar success (Ubel, Comerford, and Johnson 2015).

Intranet
Computer network using Internet protocol technology to share information, operational systems, or computer services internally in an organization.

ambassadors for the organization and its new services in the community. One useful tool is the **intranet**, which most organizations use as an online method of communicating with employees, secure from external audiences. Each individual's desktop can serve as a consistent location for important topics and communication of the organization's mission, vision, and values. A health system's intranet can serve as an important integration tool.

Clear communication with internal audiences is essential—withholding or poorly communicating key information on finances, operations, or healthcare quality can have negative consequences for staff. To improve communication with managers, leadership staff should avoid using technical jargon. Leaders should educate department heads on accounting, finance, ratios, and benchmarks and make sure they have the financial reports they need to present the strategic plan and then measure operating performance over time. Management communications should balance operational, clinical, and financial performance to ease the decision-making process. When they note deficiencies in internal communication, organizations should invest in courses and books that employees can use to improve their skills.

VERBAL COMMUNICATION

Verbally communicating in a way that motivates others to do things they normally would not do, overcome barriers, and perform to the best of their abilities is a major part of a healthcare leader's job. By communicating the strategic plan to stakeholders, a leader can generate grassroots support for new business initiatives and enhance acceptance in the community. When a leader has an idea to communicate, developing a message that is true and correct, well-reasoned, and substantiated—by solid business logic that is specific, consistent, clear, and accurate—is key. Communication is not about the presenter, his opinions, or his position. It is about helping others understand and, in turn, understanding their concerns and needs (Myatt 2012).

A good verbal presentation generates **motivation**, the act or process of energizing people to overcome barriers and achieve outstanding performance. Steve Jobs, CEO of Apple Inc., believed that a speaker can motivate an audience by connecting with it on emotional and intellectual levels to keep it focused on the message. He believed that developing a **stage charisma**—the ability of a leader to command audience attention in an impressive manner—that appeals to the audience's emotions is important; after a speaker gains its attention, he can focus on conveying the one thing an audience really needs to hear (Vesterager 2014). But to successfully motivate an audience, a leader must have a basic grasp of how to structure and deliver a persuasive verbal presentation on the strategic plan (for a summary, see Exhibit 8.1).

Content

Effective communication of the strategic plan transfers knowledge to stakeholders and garners support for new initiatives. Speakers successfully motivate by knowing their audience and focusing on meeting its needs. The purpose of a presentation is to influence an audience,

Motivation
Act or process of energizing people to overcome barriers and achieve outstanding performance.

Stage charisma
Ability of a leader to command audience attention in an impressive manner. This quality does not require hard, authoritarian, overbearing force, but rather engaging individuals on a personal level using sincerity, credibility, concern, certainty, and hope.

EXHIBIT 8.1
Giving Healthcare Presentations

Rehearsal
Practice four times, at least once before an audience.
Monitor your allotted time.

Audiovisual Support
Use leading-edge technology, interactive whiteboard, Power Point. Use 10/20/30 rule: 10 slides, 20 minutes, 30-point font size.

Preparation Is Key
Know your audience.
Arrive early to check room and audiovisuals.
Dress appropriately.

Motivating Statement
Use comedy or story as a lead-in.

Audience Interest
Show charts; use demonstrations, facts, and case studies.
If problem is encountered, do not apologize.

Question and Answer
Summarize key points.
Invite limited number of one-minute questions.

so it must satisfy the audience's self-interest. Successful presentations answer questions, overcome objections, and present information previously not considered.

Excellent presentations provide the essential facts in a concise and understandable manner. The strategic plan should present good, workable solutions; demonstrate innovation; and use outside sources that are then appropriately cited in the presentation. Identifying a viable strategy that will address the needs of the organization and reflect a realistic revenue and expense structure is also important. The financial analysis should clearly demonstrate the viability of the recommendation. The recommended solution should be realistic given the current healthcare environment and resource constraints. It should also demonstrate long-range strategic thinking and represent best practices that have worked successfully in other environments. The presentation should be logically organized; have smooth transitions between sections; and use a format that is clear, readable, appealing, and creative.

Presenters should make a final recommendation that is summarized in a persuasive conclusion. They should also incorporate feedback from the audience to gauge its understanding of the issues.

Before the Presentation: Appearance, Rehearsal, and Arrangement

A speaker's credibility begins with preparation and appearance. A professional appearance creates a positive perception during a presentation as well as respect in the workplace (Futureofworking.com 2014).

A speaker should rehearse a presentation at least four times. Family, friends, or colleagues can serve as a test audience and provide honest feedback. The rehearsals should also be designed to ensure that the presenter covers her information in the allotted time while allowing for a question-and-answer period at the end (Morgan 2012).

Early arrival at the site of the presentation is an important part of preparation. Presenters can test the audiovisual equipment, familiarize themselves with the room, and review the presentation. This extra time helps the presenter relax and reduces the chance that problems will occur. Experienced presenters also have a backup plan ready in case the equipment should fail.

Speakers should check to make sure that the arrangement of the room is tailored to the style of the presentation. U-shaped seating is ideal for a workshop based on high audience participation. Classroom format (chairs in horizontal rows facing the front) may be suitable for informational presentations but limits audience participation. Boardroom seating (chairs around a table) works well for small groups and fosters discussion among the audience. Bistro seating (randomly placed tables) is another format that encourages discussion and is useful for group work. The objective is to make the audience comfortable, provide its members with a clear view of the presenter, and facilitate participation.

Presentation Technology

The use of technology can enhance presentation delivery. While Microsoft PowerPoint is the most familiar tool, the most cutting-edge technologies, from companies such as Google and Prezi, incorporate interactive components into presentations designed to keep an audience's interest. These technologies include multicolored images, photographs, and short video clips that can be used in presentations, webinars, or videoconferences. A presentation with visual support is five times more likely to be remembered (*Presentation Magazine* 2012). To be effective, however, PowerPoint slides must be crafted carefully; otherwise, they will detract from the presentation and the audience will lose interest. Some follow the 10/20/30 PowerPoint rule, which recommends that a PowerPoint presentation contain 10 slides, last for 20 minutes, and use 30-point font for any text included.

Keep the lighting in the room in mind when choosing colors for the presentation's background text. For example, in a bright room, light text on a dark background works well. Conversely, in a dark room, a light background with dark letters may work better. Most important, text should be kept to a minimum. The audience is there to hear the presenter speak, though slides featuring high-resolution photos can help the presenter tell a compelling story. If text is used, the software has a feature that enables the presenter to display information one bullet at a time to prevent the audience from reading ahead and losing track of what the presenter is saying. Limiting the text on each slide to five words is even more effective. Alternately, laser pointers can be used to emphasize items on a slide. Unless the speaker has a booming voice, a quality microphone is essential.

Videoconferencing and **webcasts** (video broadcasts of an event transmitted across the Internet) allow a presentation to reach a broader audience than those able to attend in person. Presentations can be viewed live on the Internet and recorded for later viewing. Another use of technology, more common in classrooms than formal presentations, is an **electronic whiteboard**, a device similar to a traditional whiteboard found in schools. It transmits written information to computers. It also allows live interaction with digital objects on the screen. Electronic or interactive whiteboards offer presenters flexibility because they can present notes directly from the board and the audience can download the notes to computers and storage devices. Electronic whiteboards can also link participants to each other and to the presenter via the Internet, facilitating presentations across the world.

Webcast
Video broadcast of an event transmitted across the Internet.

Electronic whiteboard
Electronic device that looks much like a traditional whiteboard but allows content written or drawn on the screen to be transmitted to a computer.

Audience Engagement

According to Jobs's presentation strategy, capturing the audience's attention in the first few minutes is essential. Jobs believed that the key to engaging presentations is to ask important questions that speak to the audience at an emotional level. This engagement can be accomplished by using a storytelling technique in the first 30 seconds of a presentation.

These stories can include analogies, painful events, or facts that connect with the audience on an emotional level and support the main message. An outstanding presentation should also include an agenda to keep the presenter on track and the audience engaged. Most important, developing a stage charisma that is appropriate for the audience is essential.

An outstanding presentation should be free of errors, the delivery style should be effective (projected voice, good eye contact, persuasive tone), the presenter should be confident, and the presentation should end on time. Dress, body language, and the use of audiovisual support can create positive (or negative) perceptions. Good eye contact with the audience and good posture can convey confidence and professional expertise. Presenters should avoid making distracting gestures, such as jingling coins, clicking a pen, or adjusting clothing. A monotone, mispronunciations, excessive pauses, and "uhs" and "ums" are also poor technique.

A presentation comes to life with stories, facts, and examples. Storytelling is one of the most effective techniques a good communicator can use (Manion 2011). Adding a story to make a point in a strategic plan communication will help people remember an important point. Humor targeted to the audience can be effective in engaging the group as well.

When introducing a new healthcare business initiative, leaders can express the positive impact it will have on the local community, the potential for increased profitability, and the ways it will enhance quality. Appealing to the individual personally is also powerful when the program will allow employees to improve their job skills, make more money, or gain greater prestige in the community.

Maintain Audience Interest

Presenters can maintain an audience's interest by showing trends on charts, performing demonstrations, supporting statements with facts, relating anecdotes and case studies, and developing theories with visual diagrams and videos. A good graphic display can communicate the message more clearly than words can (Manion 2011). Ideally, key items should be arranged in groups of three to maintain focus and ensure that the audience understands the information being presented. Tracing all the way back to Aristotle in ancient Greece, mathematical law supports groupings of three. Examples in history include Julius Caesar's famous quote "I came, I saw, I conquered" and the Thomas Jefferson phrase "life, liberty, and the pursuit of happiness" found in the US Declaration of Independence. Individuals more easily remember items in groups of three (Gallo 2012).

Audiences will not remember groupings, however, if they are not engaged. Conversational, interactive presentations hold audiences' attention and keep them alert.

Speakers should pause periodically to ensure that the audience understands the material. Such pauses can help a presenter establish rapport with the audience and provide an opportunity for participants to ask questions.

Question-and-Answer Session

Ending a presentation approximately ten minutes before the scheduled time gives the presenter an opportunity to summarize key points and invite questions from the audience. An effective method of managing expectations is to ask everyone in the audience who has a question to raise his hand and then give each question an equal share of the remaining time. Doing so will limit the length of the question and the time for response. Questions should be repeated to the audience and answers kept to a maximum of one minute. If an expert in the audience has information relevant to one of the questions, she can also contribute. When faced with negative or inappropriate questions, listen carefully and respond in a manner relevant to the presentation. For example, rephrase a negative question in a more positive manner and then respond. When facing questions that are inappropriate or of no interest to the group, a skillful speaker thanks the individual for the question and tells them that he will address it after the presentation.

A speaker should anticipate possible questions and prepare concise responses. Give accurate and complete answers with supporting factual statements, and answer questions with confidence. When faced with a particularly difficult question, defer to other presenters or other experts, or offer to provide an answer after further research.

Outstanding presentations result from understanding the audience, identifying the key items in the material, and finding the best method of delivery.

SUMMARY

Effective communication of the strategic plan transfers knowledge to staff and stakeholders and also garners support for new initiatives. Good communications avoid using technical jargon and acronyms, limit the number of main points, and integrate the key components listed in Exhibit 8.1. Presenters should rehearse their presentations, know their audience, and arrive early to evaluate the room and ensure all equipment works. They should use audiovisual technology wisely to support the delivery of their message and engage their audience immediately with a motivating statement that captures the importance of the topic. Finally, to wrap up the discussion, effective presenters summarize their key points and allocate time to respond to questions.

EXERCISES

REVIEW QUESTIONS

1. Who are the key stakeholders in a healthcare organization? Provide an example of a motivating statement that might engage one of these groups.
2. Discuss the key components of a healthcare presentation. Highlight three items you think are most important.

COASTAL MEDICAL CENTER EXERCISE

On the basis of the business plan you developed in Chapter 7 and the outline you created in Chapter 4, present a strategic plan for Coastal Medical Center (CMC) as if you were addressing its board and senior leadership.

COASTAL MEDICAL CENTER QUESTIONS

1. Over the past two years, CMC has experienced declining performance. Develop a motivating statement that will generate support among CMC's employees for the implementation of the strategic plan. Also, make three suggestions for delivering an effective presentation on CMC's financial data.
2. In the future, when CMC allocates its resources during the strategic planning process, which is more important: developing the strategic plan or communicating the strategic plan?

INDIVIDUAL EXERCISE: DEBATING KEY HEALTHCARE ISSUES

Chapter 8 addresses the importance of effective communications. Choose one of the following topics and develop a ten-minute presentation that incorporates the key components of communication discussed in Chapter 8. Strive to engage the audience and generate support for your position.

1. Can the United States afford its current level of healthcare expenditures?
2. Does US society get good value for its healthcare expenditures?
3. Can an individual have an impact on healthcare expenditures?
4. What is the role of healthcare organizations in assessing and improving efficiency and quality?
5. Will the ACA have a positive effect on US healthcare?

REFERENCES

FutureofWorking.com. 2014. "Professional Appearance and Grooming for the Workplace." Published April 23. http://futureofworking.com/professional-appearance-and-grooming-for-the-workplace/.

Gallo, C. 2012. "Thomas Jefferson, Steve Jobs, and the Rule of 3." *Forbes Leadership*. Published July 2. www.forbes.com/sites/carminegallo/2012/07/02/thomas-jefferson-steve-jobs-and-the-rule-of-3/.

Kash, B., A. Spaulding, C. Johnson, and L. Gamm. 2014. "Success Factors for Strategic Change Initiatives: Qualitative Study of Healthcare Administrators' Perspectives." *Journal of Healthcare Management* 59 (1): 65–81.

Manion, J. 2011. *From Management to Leadership: Strategies for Transforming Health*, 4th ed. San Francisco: Jossey-Bass.

Morgan, N. 2012. "Seven Ways to Rehearse a Speech." Public Words. Published July 26. http://publicwords.com/seven-ways-to-rehearse-a-speech/.

Myatt, M. 2012. "10 Communication Secrets of Great Leaders." *Forbes.* Published April 4. www.forbes.com/sites/mikemyatt/2012/04/04/10-communication-secrets-of-great-leaders/.

Presentation Magazine. 2012. "The Seven Sins of Visual Presentations." Published March 25. www.presentationmagazine.com/the-seven-sins-of-visual-presentations-8305.htm.

Ubel, P., D. Comerford, and E. Johnson. 2015. "Healthcare.gov 3.0—Behavioral Economics and Insurance Exchanges." *New England Journal of Medicine* 372 (8): 695–98.

Vesterager, M. 2014. "How to Be a Charismatic Leader—What We Can Still Learn from Steve Jobs." *NovaLead* (blog). Published June 14. http://novalead.co/2014/06/14/how-to-be-a-charismatic-leader-lessons-learned-from-the-late-steve-jobs/.

CHAPTER 9

ACCOUNTABLE CARE ORGANIZATIONS AND PHYSICIAN JOINT VENTURES

I will continue with diligence to keep abreast of advances in medicine. I will treat without exception all who seek my ministrations, so long as the treatment of others is not compromised thereby, and I will seek the counsel of particularly skilled physicians where indicated for the benefit of my patient.

—From *The Hippocratic Oath* (modern version)

LEARNING OBJECTIVES

After you have studied this chapter, you should be able to

➤ demonstrate an understanding of the interparty relationships associated with healthcare joint ventures and accountable care organizations;

➤ understand some of the dynamics and controversies surrounding the concept of accountable care organizations as an alternative approach to the current marketplace;

➤ demonstrate a basic understanding of the patient-centered medical home with attention to how it supports network-based delivery systems;

➤ master the concept of physician–hospital alignment and health system integration, including consumer, provider, and regulatory developments; and

➤ assess the emerging role of medical groups and hospital-owned group practices across the continuum of healthcare services.

KEY TERMS AND CONCEPTS

➤ Accountable care organization

➤ Clinical integration

➤ Equity-based joint venture

➤ Hospitalist model

➤ Integrated physician model

➤ Medical foundation

➤ Patient-centered medical home

INTRODUCTION

A positive relationship between hospitals and physicians is important to the success of the US healthcare system, because hospitals and physicians can be both collaborators and competitors. Physicians play a key role because they direct clinical services and function as patients' "agents." Physicians are responsible for major decisions, including whether to admit patients, whether to perform procedures, and whether to use pharmaceuticals or other supplies. The concept of physician–hospital alignment or integration has been discussed in the healthcare field since the early 1990s (Reiboldt 2013). Many hospitals and healthcare systems have moved to various models of physician integration since that time, through which hospitals seek to capture market share and physicians pursue security and better financial footing. After the Affordable Care Act (ACA) was passed in 2010, physician–hospital alignment became driven by another factor: cost control and quality outcomes in the accountable care era (Reiboldt 2013).

Physicians work in a wide range of settings. In 2013, 26 percent of physicians were employed by hospitals, 14 percent worked in a practice owned by a hospital or health system, 22 percent had an ownership stake in a practice, 15 percent had a solo practice, 15 percent worked for physician-owned practices with no ownership stake, and 8 percent were independent contractors (Jackson Healthcare 2013).

Physicians also serve in leadership positions and have significant responsibility for the quality of care. Unfortunately, growing economic pressures, advances in technology, and increasing use of outpatient care are straining the relationship between hospitals and physicians and forcing them to compete for patients. In addition, managed care organizations routinely bargain with hospitals and physicians separately, which only exacerbates the divide.

CLINICAL INTEGRATION

Through **clinical integration**, hospitals and physicians can bridge separation and defuse competition. The accountable care organization (ACO) represents the most recent effort

Clinical integration
Coordination of patient care between hospitals and physicians across the healthcare continuum.

to integrate the clinical care delivered to patients across providers and sites of care. Clinical integration provides an opportunity to coordinate services through centralized scheduling, electronic health records, clinical pathways, management of chronic diseases, and innovative quality improvement programs.

Clinical integration across the continuum of care is necessary to delivering high-quality, affordable care in the current environment (Jacquin 2014). The ACA created the ACO, which allows primary care providers to coordinate their patients' care across the continuum of healthcare services. Moving toward evidence-based clinical practice that spans multiple settings and is appropriate for the patient's illness will likely improve the US healthcare system. This integration is an attempt by Medicare to see healthcare from the patient and payer perspectives. Healthcare is often specialized and operates in separate silos of outpatient care, hospital care, rehabilitation, home care, and so on. Communication, goals of care, and in particular, billing are separate for all the silos. From patient and payer perspectives, however, the experience is one episode of care across a continuum.

By pooling their resources, hospitals and physicians also benefit financially. Clinical integration facilitates access to expensive medical technology, allows for greater economies of scale (see Chapter 1, Highlight 1.1), and enables subsidization of unprofitable services.

Hospitals and physicians are inherently interdependent. Yet the ability to recruit and retain quality physicians is critical to a hospital's reputation, market share, and long-term profitability. Most patients are admitted to hospitals because of physician referral. Therefore, hospitals seeking to increase their market share would be wise to focus on improving their relationships with physicians (Reiboldt 2013). Conversely, physicians rely on hospitals to provide facilities, state-of-the-art technology, and high-quality clinical staff.

Total healthcare expenditures per typical family have increased from 2008 to 2013 (see Exhibit 9.1). However, spending on physicians as a percentage has decreased. For example, in 2008, hospital inpatient and outpatient services combined represented 46 percent of total healthcare spending, while physician services ranked second at 35 percent of healthcare spending and pharmacy third at 15 percent. By 2013, hospital inpatient and outpatient services combined climbed to 49 percent of total healthcare spending, while physician services dropped to 32 percent of healthcare spending. Pharmacy remained at 15 percent (Milliman 2008, 2013).

PATIENT-CENTERED MEDICAL HOME

Patient-centered medical home (PCMH)
Care delivery model whereby a primary care physician coordinates patient treatment to ensure it is timely, cost-effective, and personalized.

The **patient-centered medical home (PCMH)** is a care delivery model whereby a primary care physician coordinates patient treatment to ensure that it is timely, cost-effective, and personalized. The idea started with pediatric groups in the 1960s. Collaboration between several professional organizations expanded the model to primary care for all ages. The term *home* does not refer to a physical place for patients to live but rather medical care they feel is comfortable (because they know the team), safe (because the team is focused on safety

Service	2008		2013	
	Spending	**Percentage**	**Spending**	**Percentage**
Physician	$5,435	35	$6,990	32
Inpatient hospital	$4,724	30	$6,855	31
Outpatient facility	$2,516	16	$4,037	18
Pharmacy	$2,302	15	$3,296	15
Other	$633	4	$851	4
Total	$15,610		$22,029	

EXHIBIT 9.1
Trends in Medical-Budget Spending for Average US Family, 2008 and 2013

Source: Data from Milliman (2008, 2013).

and quality), and accessible (because it is available on demand). *Comfortable, safe,* and *accessible* are terms you could use to describe your own home.

The ACA institutionalized the concept of the PCMH as the model for an ACO that provides primary care for Medicaid patients at a lower cost. As of 2014, 41 states had developed or planned to develop demonstration projects based on this model (Phillips et al. 2014).

The PCMH was designed to focus on individual patients with complex conditions who were disconnected from the healthcare system. The PCMH program breaks down the silos that separate providers and helps patients navigate across the continuum of care (see Exhibit 9.2). The intent of the PCMH model is to shift care increasingly to outpatient settings in which providers can use a team-based approach to make optimal use of non-physician caregivers across the continuum of health services. Team members often include patient navigators, care coordinators, and advanced practice providers (nurse practitioners and physician assistants). See Highlight 9.1 for more information about the PCMH model.

The multidisciplinary approach to care should maximize the clinical outcomes for patients with complex conditions and enhance wellness and prevention. The PCMH model emphasizes ease of access, partnerships between physicians and hospitals, and the use of innovative technologies to improve patient care. Adoption has been shown to decrease readmissions, emergency department visits, and length of hospital stays. Components include an individualized (patient-specific) health plan, management of patient healthcare services, and clinical decision making to improve quality as well as reduce costs. Reimbursement penalties for poor readmission rates could reduce Medicare costs by $8.2 billion between 2010 and 2019 (CMS 2010).

HIGHLIGHT 9.1 Patient-Centered Medical Home

The Agency for Healthcare Research and Quality (AHRQ) defines a medical home not as a place but as a model for delivering the core functions of primary care (AHRQ 2015). The Institute of Medicine (IOM) fueled the early shift of the PCMH model from pediatric programs to primary care programs. In its report *Envisioning the National Healthcare Quality Report* (Hurtado, Swift, and Corrigan 2001), the IOM challenged AHRQ to develop measures for patient centeredness. The IOM definition of patient centeredness includes healthcare that establishes a partnership among practitioners, patients, and their families (when appropriate) to ensure that decisions respect patients' wants, needs, and preferences and that patients have the education and support they require to make decisions and participate in their own care. AHRQ defines a medical home according to five functions and attributes: comprehensive care, patient centeredness, coordination, accessibility of services, and quality and safety (AHRQ 2015).

Since the 2001 IOM report, many researchers and professional organizations have proved the benefits of enhancing primary care and medical homes (Starfield, Shi, and Macinko 2005; Phillips et al. 2014). In 2010, the ACA further solidified the concept of the PCMH by supporting primary care payment increases through Medicare and Medicaid; expanding insurance coverage; and significantly investing in medical home pilots, workforce development and training, prevention and wellness, community health centers, and additional care delivery innovations (PCPCC 2015).

As a result of the ACA:

- Primary care providers receive a 10 percent Medicare bonus payment for primary care services.

- A new Medicaid state option now permits certain Medicaid enrollees to designate a provider as a health home, and states taking advantage of the option receive 90 percent federal matching payments for two years for health home–related services.

- Small employers receive grants for up to five years to establish wellness programs.

- The Centers for Medicare & Medicaid Innovation has launched the Pioneer ACO model and the Advance Payment ACO model, which offers shared savings and other payment incentives for select organizations that provide efficient, coordinated, patient-centered care.

- States maintain health benefit exchanges and Small Business Health Options Program exchanges, which facilitate the purchase of insurance by individuals and small employers.

- Teaching health centers provide payments for primary care residency programs in community-based ambulatory patient care centers.

EXHIBIT 9.2
Continuum of Care

Primary Care Silo	Acute Care (Hospital) Silo	Post-acute Care (PAC) Silo
Provide preventive services and wellness	Deliver episodic care	Transition patient to appropriate PAC
Perform baseline testing and provide individualized medicine	Use evidence-based clinical protocols	Maximize patient care and limit readmission rates
Deliver episodic care	Monitor quality metrics	Use care coordination and discharge follow-up calls
Manage chronic disease	Limit readmission rates	Maximize home care and adult day care
Provide patient navigation	Provide comprehensive discharge instructions	Optimize PAC across the continuum of care

PCMH—Organizes team members to coordinate care across the continuum and prevents duplication of efforts ⟩

Benefits: Coordinated care vs. episodic care
    Reduced readmissions
    Management of chronic illness across the continuum
    Ensured high quality of care (primary care provider/team who knows the patient)

POTENTIAL STRUCTURES FOR PHYSICIAN–HOSPITAL INTEGRATION

Many healthcare leaders believe that physician–hospital alignment is one of the greatest challenges facing the US healthcare system. Hospitals and physicians are faced with the task of finding innovative ways to collaborate while taking advantage of their joint economic interests. ACOs, medical foundations, hospital-owned group practices, and joint venture initiatives are all potential solutions. Development of a formal, board-approved physician–hospital alignment plan can help hospitals achieve this goal. At a minimum, physician engagement in strategic planning, development of an organizational culture that supports physicians, improved communication with physicians, increased emphasis on physician retention, and investment in physician leadership development are useful objectives in an alignment plan (Zeis 2013).

ACCOUNTABLE CARE ORGANIZATIONS

ACOs are groups of doctors, hospitals, and other healthcare providers who come together voluntarily to give coordinated, high-quality care to the Medicare patients they serve. Coordinated care helps ensure that patients, especially the chronically ill, get the right care at the right time, with the goal of avoiding unnecessary duplication of services and preventing medical errors.

Accountable care organization (ACO)
Group of doctors, hospitals, and other healthcare providers who come together voluntarily to give coordinated, high-quality care to Medicare patients.

The Centers for Medicare & Medicaid Services (CMS) has established the Medicare Shared Savings Program, which uses a calculated benchmark as a risk-adjusted surrogate measure of what the Medicare fee-for-service (FFS) expenditures would otherwise have been in the absence of the ACO (CMS 2014b). The ACO is paid for the service as calculated, and when it succeeds in both delivering high-quality care and spending healthcare dollars more wisely, the amount paid will be greater than expenses. In other words, if the costs for treating primary care patients assigned to physicians in the ACO are expected to increase 5 percent next year in a specific geographic area, and the ACO keeps that hike to 2 percent, the providers get to keep some portion of the extra 3 percent. All organizations involved will then share in the savings it achieves for the Medicare program (CMS 2015). The following link provides a CMS video on ACOs: http://innovation.cms.gov/initiatives/aco/.

ACOs were established by the ACA, with final rules published in 2011. CMS designed the program to reward value and care coordination, rather than volume and care duplication. The ACA uses ACOs to encourage doctors, hospitals, and other healthcare providers to work together to coordinate care better, and it stresses preventive services designed to keep people healthy. This emphasis helps to reduce growth in healthcare costs and improve outcomes. ACOs become eligible to share savings with Medicare when they deliver that care more efficiently than others providing the same care while meeting or exceeding performance benchmarks for quality of care (CMS 2014a).

Under fully capitated ACOs, the provider assumes the highest risk and receives global payment for services. A capitated payment is a fixed, prearranged payment received by a physician, clinic, or hospital per patient enrolled in a health plan. This system differs from the traditional FFS model that pays for whatever charges are presented. Under other ACO models, if the provider reduces Medicare charges by 10 percent, Medicare gives back 50 percent of the savings, which represent 5 percent savings to be shared with all partners in the ACO.

CMS sponsored the Pioneer ACO model starting January 1, 2012, and initially included 32 organizations. After some organizations dropped out of the experiment, 19 ACOs remained and were compared to similar populations of Medicare beneficiaries (in terms of age, race, and chronic illness). During Pioneer's first two performance years, total spending for beneficiaries was compared to similar FFS beneficiaries. CMS found that the Pioneer spending increase was approximately $385 million less than the spending of similar FFS beneficiaries. This outcome was primarily because of decreased hospitalization, although there were also greater decreases in primary care evaluation and office visits and smaller increases in the use of tests, procedures, and imaging services. CMS observed no difference in all-cause readmissions within 30 days of discharge, but follow-up visits after hospital discharge increased more for ACO-aligned beneficiaries. Patients registered no difference in satisfaction scores (Nyweide et al. 2015).

ACOs do have potential downsides (Herzberg and Fawson 2012). ACOs cannot require patients to use a particular set of providers. Patients are free to seek care from any Medicare provider, in or out of the network. Patients are retroactively assigned to an organization based on where they received the most primary care from the ACO. Regulators worried that providers would game the system by denying costly care. In reality, providers do not know if they might have overusers or noncompliant patients, nor can they focus additional incentives or resources on participants to influence their health behavior. As a result, providers face added financial risks that may be impossible to control. Regulators were also concerned about the requirement to meet benchmarks for quality measurement, governing structure, and information transmission. The administrative costs could add millions to expenses, and whether the expected savings will offset the additional costs is unclear. An organization must weigh these pros and cons before proceeding with enrollment in an ACO (Herzberg and Fawson 2012).

In spite of some concerns, there were 585 ACOs in 2015, up 12 percent from the previous year. In 2015, 5.6 million patients, representing 11 percent of Medicare beneficiaries, received care from ACOs. An additional 35 million non-Medicare patients received care from ACOs, up 6 percent from the previous year. Collectively, ACOs serve between 49 million and 59 million Americans, representing 15–17 percent of the US population (Oliver Wyman 2015).

MEDICAL FOUNDATIONS

One solution to physician–hospital competition is the implementation of the **medical foundation** model, under which independent physicians sell their practices to a medical foundation and then contract with the foundation to provide professional services at the foundation's practice sites. This arrangement allows hospitals and health systems to create nonprofit legal entities to employ physicians. Medical foundations provide flexibility for hospitals seeking to employ physicians and other providers directly. The medical foundation model allows physicians to be more independent than hospital-employed physicians and is a strategy for improving physician–hospital relationships.

Some states—for example, California, Texas, and New York—do not allow hospitals to employ physicians to provide outpatient services. These states legislate what is known as the corporate practice of medicine doctrine. The rationale for prohibiting employment of physicians by hospitals is derived from the idea that individual physicians should be licensed to practice medicine, not corporations.

A foundation is typically a not-for-profit corporation affiliated with a hospital. The medical foundation model works well in states that prohibit the corporate practice of medicine because the physicians are not employed by the foundation; they only contract with it. Reimbursement for physician services is paid to the foundation, and the foundation then pays the physicians for their services.

Historically, medical foundations have been successful at recruiting physicians and establishing clinics. More recently, however, opposition to medical foundations is growing among individual physicians, small practices, and loosely affiliated independent practice associations. This opposition is growing because hospitals and physicians can jointly participate in managed care contracts under this model, thereby gaining greater market share

Medical foundation
Arrangement under which independent physicians sell their practices to a medical foundation and then contract with the foundation to provide professional services at the foundation's practice sites.

and more business. This situation increases competitive pressures on individual physicians in small-group practices because they have a limited presence in the overall marketplace. Despite this resistance, the medical foundation model remains attractive to young family-practice physicians just out of their residency training because it provides them adequate compensation, and they do not have to make significant investments in facilities and technology—the clinics furnish these essentials.

HOSPITAL-OWNED GROUP PRACTICES

Hospital acquisition of medical group practices began in the 1990s as healthcare organizations created integrated delivery systems. A primary motivator for acquiring medical practices was to gain market share in the local community. Because primary care practices could drive a large number of referrals to a hospital, these practices were the first type of physician group that hospitals sought to purchase. Today, hospitals may purchase a variety of practices, including cardiology groups, orthopedic groups, and neurosurgery groups. Hospitals that purchase medical groups can improve integration, expand patients' access to care, and foster long-term relationships with their physicians. Medical groups might wish to sell their practices as a result of the growing complexity of medical group management and increasing operating costs.

In 2015, 63 percent of physicians said they were employed by hospital-owned medical groups, and less than a third (32 percent) were in private practice. These figures illustrate the growing trend toward employment in hospital-owned groups. Employment can be a good deal for physicians—compensation includes salary, bonus, and profit-sharing contributions. For physicians in private practice, compensation includes earnings after taxes and deductible business expenses.

In 2015, the average compensation for a primary care physician was $195,000 and the compensation for a specialist was $284,000. Among specialists, the top four earners were orthopedists ($421,000), cardiologists ($376,000), gastroenterologists ($370,000), and anesthesiologists ($358,000). The lowest earners were pediatricians ($189,000), family physicians ($195,000), and endocrinologists and internists (both at $196,000) (Peckham 2015). If employing physicians is part of the business plan, strategic planners must take into account their salaries.

HOSPITALISTS

Another possibility for closer cooperation between physicians and hospitals is the **hospitalist model**, in which a patient's regular outpatient physician transfers complete responsibility for the patient's care to a dedicated inpatient physician when the patient is hospitalized. This physician supervises all of the patient's inpatient care until discharge. Hospitalist physicians can be hospital employees or members of an independent hospitalist physician

Hospitalist model
Arrangement under which an inpatient physician assumes primary responsibility for managing a patient on admission to the hospital and supervising all inpatient care until the patient is discharged from the hospital.

group. In 2012, there were approximately 30,000 hospitalists in the United States, an increase from 20,000 in 2008, making hospitalists members of the fastest-growing medical specialty (AAMC 2012).

Use of the hospitalist model has had a positive impact on hospitals' profitability. Hospitals using the hospitalist model had a return on assets of 3.1 percent, whereas those not using the hospitalist model took a loss, with a return on assets of –1 percent (Harrison and Ogniewski 2004). One study done in public teaching hospitals showed the hospitalist model decreased length of stay, decreased payment denial by 2 percent in spite of increased admissions, and increased average reimbursement per patient day by 22 percent (Lundberg et al. 2010). The rapid growth in hospitalist physicians shows that organizations that have implemented a hospitalist program believe it enhances the quality of care they provide.

While choosing a physician model, strategic planners need to consider hospital size to determine whether a given model is appropriate or feasible. Hospitalists are more prevalent in large, complex hospitals that offer a wide range of clinical services. In this setting, hospitalist physicians may be critical to the coordination of care across multiple clinical service areas. Smaller hospitals offering fewer services may have a smaller need for hospitalists and may best operate under a different physician model. On the other hand, hospitalists can help manage inpatient workload when a limited number of specialists are available, as may be the case in a smaller hospital.

JOINT VENTURE INITIATIVES

As discussed in Chapter 1, joint ventures are created when two organizations create a legal entity to participate in an economic activity. Each party contributes money to the venture and shares in its profits. The combining organizations share control of the joint entity, and the joint entity gains a larger customer base through the combination of each organization's customers (patients in the case of healthcare), giving the joint venture a competitive advantage in the marketplace.

By supporting vertical integration, the ACA has created an environment in which hospital and physician joint ventures will continue to grow. The new generation of physicians will likely be receptive to business initiatives that provide incentives and measures of success designed to reward improved patient care (Moses et al. 2013). The value of their clinical judgment and their ability to engage patients in the decision-making process have the potential to improve both patient satisfaction and the value of healthcare services. As a result, physicians, nurses, and other clinical providers could become the main sources for clinical innovation. This shift will provide opportunities for joint ventures that more effectively use people, information, and technology.

Increased innovation combined with new hospital–physician enterprises allows synergistic benefits such as shared technology, collaborative research, shared expertise, and increased market share. By combining resources and patient populations, organizations can also expand their product lines to increase the availability of healthcare services in the local community. Exhibit 9.3 shows potential joint ventures between healthcare services, including ambulatory surgery centers, labs, clinics, and hospitals. The legal processes required to establish joint ventures fall on a continuum ranging from merger to affiliation. In the exhibit, the boxes above the arrow reflect the common characteristics required between the joint venture partners for optimum success. On the left side of the continuum, for mergers and acquisitions, these characteristics are less important because one party is usually the controlling party. However, the characteristics' similarity should be considered in the course of change management if they are not congruent. On the right side of the continuum, there must be similarity in those characteristics (from strategy and vision to operational and financial goals), or the chance of eventual breakdown or failure of the joint venture increases.

Equity-based joint venture
Organization whose ownership is divided between a hospital and physicians on the basis of their contributions to the enterprise.

Equity-Based Joint Ventures

Equity-based joint ventures, which are based on a new model of business cooperation, move beyond the traditional win–lose business mentality and focus on complementary relationships among physicians, hospitals, and suppliers. The philosophy of such ventures is to absorb new individuals into an organization for purposes of defusing the threat of challenging groups.

EXHIBIT 9.3
Hospital–Physician
Joint Ventures

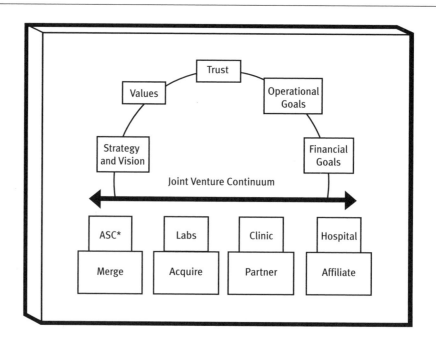

* Ambulatory surgery center

In equity-based joint ventures, ownership is divided between the hospital and the participating physicians. The hospital and physicians create a new organization and contribute funds, facilities, or services equal to their ownership proportion. For an equity-based joint venture to succeed, there must be positive relationships among the owners and mutual benefits. For physicians, joint ventures present an opportunity to gain ownership in an organization, have a positive impact on the community, and sustain their practice over the long term.

From a hospital's perspective, a joint venture does not always have to generate a profit because other benefits may accrue to the organization. For example, the joint venture may enhance recruitment of physicians, increase hospital admissions, or improve access to managed care contracts. Even for-profit hospitals sometimes are willing to participate in unprofitable joint ventures because they may increase revenue farther down the continuum of care or increase hospitals' percentage of market share, which then becomes a barrier to potential new competitors.

Equity-based joint ventures between hospitals and physicians have demonstrated that they improve clinical treatment and enhance communication between hospitals and physicians. However, potential roadblocks are abundant. Where hospital–physician joint ventures have not succeeded, the greatest problems were lack of trust, unequal contribution of capital, and disagreement on overall control (Zasa 2011). To prevent such problems, all parties must agree on the goal, strategic direction, and anticipated financial performance of the joint venture before embarking on it. Board regulation and hospital policy also deter such issues.

Joint Ventures and Profitability

Hospitals engaging in joint ventures with physicians had occupancy rates of 55 percent, compared with 53 percent for hospitals not engaged in physician joint ventures. In terms of scope, hospital–physician joint ventures offered an average of 32 clinical services, whereas hospitals without physician joint ventures averaged 26 clinical services. In financial terms, hospitals with physician joint ventures had a return on assets of 2.5 percent, compared with 1.9 percent for those not participating (Harrison 2006).

PHYSICIAN EMPLOYMENT

Instead of pursuing joint ventures or implementing one of the models discussed earlier, hospital strategists may opt to directly hire physicians. As employees, physicians are exempt from the Stark laws (see Chapter 7, Highlight 7.2) and can therefore refer patients for other services in the same hospital. Physician employees are more likely than independent physicians to stay with their employer hospital over the long term, which provides the hospital with a consistent workforce possessing critical clinical skills. Employed physicians' referral patterns are also more predictable. The disadvantages of physician employment include the high cost of recruitment and increased ongoing costs for salary and benefits.

INTEGRATED PHYSICIAN MODEL

An **integrated physician model** is the result of a series of partnerships between hospitals and physicians developed over time. Essentially, it is a joint venture that has become many joint ventures, and all of these joint ventures are connected through congruent goals. For example, an organization following an integrated physician model could include acute care hospitals, nursing homes, affiliated medical groups, primary care clinics, employed physicians, and independent medical groups.

PHYSICIAN ENGAGEMENT IN STRATEGIC PLANNING

When physicians are involved in a hospital's decision-making process, the hospital and physicians can more easily reach agreement on the values, ethics, and culture of a new business initiative. Physician empowerment is key to increasing physicians' engagement in the hospital's future. Empowerment begins with physician participation on the hospital board of directors and on key board committees. The president of the medical staff should be a voting member of the board, and physicians should be members of the strategic planning and finance committees. By soliciting their input, including them in focus groups about new business initiatives, involving them in the creation of the strategic plan and work schedules, and granting them the opportunity to become co-owners of the organization, hospitals can inspire physicians to commit to new business ventures. For example, if physicians are involved in the development of metrics to be used to evaluate the quality of care the organization provides, they will respond in a positive manner and be less likely to feel resentment if the data show a need for improvement.

SUMMARY

Hospital–physician integration can take many forms. Hospitals can contract with physician group practices and gain greater market share through managed care networks. Such relationships can lead to joint ventures in which hospitals share ownership of the enterprise with physicians. Finally, employment of physicians by hospitals and health systems is a growing trend. This arrangement frees physicians from the frustrations associated with managing a practice and allows them to focus on providing clinical care.

Historically, the US healthcare system has been fragmented, reducing the quality of healthcare services provided. Innovations such as PCMHs and ACOs illustrate Medicare's commitment to managing across the continuum of care. Outside of the government sector, many healthcare leaders believe that increasing clinical integration and coordinating strategic planning between hospitals and physicians is necessary to improving healthcare. Large, integrated healthcare delivery systems will be better able to deal with future healthcare needs because they have greater access to capital and deliver clinically integrated care.

EXERCISES

REVIEW QUESTIONS

1. How does involving physicians in the strategic planning process help a hospital reach its goals?
2. Why is clinical integration important in the current healthcare environment?
3. Choose one of the models for hospital–physician integration discussed in the chapter and list the advantages and disadvantages for hospitals and physicians under this model.

COASTAL MEDICAL CENTER EXERCISE

According to Chapter 9 and the Coastal Medical Center (CMC) case study, is adoption of the ACO model a viable strategy for CMC?

COASTAL MEDICAL CENTER QUESTIONS

1. How would you assess physician engagement at CMC?
2. How should physicians be involved in strategic planning at CMC, and at what point should you involve them?
3. What do you see as the future of physician involvement at CMC?

INDIVIDUAL EXERCISE: SOLO PHYSICIAN MEDICAL PRACTICE AND ITS EXPANSION TO A MULTIPHYSICIAN GROUP PRACTICE

After graduation, Dr. Debra Johnson founded a solo medical practice that she incorporated under the name Primary Care Medical Specialists. Now, five years after her graduation from medical school, she is experiencing significant growth in her patient volume. During this time, she has been a primary care physician and has admitting privileges at CMC.

Dr. Johnson's practice is located in Ocean County, which is anticipating an 18 percent population growth rate over the next five years. Her schedule is already fully booked, and she has stopped taking new patients. She is considering expansion. Because Dr. Johnson has no formal business education, she has approached CMC leadership to assist her with some strategic planning. As part of the planning process, Dr. Johnson shared her most recent business tax return, which includes the following income statement.

Income Statement, 2014

Revenue ($)	
Medicare/Medicaid	351,022
Commercial insurance	310,949
Other patient service revenue	301,179
Ancillary revenue	10,577
Investment income	10,000
Contributions and grants	6,185
Total	989,912
Expenses ($)	
Salaries	500,000
Operating expenses	244,165
Benefits	125,000
Facility expenses	84,000
Supplies	54,000
Insurance	7,410
Professional fees	1,190
Total	1,015,765
Net income	**−25,853**

According to her appointment system, Dr. Johnson currently sees an average of 20 patients per day, which over a 250-day annual work schedule represents 5,000 patient visits. Based on the 18 percent population growth in Ocean County, Dr. Johnson's primary care practice could grow to 10 providers over the next five years.

During the strategic planning process, CMC evaluated potential downstream revenue that could be generated from Dr. Johnson's referrals (see the following data).

CMC Downstream Revenue

Service Line	Service Volume × Fee	Revenue
Inpatient admissions	(5,000 patients × .025 admission rate) × $1,000 profit per admission	$125,000
Laboratory	(5,000 patients × .25 laboratory rate) × $50 per laboratory test	$65,000
Radiology	(5,000 patients × .10 radiology rate) × $75 per radiology image	$37,500
Pharmacy	(5,000 patients × .50 pharmacy rate) × $100 per prescription	$250,000
Total revenue		$815,000

Based on this information, answer the following questions:

1. Is Dr. Johnson's solo practice viable for the future?
2. Should Dr. Johnson recruit new providers or merge with another practice?
3. Should Dr. Johnson do just primary care or consider a multispecialty group? Identify pros and cons.
4. Can expanding practice size reduce expenses, increase net income, maintain independence, and increase contracting power?
5. Should Dr. Johnson sell her practice to CMC and become an employee?
6. How many years should the contract be guaranteed if she sells to CMC?
7. What compensation model is appropriate, including base salary and increases based on productivity or downstream revenue?

Assume Dr. Johnson decides to expand her practice by two providers annually for the next five years.

- Complete a five-year pro forma income statement for Primary Care Medical Specialists by including the additional providers. Plan on two providers total in year 1, four providers in year 2, six providers in year 3, eight providers in year 4, and ten providers in year 5. Also, budget for a second office location in years 4 and 5.
- Complete a five-year pro forma income statement for CMC's downstream revenue by including the additional primary care providers in Primary Care Medical Specialists.

REFERENCES

Agency for Healthcare Research and Quality (AHRQ). 2015. "Defining the PCMH." Accessed September 7. https://pcmh.ahrq.gov/page/defining-pcmh.

Association of American Medical Colleges (AAMC). 2012. "Estimating the Number and Characteristics of Hospitalist Physicians in the United States and Their Possible Workforce Implications." *Association of American Medical Colleges* 12 (3): 1–2.

Centers for Medicare & Medicaid Services (CMS). 2015. "Accountable Care Organizations (ACOs): General Information." Updated August 31. http://innovation.cms.gov/initiatives/aco/.

———. 2014a. "CMS Releases New Proposal to Improve Accountable Care Organizations." Published December 1. www.cms.gov/Newsroom/MediaReleaseDatabase/Press-releases/2014-Press-releases-items/2014-12-01.html.

———. 2014b. "Methodology for Determining Shared Savings and Losses Under the Medicare Shared Savings Program." Published April. www.cms.gov/Medicare/Medicare-Fee-for-Service-Payment/sharedsavingsprogram/Downloads/ACO_Methodology_Factsheet_ICN907405.pdf.

———. 2010. "Affordable Care Act Update: Implementing Medicare Cost Savings." Accessed September 7, 2015. www.cms.gov/apps/docs/aca-update-implementing-medicare-costs-savings.pdf.

Harrison, J. 2006. "The Impact of Joint Ventures on US Hospitals." *Journal of Health Care Finance* 32 (3): 28–38.

Harrison, J., and R. Ogniewski. 2004. "The Hospitalist Model: A Strategy for Success in US Hospitals?" *Health Care Manager* 23 (3): 310–17.

Herzberg, R., and C. Fawson. 2012. "Accountable Care Organizations: Panacea or Train Wreck?" National Center for Policy Analysis. Published August 14. www.ncpa.org/pub/ba769.

Hurtado, M., E. Swift, and J. Corrigan (eds.). 2001. *Envisioning the National Health Care Quality Report*. Washington, DC: National Academies Press.

Jackson Healthcare. 2013. *Filling the Void: 2013 Physician Outlook and Practice Trends*. Accessed December 22, 2014. www.jacksonhealthcare.com/physiciantrends2013.

Jacquin, L. 2014. "A Strategic Approach to Healthcare Transformation." *Healthcare Financial Management* 68 (4): 74–79.

Lundberg, S., P. Balingit, S. Wali, and D. Cope. 2010. "Cost-Effectiveness of a Hospitalist Service in a Public Teaching Hospital." *Academic Medicine* 85 (8): 1312–15.

Milliman. 2013. "2013 Milliman Medical Index." Published May 22. http://us.milliman.com/uploadedFiles/insight/Periodicals/mmi/pdfs/mmi-2013.pdf.

———. 2008. "2008 Milliman Medical Index." Published May 1. http://us.milliman.com/insight/Periodicals/mmi/pdfs/2008-Milliman-Medical-Index/.

Moses, H., D. H. Matheson, E. R. Dorsey, B. P. George, D. Sadoff, and S. Yoshimura. 2013. "The Anatomy of Health Care in the United States." *Journal of the American Medical Association* 310 (18): 1947–63.

Nyweide D. J., W. Lee, T. T. Cuerdon, H. H. Pham, M. Cox, R. Rajkumar, and P. H. Conway. 2015. "Association of Pioneer Accountable Care Organizations vs Traditional Medicare Fee for Service with Spending, Utilization, and Patient Experience." *Journal of the American Medical Association* 313 (21): 2152–61.

Oliver Wyman. 2015. "Accountable Care Organizations Now Serve Between 15 and 17 Percent of the United States, According to New Research from Oliver Wyman." *Business Wire*. Published April 22. www.oliverwyman.com/who-we-are/press-releases/2015/accountable-care-organizations-now-serve-between-15-and-17-perce.html.

Patient-Centered Primary Care Collaborative (PCPCC). 2015. "History: Major Milestones for Primary Care and the Medical Home." Accessed September 7. www.pcpcc.org/content/history-0.

Peckham, C. 2015. *Medscape Physician Compensation Report 2015*. Published April 21. www.medscape.com/features/slideshow/compensation/2015/public/overview#page=1.

Phillips, R. L., M. Han, S. M. Petterson, L. A. Makaroff, and W. R. Liaw. 2014. "Cost, Utilization, and Quality of Care: An Evaluation of Illinois' Medicaid Primary Care Case Management Program." *Annals of Family Medicine* 12 (5): 408–17.

Reiboldt, M. 2013. "Physician-Hospital Alignment in 2013: 17 Trends." *Becker's Hospital Review*. Published August 30. www.beckershospitalreview.com/hospital-physician-relationships/physician-hospital-alignment-in-2013-17-trends.html.

Starfield, B., L. Shi, and J. Macinko. 2005. "Contribution of Primary Care to Health Systems and Health." *The Milbank Quarterly* 83 (3): 457–502.

Zasa, R. J. 2011. "Physician-Hospital Joint Ventures; Alignment of Physicians with Hospitals." *Becker's Hospital Review*. Published September 8. www.beckershospitalreview.com/hospital-physician-relationships/physician-hospital-joint-ventures-alignment-of-physicians-with-hospitals.html.

Zeis, M. 2013. "How the Dynamics of Physician Alignment Are Changing." *HealthLeaders Media*. Published September 13. http://healthleadersmedia.com/page-3/FIN-296271/How-the-Dynamics-of-Physician-Alignment-Are-Changing.

CHAPTER 10

STRATEGIC PLANNING AND POST-ACUTE CARE SERVICES

A population that does not take care of the elderly and of children and the young has no future, because it abuses both its memory and its promise.

—Pope Francis

In a culture where there is trust, respect, and a moral foundation, the young can grow and the elderly thrive.

—Dr. Debra Harrison

LEARNING OBJECTIVES

After you have studied this chapter, you should be able to

➤ evaluate the availability of post-acute care services in local communities,

➤ identify the appropriate post-acute care interventions to meet the healthcare needs of older adults,

➤ identify quality issues impacting the provision of post-acute care,

➤ discuss the challenges faced by healthcare executives as they develop a strategy to meet post-acute care needs, and

➤ understand the sources of financing for post-acute care services as well as opportunities for increased efficiency across the continuum of care.

➤ Adult health day care center

➤ Comorbidity

➤ End-of-life care

➤ Hospice care

➤ Inpatient rehabilitation facility

➤ Palliative care

➤ Post-acute care

➤ Prospective payment system

➤ Skilled nursing facility

INTRODUCTION

Post-acute care (PAC)
Services provided after
discharge from an
acute care hospital.

This chapter discusses trends and factors affecting strategic planning in the **post-acute care** **(PAC)** industry. PAC providers offer important recuperation and rehabilitation services to Medicare beneficiaries after discharge from an acute care hospital. PAC providers include skilled nursing facilities (SNFs), home health agencies (HHAs), inpatient rehabilitation facilities (IRFs), and long-term care hospitals (LTCHs). In 2013, Medicare's payments to more than 29,000 PAC providers totaled $59 billion, more than doubling since 2001. Medicare has a responsibility to ensure access for beneficiaries, appropriately reimburse providers for the patients they treat, and control costs for the beneficiary and taxpayer alike. Patient utilization of PAC is affected by local practice patterns, the availability of PAC in a market, patient and family preferences, and financial arrangements between a PAC provider and the referring hospital. Because PAC can be appropriately provided in a variety of settings, Medicare ideally would pay for PAC using one payment system with payments based on patient characteristics rather than on the site of service. This system would lend itself well to a Medicare bundled payment strategy by aligning payments across settings for select conditions (MedPAC 2015).

As the longevity of Americans increases and the number of baby boomers reaching retirement grows, the demand for PAC and similar services will increase. These developments offer strategic planning opportunities and business growth potential for a wide range of healthcare providers.

Post-acute services also have the potential to significantly increase federal expenditures on the Medicare program. The Centers for Medicare & Medicaid Services (CMS) is concerned that a fragmented PAC system will increase costs and adversely affect the quality of care. To reduce expenditures and prevent fragmentation of services, CMS is considering bundling the payment for all PAC services that a Medicare patient receives after being discharged from an acute care hospital. Such a bundled payment would require IRFs, SNFs, adult health day care centers, and hospice facilities to work closely together to assume the risk associated with bundled Medicare payment for PAC. CMS views this bundling as a better approach to managing Medicare patients across the continuum of PAC services (Morley et al. 2014). A bundled payment approach also opens up opportunities for PAC providers to acquire or merge with other organizations or to pursue joint ventures with other PAC providers.

Chronic conditions are the leading cause of illness, disability, and death in the United States and account for the majority of US healthcare expenditures. Although chronic diseases can affect people in any age group, a high incidence of such conditions occurs among the elderly. As the US population ages, more people will require chronic-disease management and end-of-life care. In addition, because of advances in trauma care, use of evidence-based medicine, and proven public health initiatives, more Americans will survive major illnesses and live well into old age. Life expectancy in the United States was 78 years in 2009 and increased to 79 years in 2013 (Moses et al. 2013). However, though Americans are living longer, chronic disease and a period of significant disability now precede most deaths. Unfortunately, the US healthcare system focuses on curing disease and prolonging life but is poorly designed to provide end-of-life care.

Care for elderly patients in acute care hospitals, IRFs, and hospice facilities is paid for by Medicare Part A. Medicare's reimbursement for SNF care is limited to 20 days after hospitalization and has a lifetime limitation of 100 days of reimbursement for skilled nursing care. In contrast, Medicaid has no such limitation, so the majority of the care for skilled nursing patients is paid for by Medicaid. However, Medicaid's reimbursement rate is the lowest of all payers.

As part of its cost-cutting strategy, Medicare is attempting to shift PAC into less expensive outpatient treatment and hospice settings. Medicare spent $25 billion on PAC in 1999, $42 billion in 2005, and $59 billion in 2013, which represents an increase of $34 billion since 1999. In 2013, 42 percent of Medicare patients discharged from an acute care hospital moved to PAC; of these, 20 percent were discharged to an SNF, 17 percent to an HHA, 4 percent to an IRF, and 1 percent to an LTCH. Expenditures on skilled nursing care, which have been increasing at a rate of 9 percent annually, account for the largest proportion of Medicare spending on PAC (MedPAC 2015).

DEFINITIONS

In most cases, PAC planning is a joint decision-making process involving the patient, the patient's family, the patient's physician, and a hospital case manager. The three patient groups with the highest rate of PAC utilization are stroke patients, patients with hip fractures, and patients undergoing joint replacement. Other chronic conditions frequently requiring PAC are cancer, pulmonary disease, congestive heart failure, liver disease, diabetes, renal failure, dementia, Alzheimer's disease, and Parkinson's disease.

End-of-life care (EoLC) is a type of PAC provided when a patient is not expected to recover from his condition and further treatment is futile. EoLC does not focus on

End-of-life care (EoLC)
Care provided to improve the quality of life of patients who are facing life-threatening disease or disability and are not expected to recover.

Palliative care

Healthcare approach that improves the quality of life of patients and their families facing life-threatening illness through the prevention and relief of suffering.

life-sustaining treatments but is designed to maximize patient comfort. Such end-of-life treatment includes hospice care and components of **palliative care**, which improves the quality of life of patients and their families facing life-threatening illness through the prevention and relief of suffering (WHO 2015). Key to this process is the involvement of a multidisciplinary clinical team that manages a family-centric approach to treatment based on the needs and desires of the patient and family.

EoLC includes access to **hospice care**, services that provide EoLC or palliative care to a patient and her family when the patient is no longer responding to treatment. Hospice services focus on pain relief and help the patient and family cope during the time leading up to the patient's death. In addition to pain management, hospice offerings encompass a comprehensive mix of services, including bereavement counseling, home health care, hospital services, skilled nursing services, and other residential care services.

Hospice care

Services that provide EoLC or palliative care to a patient and her family when the patient is no longer responding to treatment.

HEALTHCARE AND US POPULATION DEMOGRAPHICS

In the United States, an aging population and an increasing proportion of international immigrants will result in substantial changes over the course of the twenty-first century. Between 2014 and 2060, the US population is projected to increase from 319 million to 417 million. By 2030, it is projected that 1 in 5 Americans will be 65 years or older. Minorities (any group other than non-Hispanic whites) will make up half of all Americans by 2044, and by 2060, 1 in 5 Americans will be foreign born (Colby and Ortman 2015).

Under the assumption of a high level of international migration, the total US population is expected to grow to 458 million by 2050. The level of international migration will play an important role in shaping changes in the size, growth rate, age structure, and racial and ethnic composition of the US population (Ortman and Guarneri 2015). The US healthcare system is facing the challenge of meeting their need for chronic care.

The Affordable Care Act has expanded the insurance coverage and access to healthcare for many Americans; however, most women and men in the United States are covered by insurance obtained through the workplace. Women are more susceptible to losing coverage because they are almost twice as likely as men to be covered as dependents—if they become widowed or divorced or their husbands become unemployed, they also lose insurance coverage. A little more than one-third (35 percent) of women receive health coverage through their jobs, compared to 44 percent of men.

Affordability of care is also a key issue for women, who are disproportionately low income. More women than men report skipping needed care and forgoing prescription medicines because of the out-of-pocket costs for premiums and copayments (Kaiser Family Foundation 2013).

Their lower incomes and eligibility for the Women, Infants, and Children program have historically meant more women than men qualify for Medicaid. In 2013, 12 percent of women were covered under Medicaid and comprised more than two-thirds of adult Medicaid beneficiaries (Kaiser Family Foundation 2013).

For frail and elderly women and their families, long-term care is a crucial concern. Women are more likely than men to need long-term care services; as a result, women comprise 73 percent of nursing home residents and home health care clients. Women who need long-term care services often pay large out-of-pocket costs for nursing home and community-based care, as a result of the limited coverage for long-term care under both Medicare and private policies (Kaiser Family Foundation 2013).

INPATIENT REHABILITATION FACILITIES

Inpatient rehabilitation facilities (IRFs) are growing in importance as the need for restorative services for traumatic injuries, acute illnesses, and chronic conditions increases. To qualify as a Medicare IRF, 75 percent of admitted patients must require intensive rehabilitation for one of ten specified physical conditions, such as stroke, spinal cord injury, head trauma, burns, hip fracture, and amputation. In 2013, about 79 percent of IRFs were hospital-based units and the remaining 21 percent were freestanding facilities. However, although the total number of facilities is greater, hospital-based IRFs usually have fewer inpatient rehabilitation beds than freestanding IRFs, so they only account for 53 percent of patients going to IRFs after acute hospital discharge (MedPAC 2015).

Large payment differences exist for the patients treated in IRFs versus **skilled nursing facilities (SNFs)** for the same conditions because they use different Medicare payment models. As part of Medicare's Conditions of Participation, at least 60 percent of an IRF's patient population must fall in the "complex rehabilitation need" category. The intensity of such rehabilitation requires a higher cost structure, and as a result, reimbursement is higher. Total Medicare payments per stay in 2012 (including the add-on payments made to many IRFs for having a teaching program or treating low-income patients or high-cost outlier cases) averaged 64 percent more for patients treated in IRFs than for those treated in SNFs. The average occupancy rate at IRFs in 2012 was 63 percent (MedPAC 2015).

In communities where IRFs are located, more PAC patients are admitted to an IRF than to an SNF. PAC services are offered in numerous settings, but physicians prefer to transition patients to IRFs because they provide a minimum of three hours of intensive rehabilitation therapy per day.

IRFs are under increasing financial pressure to meet operations costs and invest in the latest healthcare technologies. In addition, Medicare is exploring a site-neutral reimbursement policy that could lower program spending relative to current policy by between $1 billion and $5 billion (MedPAC 2015). As a result, IRFs are being forced to redefine their roles in the spectrum of PAC services as the requirement for quality rehabilitation services becomes a local and national concern (see Exhibit 10.1). Specifically, IRFs are evaluating

Inpatient rehabilitation facility (IRF)
Facility that provides restorative services for traumatic injury, acute illness, and chronic conditions.

Skilled nursing facility (SNF)
Facility that treats elderly patients with chronic diseases who need nursing care, rehabilitation, and other healthcare services.

expanding their service lines to include home health care, outpatient rehabilitation, and telemedicine to provide cost-effective care to the growing elderly population.

HealthSouth is one of the nation's largest providers of PAC services, offering both facility-based and home-based post-acute services in 33 states and Puerto Rico through its network of IRFs, HHAs, and hospice agencies. HealthSouth's hospitals provide rehabilitative care to patients who are recovering from conditions such as stroke and other neurological disorders; orthopedic, cardiac, and pulmonary conditions; brain and spinal cord injuries; and amputations.

In 2014, HealthSouth provided care to patients through 107 IRFs (32 of which operate as joint ventures with acute care hospitals) and 25 hospital-based HHAs. Health-South acquired Encompass Home Health and Hospice in 2014, which added 107 home health care locations and 20 hospice locations. The existing 25 HealthSouth HHAs were integrated into Encompass during 2015.

EXHIBIT 10.1
The Network of
Post-acute Care
Services

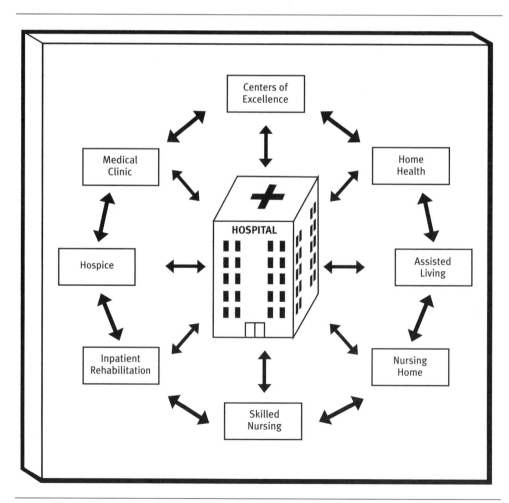

In 2014, these HealthSouth facilities generated $2.4 billion in revenue from 134,515 inpatient discharges and 739,227 outpatient visits. Nationally, HealthSouth represents 9 percent of the IRF market share, 18 percent of licensed beds, and approximately 21 percent of patients (HealthSouth 2014).

MEDICARE REIMBURSEMENT OF INPATIENT REHABILITATION FACILITIES

Medicare reimburses IRFs through its **prospective payment system (PPS)**. The PPS motivates IRFs to control costs by offering a predetermined fixed payment per patient case, regardless of the costs the IRF incurs in rehabilitating the patient. PPS has established payment rates for 385 rehabilitation services, called *case-mix groups*. Patients are assigned to these categories on the basis of their diagnosis, age, level of functional or cognitive impairment, and **comorbidity**. PPS incorporates the conversion factor, which adjusts payment levels on the basis of comorbidity, local wage rates, rural status, and income. More recently, CMS has implemented new payment methodologies that allow IRFs to assume financial risk through ACOs and to participate in CMS's bundled payment initiatives, which allow beneficiaries the freedom to select the provider of their choice. Some ACOs have established partnerships with selected PAC providers. Under this arrangement, ACOs select PAC partners by reviewing the cost and quality metrics for each provider and its geographic coverage. Hospital discharge-planning teams then choose from the selected pool of PAC providers when referring patients. Because some ACOs are at financial risk for the cost of care, CMS could consider allowing those ACOs to establish formal networks to direct beneficiaries to high-value providers (MedPAC 2015).

Prospective payment system (PPS)
Reimbursement mechanism for inpatient healthcare services that pays a predetermined rate for treatment of specific illnesses.

Comorbidity
Coexistence of one or more medical conditions in addition to the initial diagnosis.

REHABILITATION SERVICES IN ACUTE CARE HOSPITALS

Inpatient rehabilitation is the most frequently opened new clinical service in acute care hospitals. In 2015, 900 hospitals had an IRF and 185 also had an SNF (MedPAC 2015). These organizations may have an advantage over other providers because of their ability to transition patients into PAC care to improve quality and maximize total facility revenue.

In 2013, approximately 35 IRFs closed; 80 percent were hospital-based units. However, at the same time, almost two-thirds of new IRFs that year were hospital-based units. This statistic suggests that there are challenges related to hospital-based units, most likely related to reimbursement and cost, whereas some acute care hospitals with high census may find that IRF units help reduce inpatient lengths of stay and free up hospital beds for additional admissions (MedPAC 2015).

SKILLED NURSING FACILITIES

TRENDS

While acute care hospitals are experiencing increasing pressure to reduce length of stay, SNFs are experiencing strategic opportunities to work collaboratively with acute care hospitals to place discharged patients. In 2012, the average SNF occupancy rate was high at 82 percent. The average annual compensation for a nursing home administrator in 2015 was $99,566, with the top 10 percent earning $120,667 (Salary.com 2015).

Acute care hospitals are increasingly discharging orthopedic surgical patients to SNFs for rehabilitation services. To meet this increased demand, the number of SNFs has been growing at a rate of 12 percent annually—in 1995, a Medicare census found 13,945 SNFs, but by 2013, 15,632 SNFs furnished 2.4 million Medicare-covered stays to 1.7 million fee-for-service beneficiaries. In addition, Medicare expenditures for SNF services increased from $10.9 billion in 1999 to $15.7 billion in 2004 and to $28.8 billion in 2013. The data show that 67 percent of Medicare beneficiaries discharged from acute care hospitals go home, with the remainder discharged to PAC facilities. SNFs receive the largest number of PAC patients, specifically 13 percent of Medicare acute care hospital discharges (MedPAC 2015).

PALLIATIVE CARE

To *palliate* means to make comfortable by treating a person's symptoms from an illness. Hospice and palliative care both focus on helping a person be comfortable by addressing issues causing physical or emotional pain or suffering. Hospice and other palliative care providers have teams of people working together to provide care. The goals of palliative care are to improve the quality of a seriously ill person's life and to support that person and his family during and after treatment (CaringInfo 2015b).

When healthcare organizations provide palliative care services, patients have the opportunity to request information related to EoLC. Informed patients and families are allowed to participate in a care plan that includes hospital admissions, outpatient services, home health care, and PAC. These palliative care plans can reduce costs by decreasing patients' length of stay; reducing unnecessary tests, treatments, and medications; and incorporating PAC services. Palliative care allows patients and families to discuss the most appropriate healthcare options and incorporate advance care planning (see Highlight 10.1). This accommodation may help provide a sense of reassurance knowing their values and wishes were addressed.

The majority of US hospitals have palliative care programs supported by outpatient services, nursing homes, and home health care agencies. The optimal model for providing palliative care is an interdisciplinary care team that integrates healthcare providers from different backgrounds and skill sets who work collaboratively to meet the complex needs of palliative care patients. This interdisciplinary team is composed of credentialed physicians, nurses, social workers, spiritual counselors, and other healthcare practitioners whose expertise could optimize the quality of life for those patients (Hospitals in Pursuit of Excellence 2012). The following link from Allison Cuff Shimooka (2014) at The Advisory Board Company leads to a video on palliative care: http://www.advisory.com/research/physician-executive-council/multimedia/video/2014/misconceptions-about-palliative-care.

> ⊛ **Highlight 10.1** Advance Care Planning
>
> *Advance care planning* is about making decisions about the healthcare a person wants to receive if she becomes unable to speak for herself. It allows a patient time to speak to her family about her wishes and plan for the future. It includes the following (CaringInfo 2015a):
>
> - Getting information on the types of life-sustaining treatments available
>
> - Deciding what types of treatment a person would or would not want should she be diagnosed with a life-limiting illness
>
> - Sharing personal values with loved ones
>
> - Completing advance directives to put into writing what types of treatment a patient would or would not want and whom she chooses to speak for her should she be unable to speak for herself
>
> For more information, consult the National Hospice and Palliative Care Organization's website: www.caringinfo.org/i4a/pages/index.cfm?pageid=3277.

The palliative care team is responsible for conducting education and evaluating a patient's medical condition. Some palliative care team members address the patient's physical needs, such as managing pain and other symptoms; some manage referrals or coordinate discharge planning; and a chaplain can provide spiritual support and counseling to patients. The entire team works together to develop and revise care plans to ensure the patient's goals are met.

Hospice

Patients' Use of End-of-Life Care

Recognizing that a high percentage of total healthcare dollars is spent on EoLC, CMS created a unique hospice benefit designed to improve the quality of EoLC while also reducing its cost. This benefit, combined with a growing elderly population, creates a significant strategic opportunity to expand hospice services across the United States.

Role of Hospice

Hospice care contrasts with curative care in that it is not designed to cure an illness or lengthen life but emphasizes the management of pain. Hospice focuses on relieving symptoms and supporting patients with a life expectancy of months, not years, and their families. However, palliative care may be given at any time during a person's illness, from diagnosis through curative or noncurative treatment. Most hospices have a set of defined services, team members, rules, and regulations. Hospice services help the patient and family members handle the emotional, social, and spiritual aspects of terminal illness and help preserve the patient's dignity (CaringInfo 2015b).

Most hospice programs are run by not-for-profit organizations. Some are affiliated with hospitals, nursing homes, or home health care agencies. The first hospice was established in 1974 in New Haven, Connecticut. In 2013, more than 1.3 million Medicare beneficiaries received hospice services from more than 3,900 providers, and Medicare hospice expenditures totaled about $15.1 billion (MedPAC 2015).

To be admitted into a hospice program, the patient must have a physician's referral and a life expectancy of six months or less. Most hospice care is provided in the home by a family caregiver; however, inpatient hospice care is available for pain and symptom management for periods of up to five days. During the referral process, a member of the hospice staff meets with the patient's physician to talk about the patient's medical history, symptoms, and life expectancy. They also develop a plan of care for the patient and discuss the hospice philosophy and the patient's expectations.

THE MEDICARE HOSPICE BENEFIT

The Medicare hospice benefit was established in 1982 and was designed to provide families with the resources to care for their dying loved ones at home or in a hospice inpatient setting. The benefit covers palliative and support services for terminally ill Medicare beneficiaries who have a life expectancy of six months or less if the terminal illness follows its normal course. Medicare spending for hospice care increased dramatically from $2.9 billion in 2000 to $15.1 billion in 2012, an increase of 400 percent. This jump was driven by an increase in the number of people electing hospice care and increasingly lengthy stays in hospice facilities. In 2013, more than 1.3 million Medicare beneficiaries received hospice services, and Medicare expenditures totaled about $15.1 billion—which constituted no increase from 2012 (MedPAC 2015).

When a person uses the Medicare hospice benefit, his condition must be certified by a hospice physician or personal physician. A written plan of care must be established and maintained by an interdisciplinary group (which must include a hospice physician, a registered nurse, a social worker, and a counselor) in consultation with the patient's attending physician, if any. A broad set of services is included, such as nursing care, physician services, counseling and social work services, hospice aide (also referred to as home health aide) and homemaker services, short-term hospice inpatient care (including respite care), drugs to control pain and nausea, medical supplies, home medical equipment, bereavement services for the patient's family, and other services for palliation of the terminal condition (MedPAC 2015).

HOSPICE AND THE CONTINUUM OF CARE

Healthcare providers across the continuum of care benefit from cooperating with hospices to provide EoLC. Hospitals with a hospice program have higher occupancy and shorter lengths of stay and are more profitable. In a research study of almost 40,000 patients who died in 2011 of poor-prognosis cancer comparing a control group with those receiving hospice care, the latter had significantly lower rates of hospitalization, intensive care unit admission, and invasive procedures at the end of life, as well as significantly lower total costs during the last year of life (Obermeyer et al. 2014). An effective hospice program can improve acute care hospital performance by decreasing length of stay, reducing ancillary charges, and preventing unnecessary inpatient utilization by reducing hospital readmission rates and emergency department visits.

This author cowrote a research study in 2005 that showed hospitals that had a hospice program were generally larger and had more clinically complex patients. We also found that hospitals with a hospice had an average length of stay of 10.5 days, while those without a hospice had an average length of stay of 12.8 days. These statistics show that hospitals without hospice programs may be missing an opportunity to reduce costs and improve efficiency (Harrison, Ford, and Wilson 2005).

However, the provision of hospice care can be a complex challenge for healthcare organizations. Typically, hospital-based inpatient hospice care is provided, through a contract, by outside hospice services. Patients transferred to hospitals from their homes are protected by Medicare regulations that mandate service levels and visits be congruent across care sites. This standard usually requires a minimum of one interdisciplinary hospice team member contact per day in the hospital (primarily visits), supplemented with volunteer visits and 24-hour nursing care. In spite of this requirement, the hospice must use most of its Medicare payment to reimburse the hospital for patient costs. In addition, having the patient in the hospital can increase the likelihood that a patient will choose to quit hospice and switch to curative treatment because the hospital staff are most comfortable with the latter level of care. This shift may defeat the purpose of moving to hospice care and add to the overall cost of care. Leaders cannot ignore hospice services in the planning process, both because hospice care may constitute a gap in community services and because service provision may require collaboration with an outside agency.

CULTURAL DIVERSITY AND HOSPICE SERVICES

A 2011 study found that, of patients who received hospice care in the United States, 82.8 percent were white, 8.5 percent were African American, and 6.2 percent were Hispanic. When compared to overall population rates, these statistics reveal an underutilization of hospice services among minority groups. Local initiatives, such as providing education on hospice services to culturally diverse groups, can increase hospice and other EoLC utilization rates among these culturally diverse populations (NHPCO 2012).

Between 2010 and 2050, the share of the non-Hispanic white US population will decline substantially. The African American, American Indian, Alaska Native, and Native Hawaiian and other Pacific Islander populations will maintain their shares of the population. The Asian population will increase. The Hispanic population will increase substantially (Ortman and Guarneri 2015). This important demographic trend will affect the utilization of hospice and other healthcare services.

ADULT HEALTH DAY CARE CENTERS

Adult health day care centers, which provide a combination of social and medical services, are designed to keep senior citizens in the community as long as possible, thereby reducing admissions to nursing homes. These centers also provide services to patients who require PAC and assist their family caregivers. For example, an adult health day care center can provide meals, transportation, socialization, therapeutic activities, healthcare treatment, and health referrals. Respite services for caregivers include time to rest and self-esteem or family-relations improvement programs, both designed to improve the caregiver's psychological attitude. To be effective, adult health day care centers need to incorporate activities and offer services specific to the culture of their patient and caregiver population and have been found to decrease caregiver stress (Klein et al. 2014).

Adult health day care center
Facility that provides services to patients requiring long-term care and helps family caregivers with their responsibilities.

The cost of adult health day care centers varies widely. It ranges from $40 a day to more than $100 per day depending on the services offered, reimbursement, and region. The average cited by the National Adult Day Services Association is $61 per day (Senior*resource*.com 2015). Adult health day care is not usually covered by Medicare. Some coverage may be available through state or federal programs (e.g., Medicaid, Older Americans Act, Veterans Administration). The inclusion of "health" in the type of day care center indicates that it provides elements of healthcare and not just socialization and babysitting for seniors. The designation of adult day healthcare in many states is reserved for those centers that have been licensed by their states to provide medical care similar to what might be provided by a state-licensed assisted-living community or by a state-licensed nursing home (Senior*resource*.com 2015).

Norway has a unique and comprehensive system for elder care that includes adult health day care. Norway spends more per capita on caring for its elderly than any other developed nation. Nearly 10 percent of its annual budget goes toward the provision of facilities and services to fulfill the government's guarantee to its citizens that all will have a cost-free private apartment after retirement in addition to the assistance and care that they might need. Services are provided locally and provide various levels of care based on individual needs. They include home visits, home care systems, day care systems, residential apartments, and nursing homes. Day care may be considered if an elder needs more than just periodic visits to his home. For example, he may need daily help in preparing meals, dressing, attending social activities, and so on. Day care services are provided and buses are used for pickup and return between homes and day care centers, all free of cost (Gupta 2013).

Strategic planners should consider the approaches that countries around the world are taking to deal with the growing elderly population. In Norway, communities are required to provide a child care center within walking distance of parents' homes. This system has been replicated to provide adult health day care centers in similar locations. Elderly people living at home with their families can walk to these senior centers during the day and engage in a wide range of activities. Despite the fact that adult day care centers were developed with the intention of reducing admissions to nursing homes, they currently pose no threat to nursing homes.

More than 1.62 million patients used Medicaid-financed nursing home services in 2011, a small increase from 2010 but a 4.9 percent decline from 2000. The number of nursing home facilities also declined slightly between 2013 and 2014. The decline in facilities most likely reflects the expansion in some states of home- and community-based services, which allow people to remain in their homes rather than in an institution—a positive move for our country (MedPAC 2015).

SUMMARY

Faced with a rapidly growing elderly population, healthcare providers have a strategic opportunity to position themselves as integrated providers of PAC. As the population ages and the prevalence of chronic disease increases, the need for PAC in IRFs, SNFs, adult health day care centers, and patients' homes will grow significantly. More important, acute care hospitals have an opportunity to develop an integrated model of PAC services and implement EoLC or hospice programs. When exploring any new business venture, strategic planners need to ensure that the reimbursement they will receive for providing services is sufficient to make the venture profitable. Given the reality of ACOs and the bundled payment system, and given that Medicare and Medicaid reimbursement for PAC services is often less than the amount the provider will need to spend to deliver the services, this factor is especially important to consider when exploring PAC ventures.

EXERCISES

REVIEW QUESTIONS

1. Many elderly patients are being discharged from acute care hospitals after undergoing procedures such as knee-replacement surgery. They need extensive rehabilitation services. From a strategic planning perspective, investment in what type of PAC facility would be best to pursue, given these circumstances?
2. Research shows the number of elderly Americans with chronic health conditions is growing significantly. What strategic implications does the increasing demand for skilled nursing care have for the nursing home industry?

3. Given the demographics of the US population, what do you see as strategic planning opportunities in the area of hospice services?

Coastal Medical Center Exercise

What type of PAC does Coastal Medical Center (CMC) provide? What is its competition in this area?

Coastal Medical Center Questions

1. Outline a PAC plan appropriate for CMC.
2. Who should be involved in strategic planning for PAC services, and at what point should strategic planners involve them?
3. How will you know if CMC's PAC plan is a success?

Individual Exercise: Nursing Home Selection

Your grandmother is being discharged from an acute care hospital in your local community, and her physician has determined she needs to be admitted to a nursing home. Using the Nursing Home Compare website (www.medicare.gov/nursinghomecompare/search.html), answer the following questions.

1. Which three nursing homes would you recommend in your local community?
2. Of these three, which one would you choose and why?
3. Because your grandmother is a Medicare patient, what payer would pay for her nursing home care and for how long?
4. Does this payment rate make your grandmother an attractive nursing home patient?
5. What are the financial implications if your grandmother cannot return home to her independent living facility and becomes a long-term nursing home resident?

References

CaringInfo. 2015a. "Advance Care Planning." National Hospice and Palliative Care Organization. Accessed September 11. www.caringinfo.org/i4a/pages/index.cfm?pageid=3277.

————. 2015b. "Palliative Care." National Hospice and Palliative Care Organization. Accessed April 29. www.caringinfo.org/i4a/pages/index.cfm?pageid=3354.

Colby, S. L., and J. M. Ortman. 2015. *Projections of the Size and Composition of the U.S. Population: 2014 to 2060*. US Census Bureau. Published March. www.census.gov/content/dam/Census/library/publications/2015/demo/p25-1143.pdf.

Gupta, N. 2013. "Models of Social and Health Care for Elderly in Norway." *Indian Journal of Gerontology* 27 (4): 574–87.

Harrison, J. P., D. Ford, and K. Wilson. 2005. "The Impact of Hospice Programs on US Hospitals." *Nursing Economics* 23 (2): 78–84.

HealthSouth. 2014. *HealthSouth 2014 Annual Report*. Accessed April 30, 2015. http://investor.healthsouth.com/files/doc_financials/annual/2014-Annual-Report_v001_t9qefo.pdf.

Hospitals in Pursuit of Excellence. 2012. *Palliative Care Services: Solutions for Better Patient Care and Today's Health Care Delivery Challenges*. Published November. www.hpoe.org/palliative-care-services.

Kaiser Family Foundation. 2013. "Health Reform: Implications for Women's Access to Coverage and Care." Issue brief. Published August. https://kaiserfamilyfoundation.files.wordpress.com/2012/03/7987-03-health-reform-implications-for-women_s-access-to-coverage-and-care.pdf.

Klein, L. C., K. Kim, D. M. Almeida, E. E. Femia, M. J. Rovine, and S. H. Zarit. 2014. "Anticipating an Easier Day: Effects of Adult Day Services on Daily Cortisol and Stress." *The Gerontologist*. Published July 4. http://gerontologist.oxfordjournals.org/content/early/2014/07/01/geront.gnu060.full.

Medicare Payment Advisory Commission (MedPAC). 2015. *Report to the Congress: Medicare Payment Policy*. Accessed April 29. www.medpac.gov/documents/reports/march-2015-report-to-the-congress-medicare-payment-policy.pdf.

Morley, M., S. Bogasky, B. Gage, S. Flood, and M. J. Ingber. 2014. "Medicare Post-acute Care Episodes and Payment Bundling." *Medicare & Medicaid Research Review* 4 (1): E1–E12.

Moses, H., D. Matheson, R. Dorsey, B. George, D. Sadoff, and S. Yoshimura. 2013. "The Anatomy of Health Care in the United States." *Journal of the American Medical Association* 310 (18): 1947–64.

National Hospice and Palliative Care Organization (NHPCO). 2012. *NHPCO Facts and Figures: Hospice Care in America.* Accessed September 13, 2015. www.nhpco.org/sites/default/files/public/Statistics_Research/2012_Facts_Figures.pdf.

Obermeyer, Z., M. Makar, S. Abujaber, F. Dominici, S. Block, and D. M. Cutler. 2014. "Association Between the Medicare Hospice Benefit and Health Care Utilization and Costs for Patients with Poor-Prognosis Cancer." *Journal of the American Medical Association* 312 (18): 1888–96.

Ortman, J. M., and C. E. Guarneri. 2015. "United States Population Projections: 2000 to 2050." US Census Bureau. Accessed May 1. www.census.gov/population/projections/files/analytical-document09.pdf.

Salary.com. 2015. "Nursing Home Administrator Salaries." Accessed March 24. www1.salary.com/Nursing-Home-Administrator-Salary.html.

Senior*resource*.com. 2015. "Adult Day Care and Adult Day Health Care." Accessed May 1. www.seniorresource.com/hsdc.htm.

Shimooka, A. C. 2014. "The Win-Win of Palliative Care." Advisory Board Company video. Published May 5. www.advisory.com/research/physician-executive-council/multimedia/video/2014/misconceptions-about-palliative-care.

World Health Organization (WHO). 2015. "WHO Definition of Palliative Care." Accessed March 29. www.who.int/cancer/palliative/definition/en/.

CHAPTER 11

STRATEGIC PLANNING IN HEALTH SYSTEMS

By a wide margin, the biggest threat to our nation's balance sheet is the skyrocketing cost of healthcare.

—President Barack Obama

LEARNING OBJECTIVES

After you have studied this chapter, you should be able to

➤ discuss political, business, and ethical issues related to the growth in the US healthcare system;

➤ discuss the structures and governance of for-profit and not-for-profit healthcare systems;

➤ describe the key factors that affect organizational strategy and performance among healthcare systems;

➤ diagnose the differences in organizational culture between for-profit and not-for-profit healthcare systems; and

➤ relate the concept of healthcare consolidation to the development, assessment, and redesign of healthcare systems.

➤ For-profit health system

➤ Hospital acquisition

➤ Hospital merger

➤ Integrated delivery system

➤ Not-for-profit health system

➤ Virtual health system

INTRODUCTION

The number of US hospitals operating as part of a health system grew from 2,542 in 2000 to 2,868 in 2008 and to 3,144 in 2014—a 24 percent increase since the year 2000 (AHA 2015). In addition, 55 percent of all US hospitals now are part of a health system. These data indicate that the majority of strategic planners in the healthcare field must consider not just the individual hospital but the overall health system in which the hospital operates. Likewise, independently operated US hospitals, which are now in the minority, must consider future health system affiliation as part of their long-term survival plan.

In 2015, almost 90 percent of US hospitals were considering a merger or an acquisition (LeMaster and Aygun 2015). Hospital mergers and acquisitions had reached their highest levels in more than 15 years, and hospital consolidations amounted to more than 130 mergers or acquisitions annually.

Declining reimbursement and provider competition are driving this trend. Many medical groups are joining with hospitals to form affiliations, confederations, or shared economic models such as **integrated delivery systems (IDSs)**. IDSs enable better use of staff and financial resources and can lead to greater operational efficiencies across the continuum of healthcare services. They may also gain a competitive advantage by negotiating better reimbursement rates with insurers. Furthermore, IDSs bring together a wider array of clinical services and deliver them in a more coordinated manner than fragmented hospitals can. This chapter discusses the important role health systems have in positioning an organization in an environment of growing uncertainty.

Integrated delivery system (IDS)
Network of hospitals that enables better use of staff and financial resources and promotes greater operational efficiencies across the continuum of healthcare services.

HOSPITAL MERGERS AND ACQUISITIONS

In the 1990s, healthcare was characterized by the restructuring of hospitals, medical groups, and long-term care providers. These restructuring initiatives included the development of IDSs formed by a combination of acquisitions, mergers, joint ventures, and other alliances.

A **hospital acquisition** is the purchase of a hospital by another facility or multihospital system.

The number of hospitals has only marginally increased since 1999—up less than 1 percent. However, the number of hospitals affiliated with a system has increased 16

Hospital acquisition
Purchase of a hospital by another facility or multihospital system.

percent (2,524 to 2,941). This suggests a trend toward health system affiliations most likely increased by preparation for the impact of the Affordable Care Act (ACA) of 2010 (Yanci, Wolford, and Young 2013).

Not-for-profit health systems typically evaluate potential acquisitions on the basis of mission, outreach, services, and geographic location. In addition to these factors, for-profit systems evaluate opportunities to maximize profits—for example, purchasing a hospital when its sale price is below the net present value of its cash flow stream. For for-profit health systems, the advantages of acquiring a hospital include increased market share in the community, greater total revenue, and an improved referral base as a result of greater patient volume. Potential disadvantages include the major capital investment required for the purchase and the possibility of an antitrust violation caused by the increased presence in a local market (i.e., the system comes to monopolize the local market).

A **hospital merger** is a combining of two or more hospitals, often through a pooling of interests. When it constitutes a pooling of interests, a merger often requires no capital outlay. An organization may choose to merge when low profits and weak markets do not support acquisition. In other words, many hospitals choose to merge with another hospital because neither hospital has sufficient financial resources to acquire an organization. By combining their resources, organizations can pursue business and other strategic opportunities together that they could not afford to pursue on their own.

Hospital merger
Combining of two or more hospitals.

Research shows that hospital mergers tend to be horizontal, meaning the merging hospitals are competitors looking for increased operating efficiency and improved market share. By combining their services, the merged entities can offer more services than each could independently, and with more services comes more revenue. Instead of drawing from one patient base, the combined entity draws from two. Just as more services bring in more revenue, so do more patients bring in more revenue. In addition, managed care organizations (i.e., healthcare insurance companies) tend to favor contracting with larger, more complex hospitals, forcing smaller hospitals to become part of a health system (Cutler and Morton 2013).

Additional reasons for merging are to eliminate unnecessary services, reduce overhead through consolidation, and provide a more rational mix of services designed to better meet the community's needs. For example, many mergers involve hospitals located in the same community. If both hospitals offer some of the same services—say, both hospitals provide obstetrics services—the merged hospitals can close the duplicated services at one site because providing the service at a single location is more efficient. While increased efficiency through consolidation benefits the merged organization as a whole, some staff may be adversely affected when, for example, administrative functions such as human resources are combined and streamlined, leading to involuntary reductions in staff.

In a merger, similarity of the mission, vision, and culture between the two organizations is important. In an acquisition situation, organized fit is preferable, but similarity is not necessary because the acquiring organization will have dominance, and the acquired entity's assets are transferred to the purchasing entity.

INTEGRATED DELIVERY SYSTEMS

In healthcare, mergers and acquisitions are a part of horizontal integration, in which a for-profit hospital system purchases other hospitals to increase its size (Harrison, Spaulding, and Mouhalis 2015). Conversely, vertical integration results in IDSs designed to gain access to scarce resources across the continuum of care by acquiring an organization that controls those resources. During the health reform debate, many health policy experts have called for the country to reorganize healthcare providers and delivery systems through integration. IDSs have garnered considerable interest. Research shows a positive correlation between health system integration and quality of care (Hwang et al. 2013). No clear definition of an IDS yet exists; it could be not-for-profit or for-profit.

Mayo Clinic is an example of a large IDS, with a home base in Rochester, Minnesota; southern tertiary care sites in Florida and Arizona; and Mayo Clinic Health System in the Midwest. Mayo Clinic is a not-for-profit, academic medical institution with a mission focused primarily on patient care supported by education and research. In 2014, Mayo provided care to more than a million people from 50 states and 150 countries at the three tertiary care locations. It provided this care in its clinics and hospitals with 59,509 personnel comprising 4,158 physicians and scientists; 3,155 residents, fellows, and students; and 52,196 allied health staff. It generated $9.7 billion in total revenue, had operating income of $834 million, and received contributions from benefactors of $495 million. It has a medical school and an allied health school and, in 2014, had a research budget of $648 million from internal and external funding (Mayo Clinic 2014). The Mayo Clinic Health System is Mayo Clinic's network of community hospitals and clinics that formed in 1992 and now has 18 hospitals and more than 40 clinics, hospices, and nursing homes. It serves more than 60 communities in Iowa, Wisconsin, and Minnesota. Care is provided by 1,041 staff physicians and scientists and 14,944 allied health staff (clinic and hospital) for a total of 15,985 staff. As part of Mayo Clinic, a leading caregiver with more than 150 years of patient care, research, and medical education expertise, it offers a full spectrum of healthcare options to local neighborhoods, ranging from primary to highly specialized care (Mayo Clinic Health System 2015). At the same time, those patients have access to the tertiary care Mayo Clinic offers at the other three primary sites.

A **not-for-profit health system** is organized as a not-for-profit corporation. Based on charitable purpose and frequently affiliated with a religious denomination, not-for-profit systems are a traditional means of delivering medical care in the United States. They are distinct from government-owned public systems and privately owned for-profit systems. Ascension Health, headquartered in St. Louis, Missouri, is the largest not-for-profit health system in the United States. Ascension provides acute care, long-term care, psychiatric care, rehabilitation services, and residential care and grew substantially between 2008 and 2014. Exhibit 11.1 outlines its growth (Ascension 2014).

Geisinger Health System is a not-for-profit health system located in Pennsylvania that consists of tertiary care hospitals, community hospitals, outpatient facilities, and 60

Not-for-profit health system
Health system organized as a not-for-profit corporation. Based on charitable purpose and frequently affiliated with a religious denomination, this means of care delivery is traditional.

Exhibit 11.1
Ascension Health
Facts

	2008	**2014**	**% Increase**
Acute care hospitals	67	131	95
Employees	107,000	150,000	40
Hospital beds	18,012	21,936	22
Assets	$17.3 billion	$31.2 billion	70
Operative revenue	$13.4 billion	$20.1 billion	46
Provision of charity care	$748 million	$1.8 billion	94

Sources: Data from Ascension (2009, 2014) and Page (2010).

community practices. The system also includes an insurance company, the Geisinger Health Plan, which provides comprehensive coverage for 290,000 members who receive care from 37,000 credentialed healthcare providers. As of 2011, Geisinger Health System employed 220 primary care physicians and 654 specialty physicians. For these employed physicians, Geisinger uses a compensation plan that uses annually defined performance incentives to provide additional pay, up to 20 percent of physician base pay. Performance incentives are linked to quality, teamwork, and financial performance. These performance payment incentives support Geisinger's overall goal to improve the quality and efficiency of its patient care; in fact, Geisinger's patient-centered medical home program has shown improved outcomes for Geisinger Health Plan patients. These initiatives have allowed Geisinger to develop a national reputation as an IDS that delivers high-quality, cost-effective healthcare. In addition, Geisinger has increased its clinical services revenue by more than 10 percent annually over the past ten years. This growth is driven by increases in patient volume, number of clinicians, and clinician productivity (Lee, Bothe, and Steele 2012).

For-profit health systems are organizations that comprise hospitals owned by equity-based investors and that have a well-defined organizational goal of profit maximization, usually through efficiency measures. As a result, the management team of a for-profit hospital answers to the shareholders of the company. These shareholders want a return on their investment; therefore, the hospital must be able to consistently generate a profit. Although for-profit hospitals' mission is to make a profit, they do provide uncompensated care to the most vulnerable members of the population and thereby improve the health status of their local communities. As of 2013, an analysis of 749 large, for-profit hospitals found that they were 71 percent efficient on average (Harrison, Spaulding, and Mouhalis 2015).

For-profit health system
Organization that comprises hospitals owned by equity-based investors and that has a well-defined organizational goal of profit maximization.

A sample for-profit health system organization chart is provided in Exhibit 11.2. It illustrates one CEO or holding company, with many divisions or groups supported by a single corporate structure for departments such as Information Technology, Human Resources, Finance, Outpatient Practice, and Clinical Operations.

One of the largest for-profit health systems in the United States is Hospital Corporation of America (HCA), headquartered in Nashville, Tennessee. The system comprises locally managed facilities that include 168 hospitals and 113 freestanding surgery centers, including 5 hospitals in the United Kingdom (HCA 2015a). Exhibit 11.3 outlines HCA's growth between 2008 and 2014.

A number of important acquisitions occurred in the early part of the twenty-first century. For example, Tenet Healthcare acquired Vanguard Health Systems in October 2013. Community Health Systems completed its acquisition of Health Management Associates in January 2014 (LeMaster and Aygun 2015).

STRATEGIC PLANNING AT THE HEALTH SYSTEM LEVEL

Strategic planning at the health system level is different from planning at an individual hospital level. Health systems routinely evaluate the acquisition of hospitals or other smaller health systems with values in excess of $1 billion. The magnitude of these projects requires working with Wall Street banks and venture capital firms to negotiate capital financing packages, which are critical to determining whether these new business initiatives will be profitable. Most health systems have a dollar threshold of approximately $1 million for the local approval of new business initiatives. Any new business initiative that will cost in excess of this threshold must be approved by the health system's headquarters. At the

EXHIBIT 11.2
Sample For-Profit
Health System
Organization Chart

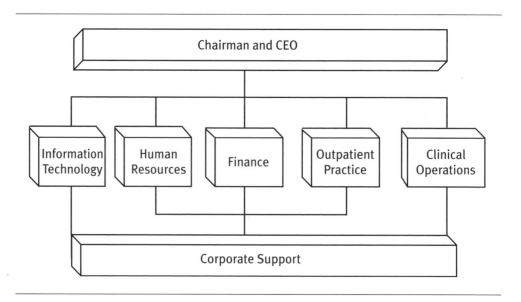

Exhibit 11.3
HCA Facts

	2008	2014	% Increase
Acute care hospitals	158	166	5
Employees	183,000	225,000	23
Hospital beds	38,504	43,356	12.6
Assets	$24 billion	$31.2 billion	30
Operative revenue	$28 billion	$36.9 billion	32
Provision of charity care	$2.1 billion	$2.5 billion	19

Source: Data from HCA (2008, 2011, 2015b).

headquarters level, these larger business initiatives compete with other business initiatives across the entire health system and are prioritized in a strategic plan for the overall health system. The number of projects funded by the health system is determined by the level of cash flow generated throughout the health system and the cost and availability of capital from banks or the equity stock markets. Health systems attempting to expand their services also must work closely with state regulatory agencies and the US Department of Justice. These agencies are responsible for ensuring that health systems do not approach monopoly status in a local community, which can have an adverse effect on competition in the marketplace. For these reasons, strategic planning at the system level requires a global perspective and additional technical skills that are not necessary when planning in local markets.

Not all systems are created equal, and many small systems (as well as some larger systems) do not really operate as a consolidated entity. These systems may comprise many facilities and have good public relations programs, but they are fragmented and do not integrate key services and functions. For example, in a small health system of five to eight hospitals distributed across a wide geographic area, there are limited opportunities for economies of scale (see Chapter 1, Highlight 1.1). The same is true for a large system of 20 hospitals located in separate parts of the world. To gain real economies of scale, multiple, large facilities must be concentrated in one geographic area (Cobb and Wry 2015). For example, suppose a small hospital system needs to buy a magnetic resonance imaging (MRI) machine. If the system's hospitals are in proximity to each other, there is no need to buy a machine for each facility. The system can buy one machine and place it in one of the facilities. If a physician at one of the other facilities orders an MRI for a patient, the patient can easily travel to the facility where the MRI machine is located. If the system's hospitals were scattered around the country, it would have to buy a machine for each facility—an exorbitant expenditure.

Health systems are attempting to lower costs by increasing their economies of scale. In addition to spreading their costs over increasing volumes of services, healthcare organizations are able to negotiate for increased revenue when they negotiate with large insurers. To date, consolidation has been primarily horizontal, meaning mergers and acquisitions in the same sector of services. These horizontal mergers allow for greater efficiencies, particularly in reducing fixed costs in areas such as facilities and health information technology. Most recently, hospitals have been limited by the Federal Trade Commission to about 30 percent of hospital beds in their market area (Moses et al. 2013).

Driven in part by the ACA, vertical integration has increased since 2010. Hospital systems that are providing insurance products recognize the need to coordinate care for their enrolled populations. This vertical integration enables better-quality care at a lower cost and can provide a competitive advantage in fragmented geographic markets. Most important, vertical integration has been explicitly sanctioned by the ACA, which supports integration by transferring some risk and management functions to individual hospitals. In addition, this vertical integration increasingly has led to the employment of physicians by health systems. By failing to leverage the economies of scale made possible by consolidated systems, fragmented systems are not in much better shape than small, stand-alone rural hospitals because the systems lack the technical expertise and facility infrastructure to operate in an increasingly complex healthcare environment (Moses et al. 2013).

INTEGRATION ACROSS THE CONTINUUM OF CARE

In the future, management of individual patients across the continuum of healthcare services will become increasingly important. US healthcare will continue to move toward further integration of clinical services and consolidation of payers and health systems (Moses et al. 2013). This consolidation is a result of the high level of complexity associated with healthcare and requires individual institutions to become part of a regional and national strategy. Affiliation and the integration of care are also strategies for achieving quality improvement goals. Health systems are in a position to manage variation across their facilities in both administrative and clinical areas. For example, the health system HCA once had a billing office and a payroll department in each of its hospitals. Each hospital also had a purchasing agent and central supply warehouse to meet its ongoing needs. This individualization led to a wide variation in performance. To reduce this range, HCA regionalized its billing and supply chain operations. These regional centers leveraged consistency across the health system, improving quality and efficiency as a result.

HCA uses the same approach to clinical quality improvement, calling on the best talent in the organization to transfer best practices across the enterprise. When protocols of care are standardized and implemented across a health system, quality scores improve, patient satisfaction increases, and fewer malpractice claims are filed.

VIRTUAL HEALTH SYSTEMS

Virtual health systems—networks of organizations created through the use of health information technology—allow independent healthcare providers to link together without having to merge with or acquire other facilities. Participation in a virtual health system may appeal to some independent hospitals because they can gain many of the advantages of health system membership without giving up operational control to the health system. Independent rural hospitals that have a long history of financial losses, old facilities, or antiquated equipment might also find participation in a virtual health system advantageous. Strategic planners of health systems often consider these hospitals "losers" and, as a result, not viable candidates for merger or acquisition. In such cases, the only possibility of affiliation for these hospitals is participation in a virtual health system.

Virtual health system
Network of organizations created through the use of health information technology.

Using affiliations to provide integrated services, rather than mergers and acquisitions, can be important (LeMaster and Aygun 2015). These clinical affiliations allow organizations to access the clinical expertise and resources of much larger systems without giving up organizational control. Virtual health systems provide particularly good opportunities to implement evidenced-based care, share resources and business services, develop coordinated information technology systems, reduce supply chain costs, and leverage telemedicine. In addition, virtual health systems can help expand an organization's geographic referral base, create accountable care organizations (ACOs), manage population health, create clinically integrated networks, and provide a framework for new service-line joint ventures.

Virtual health systems can also link hospitals with physician groups or long-term care providers to enable smooth transitions for patients from facility to facility. To make transitions even more seamless, members of virtual health systems can use a shared electronic health record so that they all have access to the same information. Virtual health systems cannot incorporate all the linkages an IDS can, but they can emulate some of the important components of a "physical" health system.

INTERNATIONAL HEALTH SYSTEMS

In recognition of the global market, many health systems are considering international healthcare. For example, high-profile organizations such as Johns Hopkins Medicine have expanded to international communities and created relationships or linkages there. They establish a clinic, provide some local healthcare services, and send inpatient referrals back to the flagship hospital in the United States. There is nothing wrong with this approach, but the scale of the enterprise is modest. A bolder approach to international healthcare is to expand a system or create a new system in the foreign country and provide comprehensive healthcare.

When considering expansion into an international market, strategic planners of health systems must ensure that a market for a new healthcare provider exists. This market is often driven by excessive waiting times for services or a perception of poor healthcare quality among the targeted international population. Once the market demand has been validated, the international strategic planner should determine whether a commercial health insurance program exists in the country to pay for services or if segments of the population have sufficient financial resources to pay for premium healthcare services.

SUMMARY

From a strategic planning perspective, what opportunities are available to small community hospitals or small systems? What do their futures look like? With limited resources, unaffiliated hospitals have few options. How will they fund new technology? How will they pay for the talent they need to move forward?

These important questions are driving the growth in the number of independent hospitals joining health systems. IDSs and ACOs are able to gain a competitive advantage in the market by negotiating higher reimbursement rates, offering a wider array of clinical services, and delivering these services in a more coordinated manner.

Also contributing to the growth of IDSs is the development of virtual health systems, a new model that allows organizations, through health information technology, to participate in a loosely structured system without having to give up operational control. This model has the potential to offer many of the advantages of a physical health system without requiring the commitment of financial resources. In addition, some US health systems are participating in international healthcare initiatives as a way to expand their market.

EXERCISES

REVIEW QUESTIONS

1. Evaluate the statement that an IDS is the wave of the future and is critical to future organizational success.
2. Identify the largest for-profit and not-for-profit health systems in the United States. Provide specific information about each, including the number of hospitals, the number of employees, and total revenue. Compare these health systems and discuss the ones you think will grow at the fastest rates.

COASTAL MEDICAL CENTER EXERCISE: DEVELOPING AN INTEGRATED DELIVERY SYSTEM

Would developing an IDS allow Coastal Medical Center (CMC) to improve the efficiency and quality of its healthcare services?

COASTAL MEDICAL CENTER QUESTIONS

1. Name five areas in which CMC has some components of an IDS in place. Next, develop a list of five new areas or activities that CMC could successfully integrate into a health system.
2. Will an IDS improve CMC's negotiating power with managed care organizations (i.e., insurers)?
3. From your perspective, does CMC need to develop an IDS, or does it just need a quick fix for its operational problems?

INDIVIDUAL EXERCISE: HEALTH SYSTEM IMPLEMENTATION OF AN ACCOUNTABLE CARE ORGANIZATION

Using Geisinger Health System and its enrollment of 290,000 members into the Geisinger Health Plan for comprehensive insurance coverage as a model, develop a plan for a potential ACO. As you develop this plan, integrate your knowledge of primary care, specialty care, and post-acute care services.

1. At a minimum, explain how you could use vertical integration as a method to build a comprehensive health system.
2. Identify those components of an ACO that will be most critical in driving future success.
3. To make an ACO successful, what types of investments and fixed costs will be necessary?
4. More broadly, what do you see as the role of ACOs in the future US healthcare system?

REFERENCES

American Hospital Association (AHA). 2015. "Fast Facts on US Hospitals." Updated January. www.aha.org/research/rc/stat-studies/fast-facts.shtml.

Ascension. 2014. *2014 Financial and Statistical Report*. Accessed March 19, 2015. http://ascension.org/~/media/files/community_investor-relations-pdfs/annual-report-2014_financials.pdf.

———. 2009. "Consolidated Financial Statements." Accessed October 1, 2015. www.ascensionhealth.org/assets/docs/AH_2009_AFS.pdf.

Cobb, A., and T. Wry. 2015. "Resource-Dependence Theory." Oxford Bibliographies in Management. Last reviewed June 18. doi: 10.1093/obo/9780199846740-0072.

Cutler, D. M., and F. S. Morton. 2013. "Hospitals, Market Share, and Consolidation." *Journal of the American Medical Association* 310 (18): 1964–70.

Harrison, J. P., A. Spaulding, and P. Mouhalis. 2015. "The Efficiency Frontier of For-Profit Hospitals." *Journal of Health Care Finance* 41 (4): 1–23.

HCA. 2015a. "HCA Facts." Published July 7. http://hcahealthcare.com/util/documents/HCA-presskit-fact-sheet.pdf.

———. 2015b. "HCA Reports Fourth Quarter 2014 Results." Published February 15. http://investor.hcahealthcare.com/press-release/hca-reports-fourth-quarter-2014-results.

———. 2011. "2011 Annual Report to Stockholders." Accessed September 26, 2015. http://investor.hcahealthcare.com/sites/hcahealthcare.investorhq.businesswire.com/files/report/file/HCA_2011_Annual_Report.pdf.

———. 2008. "HCA Fact Sheet." Accessed April 30, 2009. http://hcagulfcoast.com/util/documents/CurrentFactSheet1.pdf.

Hwang, W., J. Chang, M. LaClair, and H. Paz. 2013. "Effects of Integrated Delivery System on Cost and Quality." *American Journal of Managed Care* 19 (5): e175–e184.

Lee, T. H., A. Bothe, and G. D. Steele. 2012. "How Geisinger Structures Its Physicians' Compensation to Support Improvements in Quality, Efficiency, and Volume." *Health Affairs* 31 (9): 2068–73.

LeMaster, E., and J. Aygun. 2015. "Is Hospital M&A Waning?" *Healthcare Financial Management Association*. Published January. www.hfma.org/Content.aspx?id=27401&utmsource=Realpercentage20Magnet&utm medium=Email&utm campaign=64414373.

Mayo Clinic. 2014. "Mayo Clinic Facts." Published December. www.mayoclinic.org/about-mayo-clinic/facts-statistics.

Mayo Clinic Health System. 2015. "About Mayo Clinic Health System." Accessed September 26. http://mayoclinichealthsystem.org/about-us.

Moses, H., D. H. M. Matheson, E. R. Dorsey, B. P. George, D. Sadoff, and S. Yoshimura. 2013. "The Anatomy of Health Care in the United States." *Journal of the American Medical Association* 310 (18): 1947–64.

Page, L. 2010. "52 Not-for-Profit Hospital Systems to Know." *Becker's Hospital Review*. Published March 1. www.beckershospitalreview.com/lists-and-statistics/50-not-for-profit-hospital-systems-to-know.html.

Yanci, J., M. Wolford, and P. Young. 2013. *What Hospital Executives Should Be Considering in Hospital Mergers and Acquisitions*. Dixon Hughes Goodman LLP. Published January 1. www2.dhgllp.com/res_pubs/Hospital-Mergers-and-Acquisitions.pdf.

CHAPTER 12

PAY FOR PERFORMANCE AND THE HEALTHCARE VALUE PARADIGM

Debra A. Harrison

Price is what you pay. Value is what you get.

—Warren Buffett

Knowing is not enough; we must apply. Willing is not enough; we must do.

—Johann Wolfgang von Goethe

LEARNING OBJECTIVES

After you have studied this chapter, you should be able to

➤ analyze and discuss the evolution of quality in healthcare;

➤ discuss a range of approaches to the implementation of a total quality program in a healthcare organization, including Donabedian's model of structure, process, and outcomes;

➤ articulate the concept of value and discuss performance measures that are important in healthcare organizations;

➤ define pay for performance and discuss some of the current initiatives in healthcare reimbursement; and

➤ demonstrate the ability to link quality, efficiency, and financial decision making in an organization's strategic plan.

KEY TERMS AND CONCEPTS

➤ Donabedian framework

➤ Leapfrog Group

➤ Nurse-sensitive patient outcomes

➤ Pay-for-performance program

➤ Quality

➤ Therapeutic alliance

➤ Value

➤ Value frontier

INTRODUCTION

THE VALUE FRONTIER

In 1973, President Richard Nixon signed the Health Maintenance Organization Act, which was intended to create incentives for healthcare organizations to offer services for a prepaid healthcare premium. This healthcare arrangement posed two questions: Would healthcare organizations offer quality care at a reasonable cost after having received the premiums from the patients enrolled in the system up front? And how would the value of this new prepaid care be measured?

How has the US healthcare system addressed these questions? A paradigm shift from the efficiency frontier to a **value frontier** is occurring in healthcare. The value frontier is a benchmark that takes into account not only efficiency but also quality. Organizations on the value frontier are considered "best in class," and their levels of performance become models for improved performance in healthcare organizations everywhere. A healthcare organization is efficient if it has achieved an optimal fit between its structural characteristics and its processes. Even when an optimal fit is achieved, however, the healthcare organization struggles to maintain that fit because the healthcare environment is dynamic and requires organizations to make changes on a continuous basis.

Value frontier
Organizations that create the highest value in healthcare.

THE COST OF QUALITY

US healthcare spending grew 3.6 percent in 2013, reaching $2.9 trillion, or $9,255 per person. Health spending accounted for 17.9 percent of the nation's gross domestic product (CMS 2014c). Health spending increased by 5 percent in 2014, compared to 3.6 percent in 2013, marking the biggest jump since before the recession (Tozzi 2015). How to provide access to affordable healthcare is an ongoing philosophical discussion in modern medicine. In healthy industries, competition is not based on cost but on **value,** which is the level of consumer benefit received per dollar spent. In mathematical terms, value $(V) = Q/C$, where quality (Q) represents clinical outcomes, safety, and patient satisfaction and cost (C) represents the cost of care over time. Where value rules, innovation is rewarded, providers prosper, and efficiency increases. Value-based systems motivate providers to benchmark

Value
Level of consumer benefit received per dollar spent.

their value performance measures to improve processes of care and to meet patients' needs and expectations (Blumenthal and Stremikis 2013).

Discussion of healthcare quality is important as healthcare evolves and experiences technological advances that result in increased cost yet potentially improved value. We must consider whether increased costs limit access to healthcare (i.e., only those who can afford it have access), and we must also keep in mind the return on investment for the price of technology.

According to The Commonwealth Fund (see Highlight 12.1), waste and medical errors account for $100 billion of US healthcare expenses and may cost 150,000 lives annually. To encourage quality improvement and more efficient delivery of healthcare services, the government, insurance companies, and other groups implement **pay-for-performance (P4P) programs,** which offer financial incentives to physicians, hospitals, and other healthcare providers in exchange for meeting certain performance targets. P4P initiatives can also reduce the payments providers receive if they commit medical errors, have poor outcomes, or incur excessive costs.

An awareness of P4P offerings is important in strategic planning. To maximize an organization's income and improve quality and efficiency in the delivery of care, strategic

Pay-for-performance (P4P) program
Initiative implemented by the government, insurance companies, and other groups to reward providers for meeting certain performance targets in the delivery of healthcare services.

(✱) HIGHLIGHT 12.1 The Commonwealth Fund

The Commonwealth Fund is a private institution whose goal is to improve access to care, quality of care, and efficiency of care in the United States. The Commonwealth Fund is especially interested in helping vulnerable people receive better care: the low-income population, the uninsured, minorities, young children, and the elderly.

To achieve these goals, The Commonwealth Fund supports independent research on how care could be improved. For example, The Commonwealth Fund has published reports on such topics as asthma outcomes in minority children and reasons for patient readmission to hospitals after discharge. It also publishes reports to inform the public, such as its analysis of the different healthcare reform bills proposed by the US House of Representatives and Senate in late 2009. Many of its publications provide information and statistics about the current state of healthcare in the United States.

Financed by individuals and organizations that support its mission, The Commonwealth Fund grants money to tax-exempt organizations and public agencies to improve the provision of healthcare and to study and recommend policy changes that will improve the healthcare system. For example, some of its grants support programs that study the future of Medicare and the care of frail, elderly adults.

planners incorporate objectives into the strategic plan that are geared toward achieving P4P performance targets.

MEDICARE PAY-FOR-PERFORMANCE INITIATIVES

The Affordable Care Act (ACA) was signed into law as Public Law 111-148 on March 23, 2010. The legislation is commonly called "Obamacare" because it was signed by President Obama and because the act is a product of the healthcare reform agenda of the Democratic 111th Congress and the Obama administration. The ACA is often contested, though its constitutionality was upheld by the US Supreme Court in 2012 and supported by the public with the reelection of President Obama in 2012. Title III of the ACA mandated a financial reward to improve quality, safety, and the patient experience for Medicare patients, an initiative called value-based purchasing (VBP). It began in 2013 with reimbursements for patient discharges on or after October 1, 2012 (Piper 2013). The Centers for Medicare & Medicaid Services (CMS) automatically withholds a hospital's Medicare payments by a specified percentage each year (see Exhibit 12.1), and hospitals can earn back that percentage if they adopt quality processes and achieve certain patient satisfaction scores. Each year, the percentage of the withholding increases and the metrics change. The intent of the law is that the program be budget neutral, meaning that organizations performing in the bottom 10 percent lose the Medicare payment reduction and the top 10 percent receive the Medicare payment incentive.

As of 2015, the metrics in the incentive program included outcomes and efficiency of care. The payment is broken down as follows: clinical processes of care (20 percent), patient experience (30 percent), outcomes (30 percent), and efficiency of care (20 percent) (AHC Media 2014). See Exhibit 12.2 for a complete list of measures in the VBP initiative.

EXHIBIT 12.1
Medicare Payment Reductions for Hospitals

Year	Reduction*
2013	1%
2014	1.25%
2015	1.5%
2016	1.75%
2017+	2%

* Of the base operating diagnosis-related group payments
Source: Data from CMS (2014b).

Previously, payment was based on clinical processes (70 percent) and patient experience (30 percent). This change reflects CMS's shift in priorities, toward outcomes rather than processes. In addition, CMS measures of efficiency now include a cost metric. This metric is called the Medicare Spending per Beneficiary (MSPB) and is defined as the average Medicare Part A and B spending per patient from 3 days prior to admission to 30 days after discharge (Chen and Ackerly 2014). The MSPB encompasses the continuum of care and prevents cost shifting to healthcare providers outside of the hospital.

From the patient's perspective, the concept of "paying for value" includes high-quality healthcare at a reasonable price—hence the term *value based*. The quality of care is high when it provides excellent outcomes, patient-centric care, and high levels of patient satisfaction. VBP also means efficient care, which will require physicians to limit the number

EXHIBIT 12.2
Hospital Value-Based Purchasing Program Measures, 2016

Clinical Process of Care Domain

Fibrinolytic therapy received within 30 minutes of hospital arrival

Influenza immunization

Initial antibiotic selection for community-acquired pneumonia in immunocompetent patients

Prophylactic antibiotic selection for surgical patients

Prophylactic antibiotics discontinued within 24 hours after surgery

Urinary catheter removed on postoperative day 1 or postoperative day 2

Surgery patients on beta-blocker therapy prior to arrival who received a beta-blocker during the perioperative period

Surgery patients received appropriate venous thromboembolism prophylaxis within 24 hours prior to surgery to 24 hours after surgery

Patient Experience of Care Domain

Hospital Consumer Assessment of Healthcare Providers and Systems survey

Outcomes Domain

Catheter-associated urinary tract infection

Central line–associated bloodstream infection

Acute myocardial infarction 30-day mortality rate

Heart failure 30-day mortality rate

Pneumonia 30-day mortality rate

Complication/patient safety for selected indicators (composite)

Surgical-site infection: Colon and abdominal hysterectomy

Efficiency Domain

Medicare spending per beneficiary

Source: Data from CMS (2014b).

of tests they order that do not improve morbidity or mortality. These initiatives will also mandate that physicians provide care based on clinical protocols that were developed using evidence-based research and approved by the appropriate professional association for the clinical area in which these protocols are to be used. These quality measures are increasingly being developed jointly by private healthcare organizations and government institutions, such as the Agency for Healthcare Research and Quality (AHRQ). Hospital-specific performance is publicly reported on CMS's Hospital Compare website.

Although there was much attention to the VBP program in the 2010s, CMS has always supported initiatives to improve the quality of care in physicians' offices, ambulatory surgery centers, hospitals, nursing homes, and home health care agencies. The basis of CMS's recent P4P initiatives is a collaboration with providers to ensure that valid measures are used to achieve improved quality. CMS has explored P4P initiatives in nursing home care, home health care, dialysis, and coordination of care for patients with chronic illnesses. These initiatives include the Hospital Quality Initiative in 2002, the Premier Hospital Quality Incentive in 2003, the Physician Group Practice Demonstration in 2005, the Care Management Performance Demonstration in 2007, the Medicare Health Support Chronic Disease Pilot in 2008, and the Care Management for High-Cost Beneficiaries Demonstration in 2005–2012. Hospitals that submitted the required data received full Medicare diagnosis-related group (DRG) payments. (See Highlight 12.2 for a discussion of DRGs.)

Linking the reporting of hospital quality data with P4P is an effective strategy for improving the US healthcare system. Such a program will provide financial incentives to organizations that invest in quality improvement. Quality measures improved from 2005 to 2010 for acute myocardial infarction, heart failure, and pneumonia, and racial and ethnic equity increased (Trivedi et al. 2014). However, VBP may not appear to correlate directly with improved quality and patient safety (Spaulding, Zhao, and Haley 2014). Transparency of data and improved processes may have affected outcomes more than a system of reward and punishment. In any case, quality in the United States has been positively affected.

ADDITIONAL INITIATIVES IN PAY FOR PERFORMANCE
COMMERCIAL PAYER INITIATIVES

CMS is not the only entity offering P4P incentives. US health plans and other payers are also developing P4P programs to improve the quality of care and minimize future cost increases. In 2009, more than 250 private P4P programs existed across the nation, half of those programs targeting hospital care (Cauchi, King, and Yondorf 2010). One of the largest and longest-running private sector P4P programs is the California Pay for Performance Program, which is managed by the Integrated Health Association (headquartered in Oakland, California). It was founded in 2001 as a physician incentive program and has focused on measures related to improving quality performance by physician groups. Starting in 2014, it began to include value-based cost measures (James 2012).

> ### ✱ HIGHLIGHT 12.2 Diagnosis-Related Groups
>
> DRGs are a patient classification scheme used by hospitals to identify the diseases they treat. Each disease is grouped with similar diseases and assigned a code so that physicians, billing departments, and payers (particularly Medicare) can easily identify the diagnosis. Assigned to each code is an amount of money the payer will reimburse a provider for treatment of that diagnosis. The amount of reimbursement is based on the average cost of providing care for that illness and includes the cost of in-hospital nursing care, room and board, diagnostic treatments, and any other routine treatments that might be necessary for that illness while a patient is in the hospital. The payment does not include the physician's fees.
>
> Hospitals receive money from Medicare over and above the DRG payment. The amount is augmented by payments added to the base rate. For instance, if the hospital treats a high percentage of low-income patients, it receives an add-on applied to the DRG-adjusted base rate. If the hospital is an approved teaching hospital and a training site for medical students, it receives an add-on for each case.
>
> The DRG system was developed in the 1980s to control costs and motivate hospitals to provide care more efficiently. The hospital is paid a predetermined rate, so it will try not to spend more than that rate in treating the patient. DRGs, about 500 in all, are updated yearly by CMS (2014a).

LEAPFROG GROUP

Leapfrog Group
Independent healthcare purchaser, founded by major employers, that uses purchasing power to improve the quality and efficiency of US healthcare services.

The **Leapfrog Group**, a purchaser founded in 2000, represents many of the nation's largest corporations and public agencies that buy health benefits on behalf of their enrollees. The mission of the Leapfrog Group is to use employer purchasing power to improve the quality, efficiency, and affordability of US healthcare. Representing both private and public sector employers, Leapfrog represents more than 34 million Americans and tens of billions in healthcare expenditure (Leapfrog Group 2015a). Though the number of companies it represents has remained at about 60, its publication of hospital safety scores has been increasingly visible in the media since 2010. The twice-a-year results are cited in the *Wall Street Journal*, *USA Today*, and *AARP The Magazine*.

Leapfrog's hospital reporting initiative, implemented in 2001, assesses hospital performance on the basis of quality and safety measures developed by the National Quality Forum (NQF). Hospitals that meet or exceed NQF's benchmarks have been successful in reducing medical mistakes. Hospitals that participate receive a Hospital Safety Score of A, B, C, D, or F based on their ability to prevent errors, accidents, injuries, and infections. The Hospital Safety Score is calculated by top patient-safety experts and is peer reviewed, fully transparent, and free to the public. As part of this recognition program, the Leapfrog Group posts participating hospitals' scores on its website for use by employers and consumers. In 2015, approximately 2,500 hospitals participated. Of those, 31 percent had an A, 28 percent a B, 34 percent a C, and 6 percent a D; only 20 hospitals, or less than 1 percent, had an F (Leapfrog Group 2015b).

Leapfrog is focused on four major "leaps" to make healthcare safer: computerized physician order entry, evidence-based hospital referral, intensive care units staffed with physician specialists, and hospitals' progress on eight NQF benchmarks (called Safe Practices). A complete list of measures and scoring methodologies is available on the Leapfrog website (www.leapfroggroup.org).

Members of the Leapfrog Group (2015b) agree to educate their employees about patient safety and hospital quality, encourage their employees to seek care from hospitals that meet Leapfrog's safety standards, and base their purchase of healthcare on principles that encourage quality improvement among providers and consumer involvement in healthcare decision making. Such actions have been highly effective in moving patients to healthcare providers that meet Leapfrog's standards. Everyone benefits: Patients are steered to safer hospitals and, as a result, hospitals receive more business. Conversely, Leapfrog removes hospitals from its register of approved providers if their quality and safety scores decline.

Physicians' Attitudes Regarding Pay for Performance

Many physicians express a lack of trust in health plan and government initiatives imposing change. However, one of the first national surveys on physicians' attitudes about P4P, completed in 2005, found that 75 percent of responding physicians supported financial incentives for improved quality when the measures they were required to report were deemed "accurate" by an authority on those measures. A much smaller percentage of physicians supported public reporting for medical group quality performance (Casalino et al. 2007).

A systematic review of provider attitudes and P4P indicated that healthcare providers still have a low level of awareness about P4P and have serious concerns that P4P may have unintended consequences. They also believe that additional resources will be needed to provide adequate quality indicators and implementation of P4P. The findings of the study underscore the importance of provider education and of providing technical support to reduce provider burden. Developing more accurate quality measures to minimize any unintended consequences is also important (Lee, Lee, and Jo 2012).

Incorporating Pay for Performance into a Strategic Plan

Current and past P4P initiatives have focused on improving quality and reducing costs—two key factors in gaining a competitive advantage. Therefore, hospital planners should incorporate P4P initiatives into the strategic plan. Strategic planners should routinely monitor their CMS Hospital Compare quality scores to raise them to the level of CMS's

P4P incentives. If their scores are already at that level, they should focus on driving them up further to maximize rewards and reimbursement; the higher the quality, the greater the reward. Planners need to allocate money to invest in programs and new technology that will help the hospital increase its quality scores. In areas where quality is poor and unlikely to change, the strategic planner should consider closing the service so that patient safety is not jeopardized and the hospital is less likely to incur malpractice suits.

Mayo Clinic is an outstanding example of an organization that has incorporated P4P into its strategic planning process. It routinely evaluates new business initiatives that could enhance the quality of care it provides. Demonstrating its ability to prepare for the future well in advance, Mayo even benchmarks its quality and efficiency performance against P4P standards that have been developed but are not scheduled to be implemented until several years from now.

DONABEDIAN AND QUALITY

Avedis Donabedian (1966), a physician considered the father of quality assurance in health-care, defined **quality** as a reflection of the goals and values currently adhered to in the medical care system and the society in which it exists. This definition signifies that no one common criterion exists on which to measure healthcare quality. For this reason, he introduced the **Donabedian framework**, a model for evaluating the quality of medical care based on three criteria: structure, process, and outcomes.

Structure includes the environment in which healthcare is delivered, the instruments and equipment providers use, administrative processes, the qualifications of the medical staff, and the fiscal organization of the institution. Access to care may also be considered part of the structure component.

Process considers how care is delivered. For example, healthcare quality could be evaluated according to the appropriateness and completeness of information obtained through review of a patient's clinical history, physical examinations, and diagnostic tests; the provider's explanation of and reason for her diagnosis and recommended therapy; the physician's technical competence in performing diagnostic and therapeutic procedures, including surgery; evidence of preventive management in health and illness; coordination and continuity of care; and acceptability of the care to the patient (Donabedian 1966). By studying the process indicators of quality, judgments can be made whether medicine was practiced appropriately and addressed the patient's needs.

Outcomes, the most discussed measure of quality, include recovery, restoration of function, and survival. These quality indicators are some of the most frequently reported and widely understood. Other outcome indicators are patient satisfaction, physical disability, and rehabilitation. Although the latter are more complicated to assess, they remain the ultimate validation of healthcare quality (Donabedian 1966).

Quality
Standard of healthcare provision that reflects the goals and values currently adhered to in the medical care system and the society in which it exists.

Donabedian framework
Model for evaluating the quality of medical care based on three criteria: structure, process, and outcomes.

In 2014, scholars examined whether the VBP performance scoring system correlates with hospital-acquired conditions needing quality improvement (Spaulding, Zhao, and Haley 2014). They reported that while the VBP measures are covering process, structure, and outcomes, these measures do not correlate with an improvement in hospital-acquired conditions. This result could mean that we are not measuring the correct processes, or that the outcome measurements do not reflect the quality we are trying to achieve. Which is more important—promoting an incentive system that lacks a clear indication of the outcomes that health systems should be measuring, or changing the process measures to ensure that the outcomes organizations care about are actually being measured (Spaulding, Zhao, and Haley 2014)? Future healthcare leaders must answer this interesting question.

The three pillars of structure, process, and outcomes need to be addressed collectively to achieve optimum quality of care. As described above, each aspect influences the others. For example, a patient with a broken bone needs access to a qualified physician and an appropriate facility for treatment, and the care he receives should meet preestablished standards. A positive outcome of healing with no complications after treatment is expected but should also be measured. If that outcome is not achieved, then an examination of the structure (qualifications and experience of the physician and facility) and process (were standards followed?) is needed. If any one of these aspects is lacking, the others are negatively affected and optimum quality is not achieved.

DEFINING QUALITY

No single definition of healthcare quality exists, nor is there a single method of measuring quality in healthcare. Numerous judgments of its meaning, measurement, and value have been made. As a result, quality is difficult to define, measure, and apply in a health services setting. While scholars agree on some of the underlying quality issues in healthcare, they differ dramatically in their ideas about where these issues stem from and how to address them.

Access to healthcare for all Americans is paramount in the quality literature. The ACA was more about access and insurance reform than healthcare reform. Among other concerns, the law addresses having enough physicians for consumers, particularly in rural areas. Before any discussion about quality, physicians and hospital beds must be adequate to people's need for care.

The consumer's ability to choose a physician or care setting is another focal point. The rise of health maintenance organizations (HMOs) in the 1990s, with their limited network plans, left some consumers worried about choice. However, millions of people enroll in high-quality managed care plans such as Kaiser Permanente, which limit customers to physicians employed by these companies. Patients do not complain about a restrictive network when they always have first-rate providers. The ACA insurance exchange program gives consumers choices along a range of plans, from bronze, with a narrow network and lower premiums, and the platinum plan, with a broader network and higher premiums. Some insurance plans could offer narrow networks with poor-quality providers, but healthcare planners need to ensure that Americans receive high-quality care despite choosing a narrow network (Emanuel 2014).

COMPARATIVE OUTCOMES

In the early 1900s, Dr. Ernest Codman, a pioneer surgeon and advocate of healthcare reform, researched healthcare quality by measuring quality outcomes. His *end results theory* advocated measuring patient care to assess hospital efficiency and to identify clinical errors or problems. The American College of Surgeons adopted his theory as a minimum quality standard. On the basis of this theory, the college created the Hospital Standardization Program, which later evolved into the Joint Commission on Accreditation of Healthcare Organizations (now simply The Joint Commission). Codman also believed in public reporting of quality, a concept first taking hold today, a century later. The American Hospital Association also has encouraged providers to establish quality assurance programs to audit outcomes of care. The most comprehensive evaluation of hospital quality today is the CMS Hospital Compare report, which assesses hospital quality performance, measures changes in quality over time, and evaluates the patient experience.

The initial purpose of measuring the quality of healthcare outcomes and processes was to help patients make informed healthcare decisions. While research shows that Americans rate quality as the most important factor when choosing a health plan, studies also show that most do not understand their options well enough to make an informed choice. However, today's consumer is becoming more informed and considers the advantages and risks of recommended treatments. Healthcare organizations must understand, define, and measure quality of care as well as gather data from the patient's perspective for use in patient decision making. While patient satisfaction is not the only indicator of quality care, it is a significant goal. Providers could achieve exemplary clinical outcomes but have negative patient satisfaction scores if they have poor interpersonal skills or lack sensitivity to cultural differences among their patients.

Public and private groups, such as the National Committee for Quality Assurance (NCQA), have developed tools for measuring and reporting healthcare quality. The Hospital Consumer Assessment of Healthcare Providers and Systems (HCAHPS; see Highlight 12.3) and the Healthcare Effectiveness Data and Information Set (HEDIS; see Highlight 12.4) are two examples. Many hospitals use HCAHPS to assess patient satisfaction and HEDIS to measure clinical performance in the outpatient setting.

QUALITY METRICS

GROWING DEMAND FOR QUALITY-RELATED DATA

Demand for quantitative data on healthcare quality is growing. P4P programs use these data to recommend quality measures, design financial incentives, and create measurement systems. As with Leapfrog, some payers are using clinical quality measures while negotiating

HIGHLIGHT 12.3 Hospital Consumer Assessment of Healthcare Providers and Systems

HCAHPS (typically pronounced "H-Caps") is a survey used to measure patient experiences with healthcare providers. Use of this standardized survey allows patient experiences to be compared with those of other patients across the United States. All patients are asked the same questions, and all results are measured according to the same rating scale. Without a standardized survey, comparisons of quality of care would be inaccurate.

The survey focuses on several areas:

- How well nurses communicated with patients

- How well doctors communicated with patients

- How responsive hospital staff were to patients' needs

- How well caregivers managed patients' pain

- How well caregivers explained patients' medications to them

- How clean and quiet the hospital was

- How well the caregivers gave discharge instructions

- Overall satisfaction rating of their hospital stay

CMS implemented the HCAHPS survey in October 2006, and the first public reporting of HCAHPS results occurred in March 2008. The survey, its methodology, and the results it produces are in the public domain and can be found on the Hospital Compare website. Since July 2007, hospitals receiving Medicare payments must collect and submit HCAHPS data to receive their full annual payment. The ACA requires HCAHPS to be included among the measures used to calculate value-based incentive payments in the VBP program.

contracts and designing benefits to adjust patient cost sharing and direct patients toward higher-performing hospitals (Carrier and Cross 2013). Because chronic conditions account for 86 percent of medical costs, payers stress the importance of gathering data on chronic care. They also stress the importance of using quality measures based on peer-reviewed national standards of care. Because analysis of quality data can take more than a year, there may be delays in reporting hospital quality and paying timely P4P bonuses (CDC 2015).

However, while reporting requirements and transparency efforts have proliferated over the past 20 years, employers often find it difficult to determine what hospital quality measures are important, how to interpret and use quality information in a meaningful way,

---

⊛ **HIGHLIGHT 12.4** Healthcare Effectiveness Data and Information Set

In 1991, NCQA created the HMO Employer Data and Information Set to help measure the quality of care at healthcare institutions. HEDIS has undergone four name changes while maintaining the same acronym; the name was changed to Healthcare Effectiveness Data and Information Set in 2007.

According to NCQA (2014), 90 percent of health plans use HEDIS to monitor quality. HEDIS consists of 81 measures across five domains of care:

1. Effectiveness of care
2. Access to and availability of care
3. Experience of care
4. Utilization and relative resource use
5. Health plan descriptive information

Healthcare institutions are evaluated on how well they perform on the 81 measures. Examples include asthma medication use, persistence of beta-blocker treatment after a heart attack, control of high blood pressure, comprehensive diabetes care, breast cancer screening, antidepressant medication management, childhood and adolescent immunization status, and childhood and adult weight or body mass index assessment (NCQA 2014). NCQA collects the data from healthcare organizations and uses them to calculate national benchmarks and set standards for NCQA accreditation.

HEDIS is used by employers and consumers to compare health plans and identify those most appropriate for their needs. Because the measures reported to HEDIS are specific (all organizations report the same measurements), healthcare organizations across the nation can be easily compared.

and how to present useful information to their consumers (Carrier and Cross 2013). Use of consistent sources with transparency of measurement methods is important in developing a quality improvement plan.

As discussed previously, many public reports are using data from CMS's Hospital Compare website (www.hospitalcompare.hhs.gov). This website has a consumer orientation, providing information on how well hospitals provide recommended care to their patients. Hospital Compare allows the public to select up to three hospitals to compare quality measures related to heart attack, heart failure, pneumonia, surgery, and other conditions. These measures are organized by

◆   patient survey results;

◆   timely and effective care;

◆   readmissions, complications, and deaths;

◆   use of medical imaging;

◆   linking quality to payment; and

◆   Medicare volume.

The demand for data has pushed the implementation of electronic health records (EHRs), and meaningful use initiatives have furthered that effort. Hospitals must plan for the resources required to meet these demands. Clinicians will complain that "it's not good enough that I document it; I need to document it someplace where we can capture it for reporting" (Eisenberg et al. 2014). To minimize the burden on clinicians, a combination of clinical knowledge and technological expertise is required to implement manually intensive steps so that hospitals can begin to use EHR-specific quality measures (Amster et al. 2014).

AGENCY FOR HEALTHCARE RESEARCH AND QUALITY

AHRQ, whose mission is to produce evidence that helps make healthcare safer and higher quality—as well as more accessible, equitable, and affordable—is a division of the US Department of Health and Human Services (HHS). The agency also works with HHS and other industry partners to make sure that the evidence is understood and used (Kronick 2015). Its programs and software are free and publicly available for download on the AHRQ website (www.ahrq.gov). The Inpatient Quality Indicators are part of a set of software modules of AHRQ quality indicators developed by the Stanford University–University of California, San Francisco, Evidence-Based Practice Center and the University of California, Davis, under a contract with AHRQ. The Inpatient Quality Indicators were originally released in 2002. Hospital administrative data related to mortality, utilization, and volume reflect quality of care inside hospitals. AHRQ collects data on inpatient mortality for certain procedures and medical conditions; utilization of procedures for which there are questions of overuse, underuse, and misuse; and volume of procedures for which some evidence suggests that a higher volume of procedures is associated with lower mortality (AHRQ 2015).

PATIENT SAFETY

The Institute of Medicine (IOM) report *To Err Is Human: Building a Safer Health System*, published in 1999, described the problems surrounding patient safety. The report listed six aims designed to improve safety. Healthcare must be (1) safe, (2) effective, (3) patient centered, (4) timely, (5) efficient, and (6) equitable. These six aims underscore the fact that healthcare is a service delivered to a patient who is also the customer. While some of the IOM aims (such as safety, effectiveness, and fiscal efficiency of services) can be statistically measured on the basis of mortality and morbidity rates, other factors (such as patient centeredness, timeliness, and equitability) are best evaluated through research and patient satisfaction surveys. The Joint Commission publishes National Patient Safety Goals that it expects hospitals to address when pursuing accreditation (see Highlight 12.5).

OTHER QUALITY CONSIDERATIONS

WORKFORCE

An unintended consequence of an emphasis on quality is a rise in the cost of nursing services and ancillary staff. Studies have shown that patient outcomes improve with increased patient-to-nurse ratios (Spaulding, Zhao, and Haley 2014). Hospitals with poor nurse staffing (more than four patients per nurse) have higher rates of risk-adjusted 30-day mortality and failure to rescue in surgical patients (Wiltse Nicely, Sloane, and Aiken 2012). Each additional patient added to a nurse assignment results in a 7 percent increase in mortality (Aiken et al. 2002). Studies have shown that nursing retention is an important factor in maintaining a skilled nursing staff (Harrison and Ledbetter 2014).

Healthcare is a labor-intensive field. Healthcare organizations require a well-designed infrastructure for supporting nurses and other staff to maximize quality outcomes. But proper staffing may come at a price that is contrary to maintaining a lower expense base. How do

---

(✳) HIGHLIGHT 12.5 National Patient Safety Goals, 2015

1. Improve the accuracy of patient identification
2. Improve the effectiveness of communication among caregivers
3. Improve the safety of medication use
4. Reduce the harm associated with clinical alarm systems
5. Reduce the risk of healthcare-associated infections
6. Identify safety risks inherent in the patient population
7. Use the Universal Protocol for preventing wrong-site, wrong-procedure, and wrong-person surgery

Source: Data from The Joint Commission (2014).

healthcare leaders find the balance between quality and appropriate staffing? Research on workforce issues can help organizations determine the number of staff members, mix of expertise, and level of experience necessary to providing optimal care.

MAGNET RECOGNITION

The American Nurses Credentialing Center (ANCC) is the sponsor of the Magnet Recognition Program, which recognizes healthcare organizations for quality patient care, nursing excellence, and innovations in professional nursing practice (see Highlight 12.6). Studies have shown that organizations that pursue or achieve Magnet recognition have improved patient outcomes, patient satisfaction, and nurse satisfaction. Approximately 7 percent of all hospitals in the United States have achieved ANCC Magnet Recognition status (ANCC 2015). Organizations may consider achieving Magnet status to be a strategic goal in improving **nurse-sensitive patient outcomes**—patient outcomes that improve if there is a greater quantity or better quality of nursing care (e.g., pressure ulcers, falls, intravenous infiltrations).

Nurse-sensitive patient outcomes
Changes in health status that are dependent on nursing interventions.

PATIENT ENGAGEMENT

Research suggests that empowering patients to actively process information, to decide how that information personally affects them, and then to act on those decisions is a key driver behind healthcare improvement and cost reduction (Hibbard, Greene, and Overton 2013). A **therapeutic alliance** is a partnership between patient and providers that involves collaboration and negotiation to arrive at mutual goals.

Therapeutic alliance
Partnership between patient and providers that involves collaboration and negotiation to arrive at mutual goals.

⊛ HIGHLIGHT 12.6 Magnet Recognition Program Model Components

- Transformational leadership

- Structural empowerment

- Exemplary professional practice

- New knowledge, innovations, and improvements

- Empirical outcomes

Source: Data from ANCC (2015).

EMPLOYEE SATISFACTION

Efforts to create higher employee satisfaction have very desirable outcomes for patients, including increased patient satisfaction, improved care quality, and increased patient loyalty. Satisfied employees contribute to the growth of an organization. Employee satisfaction is measured through in-house surveys that allow employees to communicate concerns, ask questions, or evaluate their employer.

ACCREDITATION

Healthcare quality is also maintained through accreditation, which is a standardized method of ensuring that quality processes are consistent throughout healthcare. Examples of accrediting organizations include The Joint Commission, which accredits acute care hospitals; the American Society of Clinical Pathology, which accredits laboratory systems on the basis of the Clinical Laboratory Improvement Amendments passed by Congress in 1988; and the American College of Surgeons, which accredits trauma centers.

BALANCED SCORECARDS

Most organizations have established a dashboard or scorecard that reflects current quality measures along with financial performance. Balancing the two (hence the *balanced* scorecard) can improve the value frontier of the organization. Moving beyond sharing data at an organizational level to public reporting has raised the stakes in maintaining quality care. Transparency of data has become an expectation for consumers. It may be the most powerful factor in changing the behavior of healthcare providers and caregivers. Public image and competitive spirit can contribute to striving for the best outcomes (Spaulding, Zhao, and Haley 2014).

SUMMARY

Federal healthcare policymakers and state regulators have concerns about the negative impact that reduced reimbursement for healthcare services, low hospital occupancy, and poor efficiency can have on the quality of healthcare. They also recognize that the aging population, the ACA-induced increase in the number of insured patients, and investments in healthcare technology will continue to drive up healthcare costs. By operating in a manner consistent with evolving healthcare policy and the quality standards set forth by value-based purchasing programs, hospitals can receive financial and other rewards (e.g., a reputation for excellence), all of which will place them in a stronger competitive position.

EXERCISES

REVIEW QUESTIONS

1. From your own experience as a patient, provide an example of high-value healthcare.
2. Discuss the three pillars of Donabedian's model for healthcare quality assurance. Does this model have practical applications today, given the current focus on healthcare value?
3. What are the roles of the following groups in the healthcare value improvement process: boards of directors, senior leaders, physicians, employees, and payers?
4. Imagine you are a hospital executive and you want to improve your organization's value proposition. What areas do you need to assess to develop an improvement plan?

COASTAL MEDICAL CENTER EXERCISE

In Appendixes C and G of the Coastal Medical Center (CMC) comprehensive case study, Hospital Compare data are provided for CMC and its competitors in the local market. How does CMC's quality compare to that of its competitors? List five areas in which CMC's value could be improved.

COASTAL MEDICAL CENTER QUESTIONS

1. Should CMC expect to receive a P4P bonus for its quality scores?
2. Should VBP be incorporated into CMC's strategic planning process? Outline a process that will allow CMC to take advantage of future VBP initiatives.
3. What type of organizations should CMC use as benchmarks?
4. How will you know whether the CMC plan to increase healthcare value is a success?

INDIVIDUAL EXERCISE: LOCAL COMMUNITY QUALITY AND PATIENT SATISFACTION COMPARATIVE ANALYSIS

Access the Hospital Compare database for your community and find the state and national quality standards, then use the data to answer the following questions.

1. Compare three hospital organizations in your community and, based on the information, make recommendations for which hospital you would use for the following service lines: emergency care, cardiac treatment, and surgical procedures.

2. Based on the other quality and outcomes metrics discussed in Chapter 12, list other websites and databases that may provide additional information on the hospital organizations in your community.

3. Based on your analysis, does one particular organization in your community consistently exceed state, national, and local performance metrics? If so, would you recommend this organization to your family and friends?

REFERENCES

Agency for Healthcare Research and Quality (AHRQ). 2015. *Inpatient Quality Indicators: A Tool to Help Assess the Quality of Care to Adults in the Hospital*. Accessed October 11. www.qualityindicators.ahrq.gov/Downloads/Modules/IQI/V42/Inpatient_Broch_10_Update.pdf.

AHC Media. 2014. "Look Ahead to Succeed Under VBP." *Hospital Case Management*. Published July 1. www.ahcmedia.com/articles/117227-look-ahead-to-succeed-under-vbp.

Aiken, L. H., S. P. Clarke, D. M. Sloane, J. Sochalski, and J. H. Silber. 2002. "Hospital Nurse Staffing and Patient Mortality, Nurse Burnout, and Job Dissatisfaction." *Journal of the American Medical Association* 288 (16): 1987–93.

American Nurses Credentialing Center (ANCC). 2015. "Magnet Model." Accessed September 22. www.nursecredentialing.org/Magnet/ProgramOverview/New-Magnet-Model.

Amster, A., J. Jentzsch, H. Pasupuleti, and K. G. Subramanian. 2014. "Completeness, Accuracy, and Computability of National Quality Forum-Specified eMeasures." *Journal of the American Medical Informatics Association* 22 (2): 1–6.

Blumenthal, D., and K. Stremikis. 2013. "Getting Real About Health Care Value." *Harvard Business Review*. Published September 17. https://hbr.org/2013/09/getting-real-about-health-care-value.

Carrier, E., and D. Cross. 2013. *Hospital Quality Reporting: Separating the Signal from the Noise*. National Institute for Health Care Reform. Published April. www.nihcr.org/Hospital-Quality-Reporting.

Casalino, L. P., G. C. Alexander, L. Jin, and R. T. Konetzka. 2007. "General Internists' Views on Pay-for-Performance and Public Reporting of Quality Scores: A National Survey." *Health Affairs* 26 (2): 492–99.

Cauchi, R., M. King, and B. Yondorf. 2010. "Performance-Based Health Care Provider Payments." National Conference of State Legislatures brief. Published May. www.ncsl.org/portals/1/documents/health/perbenchformance-based_pay-2010.pdf.

Centers for Disease Control and Prevention (CDC). 2015. "Chronic Disease Prevention and Health Promotion." Updated October 6. www.cdc.gov/chronicdisease/.

Centers for Medicare & Medicaid Services (CMS). 2014a. "Acute Inpatient PPS." Modified August 4. www.cms.gov/Medicare/Medicare-Fee-for-Service-Payment/AcuteInpatientPPS/index.html.

———. 2014b. "Medicare Program. . . ." *Federal Register* 79 (163): 49853–50536.

———. 2014c. "National Health Expenditures 2013 Highlights." Accessed September 30. www.cms.gov/Research-Statistics-Data-and-Systems/Statistics-Trends-and-Reports/NationalHealthExpendData/Downloads/highlights.pdf.

Chen, C., and D. Ackerly. 2014. "Beyond ACOs and Bundled Payments: Medicare's Shift Toward Accountability in Fee-for-Service." *Journal of the American Medical Association* 311 (7): 673–74.

Donabedian, A. 1966. "Evaluating the Quality of Medical Care." *Milbank Quarterly* 44 (3): 166–206.

Eisenberg, F., C. Lasome, A. Advani, R. Martins, P. A. Craig, and S. Sprenger. 2014. *A Study of the Impact of Meaningful Use Clinical Quality Measures*. Accessed September 29. www.aha.org/content/13/13ehrchallenges-report.pdf.

Emanuel, E. 2014. "In Health Care, Choice Is Overrated." *New York Times*. Published March 5. www.nytimes.com/2014/03/06/opinion/in-health-care-choice-is-overrated.html.

Harrison, D., and C. Ledbetter. 2014. "Nurse Residency Programs: Outcome Comparisons to Best Practices." *Journal for Nurses in Professional Development* 30 (2): 76–82.

Hibbard, J. H., J. Greene, and V. Overton. 2013. "Patients with Lower Activation Associated with Higher Costs; Delivery Systems Should Know Their Patients' 'Scores.'" *Health Affairs* 32 (2): 216–22.

Institute of Medicine (IOM). 1999. *To Err Is Human: Building a Safer Health System*. Washington, DC: National Academies Press.

James, J. 2012. "Health Policy Brief: Pay-for-Performance." *Health Affairs*. Published October 11. www.healthaffairs.org/healthpolicybriefs/brief.php?brief_id=78.

The Joint Commission. 2014. "National Patient Safety Goals Effective January 1, 2015." Published November 14. www.jointcommission.org/assets/1/6/2015_NPSG_HAP.pdf.

Kronick, R. 2015. "AHRQ: Making Health Care Safer and Higher Quality for Every American." *AHRQ Views* (blog). Agency for Healthcare Research and Quality. Published October 2. www.ahrq.gov/news/blog/ahrqviews/100215.html.

Leapfrog Group. 2015a. "Explanation of Safety Score Grades." Published April. www.hospitalsafetyscore.org/media/file/ExplanationofSafetyScoreGrades_April2015.pdf.

———. 2015b. "The Leapfrog Group Fact Sheet." Revised April 1. www.leapfroggroup.org/about_leapfrog/leapfrog-factsheet.

Lee, J. Y., S. Lee, and M. Jo. 2012. "Lessons from Healthcare Providers' Attitudes Toward Pay-for-Performance: What Should Purchasers Consider in Designing and Implementing a Successful Program?" *Journal of Preventive Medicine and Public Health* 45 (3): 137–47.

National Committee for Quality Assurance (NCQA). 2014. "HEDIS and Performance Measurement." Accessed September 30. www.ncqa.org/HEDISQualityMeasurement.aspx.

Piper, L. E. 2013. "The Affordable Care Act: The Ethical Call for Value-Based Leadership to Transform Quality." *The Health Care Manager* 32 (3): 227–32.

Spaulding, A., M. Zhao, and D. R. Haley. 2014. "Value-Based Purchasing and Hospital Acquired Conditions: Are We Seeing Improvement?" *Health Policy* 118 (3): 413–21.

Tozzi, J. 2015. "U.S. Health-Care Spending Is on the Rise Again." *Bloomberg Business*. Published February 18. www.bloomberg.com/news/articles/2015-02-18/u-s-health-care-spending-is-on-the-rise-again.

Trivedi, A. N., W. Nsa, L. Hausmann, J. S. Lee, A. Ma, D. W. Bratzler, M. K. Mor, K. Baus, F. Larbi, and M. J. Fine. 2014. "Quality and Equity of Care in U.S. Hospitals." *New England Journal of Medicine* 371 (24): 2298–308.

Wiltse Nicely, K. L., D. M. Sloane, and L. H. Aiken. 2012. "Lower Mortality for Abdominal Aortic Aneurysm Repair in High-Volume Hospitals Is Contingent upon Nurse Staffing." *Health Services Research* 48 (3): 972–91.

CHAPTER 13

THE FUTURE OF HEALTHCARE

Debra A. Harrison

I look through a half-opened door into the future, full of interest, intriguing beyond my power to describe.

—Dr. William J. Mayo in 1910

Human genomics represents the new healthcare value paradigm. Individualized medicine will fundamentally change the structure of the healthcare industry by focusing on preventive medicine, effective treatment modalities, and medical interventions across the life span.

—Dr. Jeff Harrison in 2015

LEARNING OBJECTIVES

After you have studied this chapter, you should be able to

➤ explain the evolution of individualized medicine in healthcare;

➤ articulate the costs and potential rewards of incorporating genomics into an individual patient treatment program;

➤ discuss the fundamentals of population health, including the role of the patient-centered medical home and telemedicine; and

➤ gain insight regarding research in and the future direction of new healthcare initiatives.

KEY TERMS AND CONCEPTS

➤ Genomics

➤ Individualized medicine

➤ Population health

➤ Telemedicine

INTRODUCTION

In a speech about **genomics** research in 2000, President Bill Clinton stated, "This will revolutionize the diagnosis, prevention and treatment of most, if not all, human diseases." Since that time, society has invested $3 billion in exploring human genomics and sequencing the first human genome. The cost to sequence one individual's human genome dropped from $10 million in 2000 to under $5,000 in 2014. From an economic standpoint, every dollar invested in this research has resulted in $178 of economic activity. Genomics has created a new healthcare field with the potential to reduce costs, improve quality, and fundamentally change the healthcare value paradigm (Collins and Prabhakar 2013; Hayden 2014).

> *Genomics*
> Study of the entire genome (the complete set of DNA in an organism).

Genetics is the study of the function and effects of a single gene, but *genomics* is the term for the study of the entire genome. Deoxyribonucleic acid (DNA) is the chemical compound that directs the activities of nearly all living organisms. Most people recall from science classes that DNA molecules are made of two twisting, paired strands, or a double helix. An organism's complete set of DNA is called its genome. The estimated 20,000 to 25,000 genes in the human genome carry the instructions for making a specific protein or set of proteins. Genomics explores not only the actions of single genes but also the interactions of multiple genes with each other and with the environment. As a result, genomics has great potential for improving the health of the public (NHGRI 2015). The Centers for Disease Control and Prevention also recognizes that the interaction between our genes, behavior, infections, and the environment can lead to many diseases. Better understanding of genetic and family history information can help providers identify, develop, and evaluate screening and other interventions that can improve health and prevent disease (NHGRI 2015).

This chapter discusses the use of this research to incorporate predictive human genomics across the continuum of healthcare services. The appropriate use of this new clinical technology provides opportunities for significant improvements in healthcare quality and the enhanced use of preventive health services. The establishment of predictive human genomics services requires the creation of collaborative relationships between physicians and healthcare organizations as they develop process-focused care. This collaboration allows physicians, working with health systems, to integrate human genomics in a manner that facilitates innovation across the continuum of healthcare practice. Early implementation supports the premise that predictive human genomics will be a cost-effective approach to improving healthcare quality.

THE NEW HEALTHCARE VALUE PARADIGM

A paradigm shift from the existing value frontier to a new healthcare value paradigm is being driven by advances in genomics and individualized treatment protocols. This new paradigm builds on concepts of population health and evidence-based clinical protocols to develop an individualized healthcare life plan to maximize an individual's use of healthcare resources across his life span.

INDIVIDUALIZED MEDICINE

Based on current research, a human genome can be sequenced in about 24 hours for less than $5,000 (Collins and Hamburg 2013). This level of efficiency shows that clinicians can now selectively use their patients' genetics to implement changes in plans of care. This emerging healthcare technology enhances clinical care and further supports patient engagement.

Direct-to-consumer (DTC) genetic testing is the marketing of genetic testing by commercial laboratories to individual consumers. Many of the available at-home genetic test kits use a saliva sample that can identify ancestry, paternity, and ethnicity, as well as test for specific disease risks, with usage often driven by a person's own curiosity. DTC genetic testing lacks regulation, so the information can be misleading and lacks the fuller interpretation of healthcare providers. Genetic tests should undergo premarket review by the US Food and Drug Administration to ensure results are accurate, reliable, and clinically meaningful (Su 2013).

The American College of Medical Genetics and Genomics (ACMG) has developed recommendations for the clinical application of whole-genome sequencing. This test reports pathogenic or likely pathogenic variants in 56 genes. These 56 genes are associated with 24 genetic cardiovascular disorders or predisposition to types of cancer. Early recommendations were that if the test was done for a patient, the patient should receive all results, even those not specific to his current disease situation. Studies have shown, however, that not all patients want to know their future potential for disease. In the spirit of individualized medicine, the ACMG amended its recommendation to put more weight on shared decision making and patient autonomy. Patients have a right to decline clinical sequencing if the risk of incidental findings causing stress and anxiety outweighs the benefits of testing. More research is being done to group gene variants by disease type and to identify clinical linkages (McCormick et al. 2014). These advances will allow better discussion between the patient and provider before the test is ordered and should improve clinical results.

DTC genetic testing is projected to be a $230 million industry by 2018 (Su 2013). Of greater interest to the healthcare field is the growing number of centers of excellence in **individualized medicine**, the emerging practice of medicine that uses an individual's genetic profile to guide decisions about the prevention, diagnosis, and treatment of disease (also called *personalized medicine* or *precision medicine*). For example, Emory University,

Individualized medicine
Emerging practice of medicine that uses an individual's genetic profile to guide decisions about the prevention, diagnosis, and treatment of disease; also called *personalized medicine* or *precision medicine*.

Medical College of Wisconsin, and Mayo Clinic are leading the way in genomics research and patient care. Emory Genetics Laboratory (http://geneticslab.emory.edu) offers its patients a range of new and recently updated next-generation sequencing panels. These panels feature coverage of the entire genome and the mutation spectrum in clinically relevant genes for a particular phenotype, thereby reducing the incidence of variation across the clinical findings. Emory's Department of Human Genetics aims to bring genetic discoveries to the patient's bedside without delay. To do so, the department combines a team of basic research faculty with a comprehensive clinical genetics division of practicing physicians. In other words, the department is blending the areas of genetic discovery and patient care. This synthesis puts the Department of Human Genetics, which ranks among the top departments in the country, at the forefront of contemporary translational research and training.

Scientists at the Human and Molecular Genetics Center of the Medical College of Wisconsin (www.hmgc.mcw.edu/) work with the Children's Hospital of Wisconsin to run the biggest genetics program in the state and are national leaders in whole-genome sequencing. Approximately one-third of all pediatric hospitalizations are because of genetic disorders. The Human and Molecular Genetics Center has programs in general genomics, such as chromosomal abnormalities, evaluation of developmental delays, failure to thrive, birth defects, and skeletal dysplasias. Its scientists see children and adults with known or suspected genetic disorders.

These organizations have been joined by Mayo Clinic, through its Center for Individualized Medicine (http://mayoresearch.mayo.edu/center-for-individualized-medicine/). It has developed drug–gene alerts that are triggered in the patient's electronic health record (EHR) to guide the clinician regarding prescription choices and dosing recommendations. The center also performs pharmacogenomic testing to find out whether a medication is the most effective treatment for the individual, what the best dose might be, and what side effects could occur. The center seamlessly integrates the latest genomic and clinical sciences to transform healthcare. Mayo Clinic has a history of providing excellent individualized medical care to its patients. The center provides further innovation by integrating knowledge of genes and the human genome into personalized care, providing targeted therapies, reduced side effects, better prevention and prediction of disease, and earlier disease intervention. A video describing Mayo's Center for Individualized Medicine can be found at http://mayoresearch.mayo.edu/center-for-individualized-medicine/vision-for-individualized-medicine.asp.

POPULATION HEALTH

Population health is a critical component of accountable care organizations (ACOs; see Chapter 9). The term refers to the health outcomes of a group of individuals, including the distribution of such outcomes in the group. These groups are often geographic populations,

Population health
Health outcomes of a group of individuals, including the distribution of such outcomes in the group.

such as nations or communities, but can also be other groups such as employees, ethnic communities, disabled persons, prisoners, or any other defined population. The idea of population health gained popularity in 2007 when the Institute for Healthcare Improvement (IHI; www.ihi.org) published its concept of the Triple Aim and the Centers for Medicare & Medicaid Services adopted IHI's framework as an element of its reforms. The term *Triple Aim* refers to the simultaneous pursuit of three dimensions of improving US healthcare:

1. Improving the patient experience of care (safe, effective, patient centered, timely, efficient, and equitable)

2. Improving the health of populations

3. Reducing the per capita cost of healthcare

Though the terms *population health* and *individualized medicine* seem contradictory, the two can complement each other. If we are able to measure and store genetic and genomic information, we should be able to model the progression of a particular disease common in a population. A major scientific focus is to use data, information, and knowledge to build public health benefits. Even the US public health system has shifted its focus from public health promotion and disease prevention to predictive analytics and specific population assessment (CDC 2015). Major factors such as medical care, education, and income are outside of public health authority and responsibility, and current resources do not allow adequate attention to emerging public health priorities. Our current public health system has some data and information on populations, but more funding is needed to progress further. Hospitals and public health agencies should be partners in population health initiatives.

Heartland Regional Medical Center in St. Joseph, Missouri, was involved in setting up an ACO in 2012 to further develop its involvement in population health. It was able to identify high-risk patients—those with one or more chronic conditions not under control—and provide comprehensive care management. Its EHR system was able to identify patients who were taking six or more medications, who used the emergency department (ED) twice in a month or three times in six months, or who had a hospital admission. The hospital assigned a risk score based on predictive analytics. These patients represented about 5 percent of its Medicare population. It provided interventions (such as weight monitoring for heart failure), social assessments, nutrition and medication compliance assessments, and fall-risk assessments. Nurse practitioners visited patients in their homes to prevent readmission. Considering the bonus the hospital received from Medicare and the expenses incurred, the program broke even. But the organization also learned how to better manage that high-risk population (Larkin 2014).

Even the US Navy is on board with population health. The 2014 Military Health Innovation Award went to a multiyear program called the Integrated Health Community

Initiative. The Navy developed a patient scorecard that pulls information from hospital databases into one document that makes it easy to read and interpret. The scorecard includes the patient's chronic diseases, ED visits, hospital admissions, medical appointments, and healthcare costs. It is used by a primary care team to customize and target individual patient intervention measures to optimize health and reduce costs (Kowitz 2014).

Another example of population health is the Hispaniola case study found in Chapter 7. Although the countries share one island, they have vastly different public health needs. Studying the gaps for each will yield different strategies to improve the population's health. Population health management (PHM) has two aims that will help with the cost-reduction challenges presented by healthcare reform: better management of the chronically ill and health maintenance for the healthy through preventive care (IHTT 2012).

The implementation of PHM includes the following steps:

1. *Identify your population through a community assessment.* Determine what population or community you want to affect. If you set up a program that is not helpful to the community, the program will fail. The organization must be able to apply all three dimensions of the Triple Aim: delivering safe and effective care, improving health, and lowering total cost. Where can you make the most difference?

2. *Prioritize risk factors.* Use focus groups to complete a gap analysis. In what ways can your organization improve the care currently offered? Is it patient centered, timely, efficient, and equitable? You may not be able to tackle all community problems, but identify those that contribute to increased healthcare costs, readmissions, or patient mortality.

3. *Commit to provider education on PHM.* Physicians were primarily taught to treat individuals. Healthcare organizations can help providers master this new model by providing continuing education on the core competencies of population health. Nurse practitioners and registered nurses can benefit from new training as well.

4. *Focus on patient engagement.* Patients need to be partners in the goal of health management. Teaching them when to call the ED and when to call their primary care physician is small but important. Ensuring they have social connections or a support system will help guarantee success.

5. *Use technology to manage care.* Registries, EHRs, health information exchanges, and other technological tools for care coordination are critical to efficient and effective management. They allow one to monitor and analyze the data from specific populations and benchmark performance (Nicholson

2014). In the future, the use of mobile devices and telemedicine at home will become routine.

6. *Employ analytics to measure performance outcomes.* Three major components of strategic planning are people, data, and analytics. People are most important, but without analytics, the data are unmanageable and costly. Applying analytics tools that incorporate past medical visits and cost to project future use is key to predicting population needs (Nicholson 2014). Displaying the outcomes in a dashboard and fostering transparency also aid in performance improvement.

The future evolution of PHM will also require providers to make smarter care decisions in real time based on the data. Care teams will need to focus on proactive care, with fuller engagement from patients before and during office visits. As we shift to value-based care models, the care team will need to use EHR data in more intelligent ways that optimize care planning and improve health outcomes. In other words, the team needs to leverage data through the entire care cycle in ways that engage with patients and activate them to improve their health.

Patient-Centered Medical Homes

A key element of population health is a delivery system innovation called a patient-centered medical home (PCMH). Hospitals and health systems are moving toward this model to support PHM. The PCMH started as a demonstration project in 2006 by the American Academy of Family Physicians (see Chapter 9 for more information on PCMHs). The concept requires changing from the primary care model of seeing one patient at a time to a population-based, proactive care model focusing on prevention and high-risk, chronically ill groups of patients (Saultz et al. 2015).

The National Committee for Quality Assurance offers recognition to organizations that meet the standard for a PCMH. It describes three elements that define a PCMH:

1. Holistic, coordinated care focused on what the patient wants it to be

2. Clinician–patient relationships that expand beyond annual or periodic appointments

3. Use of information technology, such as registries, to support the Triple Aim and improve population health

The PCMH is not necessarily a single place or location. It is a model of primary care that includes team-based, coordinated, and patient-centered care supported by technology and focused on quality and safety (Nielsen et al. 2012). Accountable care reform includes a focus on health outcomes and system efficiencies; results from a review of 46 initiatives showed that PCMHs improved health outcomes, enhanced patient and provider experience, and reduced unnecessary and sometimes expensive hospital visits. The results of the PCMH model meet the goals of IHI's Triple Aim (Van Hasselt et al. 2015).

Telemedicine

Technology is at the center of individualized medicine, genomics research, and population health. The future of medicine also includes the use of **telemedicine** (remote diagnosis and treatment of patients by means of telecommunications technology; see Highlight 13.1) or nonvisit care for patients. The term *telemedicine*, meaning "healing at a distance," was developed by Thomas Bird in the 1970s. However, earlier examples of telemedicine are on record. For example, the Dutch physiologist Willem Einthoven invented the electrocardiograph in 1902. He subsequently used telephone wires to transmit the cardiac signals of patients 1.5 kilometers. In the 1920s, Norwegian physicians began providing medical assistance to ill and injured sailors via radio transmission. In 1967, Bird created an audiovisual link between Boston's Massachusetts General Hospital and Logan Airport. This link resulted in 1,000 medical consultations for airport employees and was the first modern example of telemedicine. Tele-ICU services began in the 1990s, connecting on-site healthcare providers with off-site consultants to discuss patient care (Trossman 2014).

Telemedicine
Remote diagnosis and treatment of patients by means of telecommunications technology.

(✱) HIGHLIGHT 13.1 Telemedicine Services

Telemedicine encompasses the following:

- Real-time remote patient consultations

- Remote monitoring of patients' vital signs and conditions

- The storing and forwarding of critical health information for analysis and diagnosis (e.g., magnetic resonance imaging results and EHRs)

- The provision of specialized services over long distances (e.g., teledentistry, telepharmacy, telepsychiatry, mobile health)

- The wide availability of health information to patients and caregivers

Source: Adapted from Broadband Expanded (2013).

Similarly, Mayo Clinic's entrance into the world of telemedicine during the 1960s explored the use of radio, telephone, microwave, two-way television, and computer and satellite technologies to link rural areas to specialty care. In 1967, Mayo Clinic began telephone transmission of electrocardiographic (ECG) signals between Saint Marys Hospital and Methodist Hospital in Rochester, Minnesota. In 1971, the distance was expanded when two Mayo Clinic cardiovascular physicians participated in a transoceanic transmission of ECGs from a hospital in Sydney, Australia, to Mayo Clinic. The transmission was initiated by telephone and involved cable, telephone, and satellite technologies. Continuing its leadership in telemedicine, on April 12, 1978, Mayo participated in its first two-way, live, intercontinental exchange via a 45-minute live telecast between Mayo staff in Rochester and the medical staff of a hospital in Sydney. The program was brought to Australia by the use of phone lines, microwaves, a domestic American satellite, and an international satellite over the Pacific (Mayo Clinic 2014).

Because it deploys troops across the world, the US military was an early adopter of telemedicine. About 55 percent of its telemedicine activities is devoted to treating behavioral health issues such as posttraumatic stress disorder. A HIPAA (Health Insurance Portability and Accountability Act)-compliant text-messaging system allows counselors to communicate with soldiers to track their moods. According to a study by the Affiliated Workers Association, more than 36 million Americans have already used telemedicine in some way, and it estimates as many as 70 percent of doctor visits can be handled over the phone. This innovation could be a cost-efficient solution for the future (Ehley 2014).

The following innovations are among the most cutting-edge ideas in telemedicine (Kim 2013):

◆ *A HealthSpot* is a telephone booth–type station that could be deployed at employer sites, universities, and other locations. It would provide a private, spacious (more than a telephone booth) place to have face-to-face videoconferences with a provider. A patient could take her vital signs there and transmit the information to her physician. A HealthSpot would support access to an EHR to assist with provider communication and medication prescription.

◆ *Handheld telemedicine kits* are personal take-home kits, including the medical devices needed to conduct first-line patient exams, integrated with tablet computers.

◆ *Rural school–based telehealth clinics* are telemedicine deployed in rural areas of the United States that are still home to underserved children. The use of telemedicine has given children access to basic primary care services.

◆ *iPads* enable the use of the program VSee to videoconference one-on-one with a physician. VSee provides integration with medical diagnostic tools such as stethoscopes, otoscopes, ultrasounds, X-rays, and more.

◆   *Interactive patient care* can employ telemedicine in the hospital setting, taking advantage of interactive computer screens to teach patients about upcoming procedures and their medications and to provide a mechanism to communicate electronically with their nurses about pain medications and other needs. Interactive patient care can enhance patient engagement while decreasing the need for face-to-face contact.

◆   *A telemedicine robot* links a patient and a physician in different locations. The robot can zoom in to examine the patient and allows physician-to-physician communication.

STRATEGIC PLANNING FOR HEALTHCARE VALUE

Patients, employers, and the government want high-quality, low-cost healthcare. The degree to which organizations successfully coordinate high quality with low cost reflects the value of the care they are delivering.

While planning for healthcare value, strategists must consider all of the topics presented in this book:

◆   The development of a mission, vision, and culture that support change

◆   The transformational approach to leadership

◆   Evaluation of strengths, weaknesses, opportunities, and threats through SWOT analysis

◆   The use of health information technology

◆   Examination of financial data

◆   Healthcare marketing

◆   Opportunities for joint ventures, mergers, and affiliations (with physicians and with other organizations)

◆   Compliance with pay-for-performance initiatives

The list does not end there, but guided by these basic elements, strategic planners in healthcare have a solid foundation on which to build an organization that provides the high value sought in healthcare today.

SUMMARY

With the Triple Aim, the future of healthcare has a clear direction: the field must move toward providing high-quality care at a reduced cost to a greater number of people. Using technology is a natural part of the twenty-first century, and healthcare will be a part of that through telemedicine advancements. Healthcare organizations must also continue to support research activities, such as those with genomics, working to find approaches to individual situations that zero in on a solution.

EXERCISES

REVIEW QUESTIONS

1. What is individualized medicine? What value does it bring in a competitive market?
2. Why is collaboration between physicians and health systems important in developing innovative and cost-effective processes of care for predictive genomics? Provide an example of a potential new business line.
3. Where would PHM fit in the strategic plan of a hospital, a clinic, or an integrated system? How would you go about assessing community or population needs?
4. What are the important characteristics of a PCMH? How could telemedicine be a part of the PCMH?

COASTAL MEDICAL CENTER EXERCISE

The newly hired CEO has been investigating the declining performance of Coastal Medical Center (CMC) and was given clear direction by the board of trustees to get the organization back on track. How can population health and individualized medicine help CMC move forward on a new road to success?

COASTAL MEDICAL CENTER QUESTIONS

1. If CMC decides that genomics and individualized medicine are an appropriate strategic planning focus, where would it go to find the human capital necessary to move forward?
2. How can you develop an estimate of the profitability of individualized medicine at CMC?
3. How can CMC use the concept of population health to improve performance?

INDIVIDUAL EXERCISES

1. Has someone you know experienced a treatment that incorporated individualized medicine or genomics? What was his experience? Would you want your genome mapped and the results shared with you?
2. Discuss the implementation of and technology required for telemedicine.

REFERENCES

Broadband Expanded. 2013. "Broadband and Telemedicine: Stats, Data, and Observations." Published January. www.broadbandexpanded.com/policymakerfiles/telemedicine/Telemedicine_Stats&Data.pdf.

Centers for Disease Control and Prevention (CDC). 2015. "The Public Health System and the 10 Essential Public Health Services." Updated May 29. www.cdc.gov/nphpsp/essentialservices.html.

Clinton, W. 2000. "Speech on the Completion of the First Survey of the Entire Human Genome Project." US National Archives and Records Administration. Published June 26. http://clinton5.nara.gov/WH/New/html/genome-20000626.html.

Collins, F. S., and M. A. Hamburg. 2013. "First FDA Authorization for Next-Generation Sequencer." *New England Journal of Medicine* 369 (25): 2369–71.

Collins, F. S., and A. Prabhakar. 2013. "BRAIN Initiative Challenges Researchers to Unlock Mysteries of Human Mind." *The White House* (blog). Published April 2. www.whitehouse.gov/blog/2013/04/02/brain-initiative-challenges-researchers-unlock-mysteries-human-mind.

Ehley, B. 2014. "Why Telemedicine Is the Future of the Health Care Industry." *The Week*. Published April 23. http://theweek.com/articles/447611/telemedicine-future-health-care-industry.

Hayden, E. C. 2014. "Technology: The $1,000 Genome." *Nature* 507 (7492): 294–95.

Institute for Health Technology Transformation (IHTT). 2012. *Population Health Management: A Roadmap for Provider-Based Automation in a New Era of Healthcare*. Accessed January 22, 2015. http://ihealthtran.com/pdf/PHMReport.pdf.

Kim, J. 2013. "12 Telemedicine Innovations That Will Shape Healthcare's Future." *CIO*. Published May 20. www.cio.com/article/2369849/healthcare/101906-12-Telemedicine-Innovations-That-Will-Shape-Healthcares-Future.html.

Kowitz, R. E. 2014. "Navy Medicine Initiative Receives Military Health System Innovation Award." *America's Navy*. Published December 5. www.navy.mil/submit/display.asp?story_id=84729.

Larkin, H. 2014. "Lessons for Hospitals Transitioning to Population Health Management." *Hospitals & Health Networks*. Published December 9. www.hhnmag.com/Magazine/2014/Dec/fea-pophealth-population-health-care-lessons.

Mayo Clinic. 2014. "Advances in Medicine: Telemedicine at Mayo." Accessed January 26, 2015. www.mayoclinic.org/tradition-heritage/telemedicine.html.

McCormick, J. B., R. R. Sharp, G. Farrugia, N. M. Lindor, D. Babovic-Vuksanovic, M. J. Borad, A. H. Bryce, R. J. Caselli, M. J. Ferber, K. J. Johnson, K. N. Lazaridis, R. R. McWilliams, J. A. Murray, A. S. Parker, K. A. Schahl, and E. D. Wieben. 2014. "Genomic Medicine and Incidental Findings: Balancing Actionability and Patient Autonomy." *Mayo Clinic Proceedings* 89 (6): 718–21.

National Human Genome Research Institute (NHGRI). 2015. "A Brief Guide to Genomics." National Institutes of Health. Published August 27. www.genome.gov/18016863.

Nicholson, J. 2014. "What Is the Future of Population Health Management?" *HIT Consultant*. Published January 7. http://hitconsultant.net/2014/07/07/future-of-population-health-management/.

Nielsen, M., B. Langner, C. Zema, T. Hacker, and P. Grundy. 2012. *Benefits of Implementing the Primary Care Patient-Centered Medical Home: A Review of Cost and Quality Results, 2012*. Patient-Centered Primary Care Collaborative. Published September. www.pcpcc.org/sites/default/files/media/benefits_of_implementing_the_primary_care_pcmh.pdf.

Saultz, J. W., S. M. Jones, S. H. McDaniel, B. Bagley, T. McCormally, J. E. Marker, J. A. Weida, and L. A. Green. 2015. "A New Foundation for the Delivery and Financing of American Health Care." *Family Medicine* 47 (8): 612–19.

Su, P. 2013. "Direct-to-Consumer Genetic Testing: A Comprehensive View." *Yale Journal of Biology and Medicine* 86 (3): 359–65.

Trossman, S. 2014. "Back to the Future?" *American Nurse* 46 (5): 1–6.

Van Hasselt, M., N. McCall, V. Keyes, S. G. Wensky, and K. W. Smith. 2015. "Total Cost of Care Lower Among Medicare Fee-for-Service Beneficiaries Receiving Care from Patient-Centered Medical Homes." *Health Services Research* 50 (1): 253–72.

EPILOGUE: TEN CONCEPTS FOR EFFECTIVE LEADERSHIP

R. Timothy Stack

Leadership plays an important role in promoting change in a rapidly evolving healthcare industry. The literature shows that outstanding leadership is associated with future organizational success. By incorporating the concepts shown in Exhibit E.1 into your leadership repertoire, you will position yourself and your organization for outstanding achievement.

HAVE MENTORS

Mentors are experienced leaders who can be consulted for advice on business and career planning issues. Mentoring is an opportunity for younger leaders to take advantage of the knowledge and experience of individuals who have "traveled the leadership road." Many organizations have a formal mentoring program that assigns senior executives as mentors to junior leaders. Informal mentors are equally important. Informal mentors are individuals outside the organization who can be consulted on a more personal level and serve as a sounding board for business issues, ethical dilemmas, or career planning purposes.

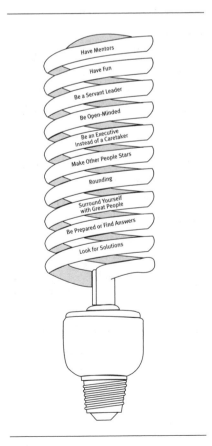

EXHIBIT E.1
Ten Concepts for Effective Leadership

- Have Mentors
- Have Fun
- Be a Servant Leader
- Be Open-Minded
- Be an Executive Instead of a Caretaker
- Make Other People Stars
- Rounding
- Surround Yourself with Great People
- Be Prepared or Find Answers
- Look for Solutions

HAVE FUN

Individuals routinely spend eight hours per day at the workplace, so having fun at work is important. As you look at your future career, select work that is meaningful and inspiring to you. You can have fun by connecting with others on a personal level and offering positive feedback. Identify individuals with negative energy early on and take steps to insulate yourself from their temperament. When your job stops being fun, consider actions you can take to reinstate the fun or think about making a career change. Remember that all people need to maintain balance in their lives. For most people, the balance involves religion, family, and work. Establish priorities. Place work after religion and family. Healthcare leaders who place a high value on broader issues such as religion, family, and community relationships can make difficult decisions from a wider perspective. History has shown that many inappropriate and unethical decisions were made on the basis of one-dimensional thinking that considered only how the organization would be affected as a result of the decision.

BE A SERVANT LEADER

A servant leader believes that each member of the organization makes a meaningful contribution toward meeting overall goals. As a servant leader, the issue is not how you can accomplish your work, but how you can assist your team in meeting the organization's goals. Servant leaders understand that their personal success and the organization's success are not driven by their individual efforts but by their team. This perspective can be liberating because it takes the pressure off the leader and puts it on the team. It also recognizes that the team's combined effort is more valuable than the contribution of any single individual.

BE OPEN-MINDED

Older senior executives tend to think they have seen it all and have all the answers. In a complex, dynamic industry, leaders need to be open-minded and create an environment that fosters communication, innovation, and change. The best ideas will percolate up from within the organization.

BE AN EXECUTIVE INSTEAD OF A CARETAKER

The authors have seen the impact that caretaker leaders, who believe their function is to safeguard resources, can have on an organization. In every case they observed, the organization stagnated, failed to take advantage of opportunities in the marketplace, and ultimately declined in profitability. Organizations whose leaders have the caretaker mentality fail to attract the best leadership and clinical talent. The best talent flocks to organizations that support innovation and are successful in the marketplace. Be an executive who can make decisions, not just a caretaker.

MAKE OTHER PEOPLE STARS

The authors have received many awards and have been humbled by the realization that, in many cases, another individual or team was responsible for the accomplishment. As a matter of personal ethics, make sure the recognition is placed where it is deserved. Rewards and recognition are part of a positive feedback loop that encourages recipients to continue their outstanding efforts.

ROUNDING

Research shows that a leadership concept called *management by walking around*, or *rounding*, is important to organizational success. It is not only a way to get to know the individuals and facilities in the organization but also a convenient method of exercising! Walking around the organization helps the leader gain a greater perspective about each individual's critical, integral role in meeting the organization's mission. Rounding also helps the leader better understand the overall healthcare system and develop interpersonal relationships with staff. Rounding also lets staff members know the organization values their contributions and that leaders are accessible.

SURROUND YOURSELF WITH GREAT PEOPLE

Academic knowledge and practical experience are important to success, but in healthcare, no one individual could possibly develop the level of knowledge or skills necessary to succeed alone. Leaders should focus their efforts on identifying, hiring, training, and motivating the best individuals healthcare has to offer. This search begins by identifying individuals who have a track record of success. Once they have been identified and have demonstrated their knowledge and outstanding performance, they should be rewarded with appropriate financial compensation and other organizational recognition. Rewards are essential to retaining the great people who will lead the organization to future success.

BE PREPARED OR FIND ANSWERS

No single individual knows all the questions or has all the answers. Be willing to commit the time and effort to find them. If you do not know the answer to someone's question, be honest and say so, and then research the issue. Close the loop by getting back to the person with the answer in a timely manner. Giving half-baked answers without supporting data may cause the organization to move forward in the decision-making process with invalid information.

LOOK FOR SOLUTIONS

The healthcare industry is dealing with manifold problems that require innovative solutions. Healthcare leaders need to proactively search for solutions that will support the organization and the community it serves; supporting the status quo is not acceptable. In short, if you are not part of the solution, you are part of the problem.

GLOSSARY

Accountable care organization (ACO). Group of doctors, hospitals, and other healthcare providers who come together voluntarily to give coordinated, high-quality care to Medicare patients.

Adjusted occupied bed. Number of inpatient occupied beds, adjusted (increased) to account for the bed occupancy attributed to outpatient services, partial hospitalization, and home services.

Adult health day care center. Facility that provides services to patients requiring long-term care and helps family caregivers with their responsibilities.

Ambulatory surgery center (ASC). Facility at which outpatient surgeries (i.e., surgeries not requiring an overnight stay) are performed, often at a price that is less than that charged by hospitals.

Balanced scorecard (BSC). Tool that allows organizations to assess their missions by evaluating specific objectives and metrics across multiple domains.

Benchmarking. Examination of other organizations' business practices and products for purposes of comparing and improving one's own company.

Big data. Data sets of such massive size that they are difficult to process using traditional computation tools.

Board of directors. Governing body appointed to hold fiduciary responsibility for the organization.

Bundled payment. Single payment made to providers or healthcare facilities (or jointly to both) for all services rendered to treat a given condition or provide a given treatment.

Charisma. Leadership charm that provokes strong emotions and loyalty in followers.

Chief executive officer (CEO). Highest-ranking executive in an organization, responsible for strategic planning, hiring senior leadership, and managing operations.

Chief financial officer (CFO). Executive responsible for planning, organizing, and directing all financial activities.

Chief information officer (CIO). Executive responsible for planning, organizing, and directing all information systems in the organization.

Chief medical officer (CMO). Executive responsible for planning and implementing programs to improve the quality of patient care.

Chief nursing officer (CNO). Nurse executive responsible for planning, organizing, and directing all nursing activities.

Churn rate. Ratio indicating the quantity of new patients relative to existing patients.

Clinical information system. Technology applied at the point of care and designed to support the acquisition of information as well as providing storage and processing capabilities.

Clinical integration. Coordination of patient care between hospitals and physicians across the healthcare continuum.

Code of ethics. Guide to standards of behavior and ethical conduct.

Community health needs assessment (CHNA). State, tribal, local, or territorial health assessment that identifies key health needs and issues through systematic, comprehensive data collection and analysis.

Comorbidity. Coexistence of one or more medical conditions in addition to the initial diagnosis.

Cost of capital. Opportunity cost of making a specific investment; that is, the rate of return an organization must achieve to make a capital investment worthwhile.

Credentialing. Process used to evaluate a physician's qualifications and practice history.

Critical access hospital (CAH). Rural hospital certified to charge a fee-for-service rate in return for providing community access to emergency department and basic hospital services.

Culture. Collection of values and norms shared by a group of individuals.

Dashboard. Tool that links strategic goals to operating performance.

Days accounts receivable. Average number of days an organization takes to collect payments on goods sold and services provided, calculated as follows: Average accounts payable (in dollars) × 365 (days per year) ÷ Sales revenue.

Debt service. Cash required over a given period for the repayment of interest and principal on a debt.

Digital media. Web-based methods of making contact with consumers.

Direct-to-consumer telehealth. Online medical services that market directly to individual patients.

Donabedian framework. Model for evaluating the quality of medical care based on three criteria: structure, process, and outcomes.

Downstream value. Revenue captured by the services a patient uses after his initial visit, such as subsequent testing or return visits.

Efficiency frontier. The best investment of resources for the best possible profits and outcomes of care.

E-health. Broad range of data processing and computer networking applications (including use of the Internet) in healthcare.

Electronic whiteboard. Electronic device that looks much like a traditional whiteboard but allows content written or drawn on the screen to be transmitted to a computer.

End-of-life care (EoLC). Care provided to improve the quality of life of patients who are facing life-threatening disease or disability and are not expected to recover.

Equity-based joint venture. Organization whose ownership is divided between a hospital and physicians on the basis of their contributions to the enterprise.

Ethics. Moral duty, values, and obligation.

External rewards. Tangible incentives outside an individual that motivate that person to perform, such as money and gifts; the threat of punishment for nonperformance could also be a motivator.

Fiduciary. An individual or a group who acts for and on behalf of another in a relationship of trust and confidence.

Financial plan. Document that analyzes financial information to demonstrate potential performance of a new business initiative.

Five Ps of healthcare marketing. Key marketing elements that are used to ensure a complete assessment of needs. In healthcare, they include people, product, price, place, and promotion.

Fixed cost. Cost incurred despite volume or use of a particular service. Examples of fixed-cost elements include buildings, equipment, and some salaried labor.

Force field analysis. Examination of the forces helping or hindering organizational change.

For-profit health system. Organization that comprises hospitals owned by equity-based investors and that has a well-defined organizational goal of profit maximization.

For-profit hospital. Investor-owned hospital that must pay federal and state taxes on its profits.

Full-time equivalent (FTE). Total number of full-time and part-time employees, which is expressed as an equivalent number of full-time employees.

Gap analysis. Comparison of an organization's current standing and its target performance.

Genomics. Study of the entire genome (the complete set of DNA in an organism).

Goals. Written objectives that can be measured to assess performance.

Groupthink. Within a group, the tendency to maintain harmony by incorporating minimal input and making rapid decisions.

Health information technology. Information and communication technology in healthcare, such as electronic health records, clinical alerts and reminders, and decision support systems.

Healthcare business plan. Method by which a healthcare organization evaluates future investment in a new business initiative.

Healthcare data analysts. Individuals hired by healthcare organizations to compile, validate, and analyze crucial medical data.

Healthcare data warehouse. Database that integrates multiple types of data, such as patient demographic information, comprehensive clinical information, and resource utilization data.

Healthy People 2020. A comprehensive analysis of the US population's healthcare needs and a statement of goals and measures by the US Department of Health & Human Services, around which local and regional planning can take place; also the name of a ten-year effort to achieve the goals it outlines.

High-performance work processes. Work processes used to systematically pursue ever-higher levels of overall organizational and individual performance (emphasizing, e.g., quality, productivity, innovation rate).

Horizontal integration. Expansion along current lines of business into new geographic areas, often through mergers with other organizations, for purposes of increasing market share.

Hospice care. Services that provide EoLC or palliative care to a patient and her family when the patient is no longer responding to treatment.

Hospital acquisition. Purchase of a hospital by another facility or multihospital system.

Hospital merger. Combining of two or more hospitals.

Hospitalist model. Arrangement under which an inpatient physician assumes primary responsibility for managing a patient on admission to the hospital and supervising all inpatient care until the patient is discharged from the hospital.

Incentive. Reward that motivates someone to take action or perform, such as a bonus payment awarded for achieving a goal.

Income statement. Summary of an organization's revenue and expenses over a certain period.

Indirect marketing. Advertising that does not directly communicate with consumers but rather leverages brand recognition and consumer awareness of an organization's presence in the marketplace.

Individualized medicine. Emerging practice of medicine that uses an individual's genetic profile to guide decisions about the prevention, diagnosis, and treatment of disease; also called *personalized medicine* or *precision medicine*.

Infrastructure. Underlying foundation or basic framework.

Inpatient rehabilitation facility (IRF). Facility that provides restorative services for traumatic injury, acute illness, and chronic conditions.

Integrated delivery system (IDS). Network of hospitals that enables better use of staff and financial resources and promotes greater operational efficiencies across the continuum of healthcare services.

Integrated physician model. Series of partnerships between hospitals and physicians developed over time.

Internal data. Information and facts that can be gathered from sources within an organization.

Internal rate of return (IRR). Interest rate at which the NPV of all the cash flows (both positive and negative) from a project or an investment equal zero. The term is used in capital budgeting to measure and compare the profitability of investments.

Internal rewards. Feelings that arise out of performing an activity and that motivate an individual to perform, such as the enjoyment from creating a work of art or playing a sport.

Intranet. Computer network using Internet protocol technology to share information, operational systems, or computer services internally in an organization.

Joint venture. Partnership formed between two or more organizations that draws on their combined resources to accomplish a specific purpose.

Leadership. Ability to guide, influence, and inspire individuals to meet organizational goals.

Leapfrog Group. Independent healthcare purchaser, founded by major employers, that uses purchasing power to improve the quality and efficiency of US healthcare services.

Magnet hospital designation. Status awarded by the American Nurses Credentialing Center to hospitals whose nursing staff meets certain criteria based on quality and professional practice.

Magnet Recognition Program. Sponsored by the American Nurses Credentialing Center, a program recognizing healthcare organizations for quality patient care, nursing excellence, and innovations in professional nursing practice.

Marketing plan. Written document guiding marketing activities by considering the competitive marketplace, the healthcare organization's capabilities, and areas with the greatest economic potential.

Meaningful use. CMS-sponsored program imposing a standard for using certified EHR technology to improve the overall quality of healthcare by providing financial incentives.

Medical foundation. Arrangement under which independent physicians sell their practices to a medical foundation and then contract with the foundation to provide professional services at the foundation's practice sites.

Medical staff. Full- and part-time physicians and dentists who are approved and given privileges to provide healthcare to patients in a hospital or another healthcare facility; may be employed by the facility or granted admitting privileges to practice.

Medical tourism. Traveling outside one's local area for higher-value or unique healthcare services; also called medical travel, health tourism, or global healthcare.

Medicare Payment Advisory Commission (MedPAC). Government agency composed of 17 members and established by the Balanced Budget Act of 1997 to advise Congress on issues that affect the Medicare program.

Mission. Written statement of an organization's fundamental purpose.

Morale. Positive emotions and sense of common purpose among members of a group.

Motivation. Act or process of energizing people to overcome barriers and achieve outstanding performance.

Net present value (NPV). Figure calculated on the basis of discounted cash flow to evaluate the financial worth of a business initiative; the amount of money a business initiative is projected to earn minus the amount of money originally invested in it.

Not-for-profit health system. Health system organized as a not-for-profit corporation. Based on charitable purpose and frequently affiliated with a religious denomination, this means of care delivery is traditional.

Not-for-profit hospital. Hospital designated as a 501(c)(3) organization by the Internal Revenue Service and eligible for tax-exempt status.

Nurse-sensitive patient outcomes. Changes in health status that are dependent on nursing interventions.

Opportunities. Significant new business initiatives available to a healthcare organization.

Organizational culture. Shared beliefs among individuals in an organization.

Palliative care. Healthcare approach that improves the quality of life of patients and their families facing life-threatening illness through the prevention and relief of suffering.

Patient portal. Secure website that gives patients 24-hour access to personal health information.

Patient-centered medical home (PCMH). Care delivery model whereby a primary care physician coordinates patient treatment to ensure it is timely, cost-effective, and personalized.

Payback period. Length of time it takes a new business initiative to recoup the cost of the original investment.

Payer mix. Percentage of revenue coming from private insurance versus government insurance versus individuals. The *mix* is important because Medicare and Medicaid often pay hospitals less than what it costs to treat patients.

Pay-for-performance (P4P) program. Initiative implemented by the government, insurance companies, and other groups to reward providers for meeting certain performance targets in the delivery of healthcare services.

Population health. Health outcomes of a group of individuals, including the distribution of such outcomes in the group.

Post-acute care (PAC). Services provided after discharge from an acute care hospital.

Print media. Newspapers, magazines, brochures, and billboards.

Pro forma financial statement. Statement prepared before a business initiative is undertaken to model the anticipated financial results of the initiative.

Profit margin. Difference between how much money the hospital brings in and how much it spends.

Prospective payment system (PPS). Reimbursement mechanism for inpatient healthcare services that pays a predetermined rate for treatment of specific illnesses.

Quality. Standard of healthcare provision that reflects the goals and values currently adhered to in the medical care system and the society in which it exists.

Radio and television media. Programming distributed via television or radio.

Regression analysis. Mathematical method of determining the relationships between variables, usually the effect of one variable on another, such as the effect of a price increase on demand.

Safety-net providers. Healthcare providers that deliver a significant amount of care to uninsured, Medicaid, and other disadvantaged patients.

Senior marketing executive. Executive responsible for developing, directing, and executing a comprehensive, systemwide marketing strategy that includes advertising, market research, production, and sales.

Servant leadership. Culture in which employees become partners in fulfilling the organization's mission.

Skilled nursing facility (SNF). Facility that treats elderly patients with chronic diseases who need nursing care, rehabilitation, and other healthcare services.

Social media. Websites and applications that enable users to create and share content or to participate in social networking sites, collaborative services, blogs, content hosting sites, and virtual communities.

Stage charisma. Ability of a leader to command audience attention in an impressive manner. This quality does not require hard, authoritarian, overbearing force, but rather engaging individuals on a personal level using sincerity, credibility, concern, certainty, and hope.

Stakeholder. One who is involved in or affected by an organization's actions.

Strategic planning. Process by which an organization determines its future direction by defining the actions that will shape it and developing objectives and techniques for measuring ongoing performance.

Strengths. Current factors that have prompted outstanding organizational performance.

SWOT analysis. Examination of an organization's internal strengths and weaknesses, its opportunities for growth and improvement, and the threats the external environment presents to its survival.

Systems approach. Management that emphasizes the interdependence of elements inside and outside an organization.

Telehealth. Use of telecommunications to deliver health services.

Telemedicine. Remote diagnosis and treatment of patients by means of telecommunications technology.

Therapeutic alliance. Partnership between patient and providers that involves collaboration and negotiation to arrive at mutual goals.

Threats. Factors that could negatively affect organizational performance.

Total cost. All hospital expenditures, including facility operating costs.

Transactional leadership. Model of leadership that emphasizes giving rewards for good performance or taking corrective action for poor performance.

Transformational leadership. Model of leadership that emphasizes flexibility, selflessness, and interpersonal motivation to maximize individual and group potential.

Value. Level of consumer benefit received per dollar spent.

Value frontier. Organizations that create the highest value in healthcare.

Value-based purchasing. Centers for Medicare & Medicaid Services initiative that rewards acute care hospitals with incentive payments for the quality of care they provide to people with Medicare.

Values. Social principles, goals, and standards of an organization.

Variable cost. Cost that changes with volume or use and can be saved by the hospital if a service is not provided. Examples include medication, test reagents, and disposable supplies.

Vertical integration. Expansion to a new line of business located somewhere along the continuum of care (e.g., a hospital that normally provides acute care opening a primary care clinic or acquiring a skilled nursing facility).

Virtual health system. Network of organizations created through the use of health information technology.

Vision. Short, inspiring statement of what an organization intends to achieve in the future.

Weaknesses. Organizational factors that increase healthcare costs or reduce healthcare quality.

Webcast. Video broadcast of an event transmitted across the Internet.

INDEX

Note: Italicized page locators refer to figures or tables in exhibits.

Accountability: digital health data and, 132

Accountable care organizations (ACOs), 43, 119, 130, 132, 163, 190, 221, 222; advent of, 81; clinical integration and, 179–80; definition of, 183; disadvantages of, 184–85; growth in number of, 185; human resources and, 155; patient-centered medical home and, 181, 182; physician–hospital integration and, 183–85; population health and, 251–52; post-acute care providers and, 203

Accreditation: healthcare quality and, 242

Acquisitions, of hospitals, 43, 53, 214–15, 216; definition of, 214; mergers *vs.,* 215

Acute care hospitals: inpatient rehabilitation services in, 203

Adjusted occupied bed, 2

Adult health day care centers, 208–9; cost of, 208

Advance care planning, 204, 205

Advertising, 116, 117, 124. *See also* Healthcare marketing

Advisory Board Company, 204

Affiliated Workers Association, 256

Affordable Care Act (ACA), 43, 135, 140, 200, 215, 237; accountable care organizations and, 180, 184; community health needs assessments and, 123; digital health data and, 132; expanded insurance coverage under, 82; healthcare communication and, 169, 170; insurance exchange program, 235–36; integrated care and, 104; joint ventures and, 187; Medicaid expansion and, 94; Medicare reimbursements and, 105; passage of, 73, 94, 229; patient-centered medical home and, 182; physician–hospital alignment and, 179; value-based service model and, 88; vertical integration and, 220

Agency for Healthcare Research and Quality (AHRQ), 231; Healthcare Cost and Utilization Project, 143; Inpatient Quality Indicators, 239; medical home functions/attributes in definition by, 182

Aging population: chronic diseases and, 199, 209; demographics of, 198, 200

Allocation of resources. *See* Resource allocation

Ambulatory surgery centers (ASCs), 83

American Academy of Family Physicians, 254

American College of Healthcare Executives (ACHE), 34; *Code of Ethics*, 68–69, 71; on diversity in healthcare management, 86

American College of Medical Genetics and Genomics (ACMG), 250

American College of Surgeons, 236, 242

American Community Survey (ACS), 141

American Hospital Association, 39, 236; *Engaging Trustees in the Redefinition of the H*, 51; position on organizational mission, 52

American Nurses Credentialing Center (ANCC), 72, 241

American Organization of Nurse Executives, 34

American Society of Clinical Pathology, 242

Anesthesiologists: average compensation for, 186

Answering questions: effective leadership and, *263*, 265–66

Aristotle, 174

Ascension Health, 45, 216, *217*

Audience: strategic plan presentations and, 171–72, 173–75

Audio/visual support, for presentations, 172

Baby boomers: demand for post-acute care and, 198

Bad debt write-offs, 46

Balanced scorecards (BSCs), 92–93, 242

Balance sheets, 21

Bankruptcy: corporate ethical problems and, 68; of hospitals, 43, 56

Bass, Bernard M., 64

Bass's Transformational Leadership Theory, 64, 65

Benchmarking: definition of, 87; National Quality Forum, 232

Bennis, Warren, 29

Bextra, 69

Big data, 134, 139; definition of, 130; optimal use of, 130–31, 140

Billboards, 119

Bird, Thomas, 255

Blogs, 121

Board of directors: definition of, 33; members of, *35*; off-site retreats for, 50; role in strategic planning, 36–37

Bond interest tax, 46

Brochures, 116, 119

Buffet, Warren, 226

Bulletin boards, digital, 122

Bundled payments, 130, 150; definition of, 104; for post-acute care services, 198–99, 209

Burns, James MacGregor, 64

Burton, Harold, 4

Business planning, effective, 150, 163. *See also* Healthcare business plan

Business planning software, 162

California: corporate practice of medicine doctrine in, 185

California Health Care Foundation, 142

California Hospitals Assessment and Reporting Taskforce, 142

California Pay for Performance Program, 231

Cancer: genetic mapping and, 137

Capital: cost of, 153, 154

Capital allocation plan, 156

Capital funding, 157

Capitated payment: definition of, 184

Cardiologists: average compensation for, 186

Caregivers: respite services for, 208

Case-mix groups, rehabilitation services and, 203

Case study of strategic planning. *See* Coastal Medical Center (CMC) case study

Center for Medicare & Medicaid Innovation: Advance Payment accountable care organization model, 182; Pioneer accountable care organization model, 182, 184

Centers for Disease Control and Prevention (CDC), 134, 249

Centers for Medicare & Medicaid Services (CMS), 43, 140–41, 143, 231, 252; accountable care organizations and, 81, 184; Care Management for High-Cost Beneficiaries Demonstration, 231; Care Management Performance Demonstration, 231; Hospital Compare reports of, 105, 231, 233, 236, 237, 238; Hospital Quality Initiative, 231; Long-Term Care Minimum Data Set, 144; meaningful use and, 131; Medicare Shared Savings Program, 184; Nursing Home Compare, 144; Online Survey, Certification, and Reporting (OSCAR) database, 144; pay-for-performance initiatives of, 229, 230; payment incentives, 163; Physician Group Practice Demonstration, 231; post-acute care services and, 198–99; Premier Hospital Quality Initiative, 231

Central Intelligence Agency, 140

Certificate-of-need (CON), 47

Change: healthcare environment and, 62, 78, 101; participative management and, 108

Charisma: definition of, 65; internal motivation and, 66; stage, 171

Charity care, 87

Chief executive officers (CEOs): compensation for, 37–38; definition of, 33; role in strategic planning, 37–38; roles and responsibilities of, 35–36; succession planning for, 37; turnover rate in US hospitals, 37

Chief financial officers (CFOs), 38

Chief information officers (CIOs), 39–40

Chief medical officers (CMOs), 41

Chief nursing officers (CNOs), 38–39; Magnet Recognition Program and, 72–74

Children's Health Insurance Program, 140

Children's Hospital of Wisconsin, 251

Chronic disease management: telehealth and, 133

Chronic diseases: aging population and, 199, 209

Churchill, Winston, 64

Churn rate: definition of, 106

Clinical informatics specialists, 139

Clinical information systems, 130; initiatives for, 135

Clinical integration: definition of, 179; physician–hospital relationships and, 180, 190

Clinical Laboratory Improvement Amendments, 242

Clinical leaders, 41

Clinton, Bill, 73, 249

Closure, of hospitals, 43, 56; corporate ethical problems and, 68; Veterans Health Administration and Department of Defense hospitals and, 54

Coastal Medical Center (CMC) case study, 1–28; balance sheet, 16, 21; case-mix index, 17; competition, 2; corporate staff, 11–12, *12*; duplication of functions, 12; executives and middle management, 11; financial ratios, 16, 21–24; general conditions, 15–16; governing board, 5–6, *6, 7*; 8, 20; healthcare costs, 1–2; highlights, 2–4; historical perspective, 4–5; Hospital Consumer Assessment of Healthcare Providers and Systems scores, 8, 20; income statement by calendar year, 20; inpatient data and, 17, 27–28; leadership surveys, 24–25; market share analysis, 3, *3*; materials management, 13; medical staff, 7–8; new business initiatives, 16; new chief executive officer, 13–15; parent corporation, 6–7; population and household data, 1, 18–19; service and professional contracts, 12–13; special projects, 13; subsidiary companies, 9–10; value-based purchasing, 17, 25–26
Code of ethics, 68
Coding, diagnosis-related group system, 232
Codman, Ernest, 236
Cofiduciary concept, organizational ethics and, 42
Common stock: sale of, 157
Commonwealth Fund, 228
Communication: of strategic plan, 169–75
Community health needs assessment (CHNA), 123
Community Health Systems, 45
Comorbidity: definition of, 203
Comparative outcomes: quality and, 236
Competency models: of leadership, 32
Competition: value-based systems and, 227–28
Complication rates, 130

Constantine I (Roman emperor), 67
Consultants, 40–41
Continuous quality improvement (CQI), 34, 35
Continuum of care, 135, 190, 230; hospice and, 207; integration across, 180, 220; patient-centered medical home model, silos, and, 181, *183*
Corporate misconduct, 68
Corporate practice of medicine doctrine, 185
Cost of capital, 153, 154
Credentialing, 41, 72–73
Critical access hospitals: Medicare-certified, 137
Crossing the Quality Chasm (Institute of Medicine), 41
Cultural competence: goal of, 86
Cultural diversity: hospice services and, 207–8
Culture: definition of, 48. *See also* Organizational culture
Curative care: hospice care *vs.*, 205
Current strategies: strategic plans and, 86, 89–90
CVS, 130
Cyber attacks, 139
Cyrus the Great of Persia, 67

Dashboards, 95; balanced scorecards and, 242; definition of, 91; hospital, *92*
Data: internal and external, 40; quality-related, growing demand for, 236–39; transparency of, 242
Data analysts, 139
Data analytics, 129, 134, 140
Data breachers, 138–39
Data capture, 140
Data management: challenges with, 129
Data provisioning, 140
Data security, 138–39
Days accounts receivable: definition of, 14
Debt service: definition of, 9

Defense Healthcare Management System Modernization initiative, 137

Delegating leadership style, 66, *67*

Demographics: demand for post-acute care and, 198; forecasting tools and, 162; healthcare and, 200–201; marketing plan and, 157; of US aging population, 198, 200

Deoxyribonucleic acid (DNA), 249

Destination medical centers, 124

Diagnosis-related groups (DRGs), 231, 232

Digital advertising, 124

Digital bulletin boards, 122

Digital media: cost-effectiveness of, 119; definition of, 120; digital bulletin boards, 122; organizational websites, 120–21; patient portals, 121–22; social media, 121; trends in, 120–22

Digital technology, 115

Directing leadership style, 66, *67*

Direct mail, 117

Direct-to-consumer advertising (DTCA), 120

Direct-to-consumer (DTC) genetic testing, 250

Direct-to-consumer telehealth, 132–33

Disaster plans: electronic documentation and, 139

Discounted cash flow, 159, 160

Discount rate, 160

Disney, Walt, 149

Disparities in healthcare: national planning and, 94

Diversity in workplace: as competitive advantage, 84, 86

Donabedian, Avedis, 234–35

Donabedian framework, 234

Downstream revenue, 109, 110

Downstream value: definition of, 109

Duplication of services: avoiding, coordinated care and, 183

Economies of scale, 219, 220; basis of, 33; clinical integration and, 180

Efficiency: strategic plans and, 86, 88

Efficiency frontier, 88

e-health, 132–35; definition of, 132; initiatives for, 134–35, 144; landscape of, 115

Einthoven, Willem, 255

Electronic health records (EHRs), 129, 134; as competitive advantage, 83–84; drug-gene alerts in, 251; Health Insurance Portability and Accountability Act and, 85; initiatives on, 135–37; interoperability of, 131; open-source software for, 137; patient portals and, 133; quality-related data and, 239; Veterans Health Administration's system, 136–37

Electronic whiteboards, 173

Emory Medical College of Wisconsin: Department of Human Genetics, 251

Employee satisfaction: patient satisfaction and, 242

Employment: in hospital-owned group practices, 186

Encompass Home Health and Hospice: HealthSouth acquisition of, 202

Endocrinologists: average compensation for, 186

End-of-life care (EoLC): definition of, 199; hospice and palliative care, 200, 204

End results theory, 236

Engaging Patients Through Social Media, 121

Engaging Trustees in the Redefinition of the H (American Hospital Association), 51

Envisioning the National Healthcare Quality Report (Institute of Medicine), 182

Equity-based joint ventures, 188–89

Equity capital, 157

Ethics: definition of, 68; strategic planning and, 68–69

Ethics in Patient Referral Act, 155

Evidence-based medicine initiatives, 137

Excel: financial planning tools in, 162, 163

Executive vs. caretaker mentality: effective leadership and, 263, 264–65

Exponential regression, 163

External environment: trends in, 81–83

External motivation, 66

External rewards, 63, 74

Facebook, 121

Facility planning, 156

Family-practice physicians: average compensation for, 186; medical foundations and, 186

Federal Bureau of Investigation, 142

Federal Trade Commission, 220

FedStats, 141

Fee-for-service model: fully capitated accountable care organizations vs., 184

Fiduciary, 33, 42

Financial analysis tools, 162

Financial modeling, 39

Financial plans, 157–62; definition of, 157; income statement, 158; internal rate of return, 161–62; net present value, 158–61; payback period, 158; pro forma financial statements, 158

Financial ratios, 21–24

Firewalls, 138

501(c)(3) organizations, 44

Fixed cost: price analysis and, 87

Florida Department of Health, 142–43

Food and Drug Administration, 250

Force field analysis, 106–8, 107, 110; definition of, 107; healthcare model for, 107

Forecasting tools, 162–63, 164

For-profit health systems, 215, 217–18, 218

For-profit hospitals: big data and, 140; definition of, 45; equity capital and, 157; specialty, 48; strategic financial planning by, 87; strategic planning by, 53

Foursquare, 121

Franklin, Benjamin, 114

Fraud, 69

Frist, Thomas, 45

Full-time equivalents (FTEs), 2, 3, 12

Fun, effective leadership and, 263, 264

Gandhi, Mohandas, 67, 128

Gap analysis, 83, 108–9, 109, 110

Gaps: definition of, 83

Gastroenterologists: average compensation for, 186

Geisinger Health System, 216, 217

Genetic mapping, 137

Genetics, 249

Genetic testing: direct-to-consumer, 250

Genghis Khan, 67

Genome, 249

Genomics, 249, 258

Global Alliance for Genomics and Health, 137

Goals: definition of, 44

Godin, Seth, 61

Goethe, Johann Wolfgang von, 226

Google, 132, 173

Government hospitals, 45–46; specialty, 48; strategic planning by, 54

Graphic displays: for presentations, 174

Great people: effective leadership and, 263, 265

Gretzky, Wayne, 100

Gross domestic product (GDP): health-care spending (United States) as percentage of, 30–31, 78, 115, 227

Group practices: hospital-owned, 186

Growth: good strategy development and, 31

GuideStar, 143

Hackers, 138

Harrison, Debra, 197

Harrison, Jeffrey, 248

Healthcare: US population demographics and, 200–201

Healthcare business plan: capital acquisition strategy for, 157–58; definition of, 150; environmental analysis, *152,* 153; financial plan, *152,* 157–62; human resources, *152,* 154–56; marketing plan, *152,* 157; physical plant, *152,* 156–57; planning tools, 162–63; planning workflow, 151, *152;* regulatory factors, *152,* 153–54; role of, 150; sample outline, *151;* Small Business Administration resources, 150–51; statement of business purpose, 152, *152;* typical, 151

Healthcare data analysts, 139

Healthcare data warehouses, 134

Healthcare Effectiveness Data and Information Set (HEDIS), 236, 238

Healthcare environment: change in, 62, 78, 101

Healthcare Financial Management Association, 34

Healthcare Information and Management Systems Society (HIMSS), 34, 131; Electronic Medical Record Adoption Model, 135, *136*

Healthcare information databases, 129–31, 144

Healthcare information resources, 140–44; hospital data, 143; international data, 140; national data, 140–42; nursing home data, 144; state data, 142–43

Healthcare Leadership Alliance (HLA), 32, 34

Healthcare management: diversity in, 86

Healthcare marketing, 124; five Ps of, 117–18, *118,* 157; local, 123; overview, 115–16; regional, 123–24; strategic, 116. *See also* Marketing media trends

Healthcare policy, US: transformational and transactional styles in history of, 73

Healthcare quality and efficiency model, *44*

Healthcare spending: in United States, 30–31, 78, 180, *181,* 227

Healthcare strategic-planning model, *79*

Healthcare value paradigm, 250–57; individualized medicine, 250–51; patient-centered medical homes, 254–55; population health, 251–54; telemedicine, 255–57

Health information: online, 115

Health information technology (HIT), 129, 130; checklist, *138;* as competitive advantage, 83–84; definition of, 34; growing workforce in, 139–40; investment in, 130; planning for, 157; strategic initiatives in, 134–37; strategic planning for, 137–39, 144; strategic value of, 129, 144

Health insurance: expanded coverage in, 82; gender and, 200

Health Insurance Portability and Accountability Act (HIPAA), 130, 153; data security and compliance with, 138; electronic health records and, 85

Health Maintenance Organization Act, 227

Health maintenance organizations (HMOs), 42, 43, 235

HealthSouth: accounting scandal, 68, 69; inpatient rehabilitation services market and, 202–3

HealthSpot, 256

Health systems: for-profit, 215, 217–18; integrated delivery systems, 214, 216–18; international, 221–22; not-for-profit, 215, 216–17; strategic planning at health system level, 218–20; virtual, 221

Healthy People 2020, 94, 95, 141

Healthy People Project, 141

Heartland Regional Medical Center, Missouri, 252

Helping forces, 107, 108

High-performance work processes: definition of, 63

Hill, Lister, 4

Hill-Burton Act, 4

Hindering forces, 107, 108

Hippocratic Oath, 178

Hispaniola case study, 165–66, 253

Home health care agencies: palliative care programs and, 204

Horizontal integration, 152, 216

Horizontal mergers, 220

Hospice: continuum of care and, 207; cultural diversity and, 207–8; definition of, 200; length of stay in, 206; Medicare coverage for, 206; role of, 205–6

Hospital-acquired infections, 130, 235

Hospital acquisitions, of medical practices, 186

Hospital Compare, 105, 143, 231, 233, 236, 237, 238

Hospital Consumer Assessment of Healthcare Providers and Systems (HCAHPS), 236, 237

Hospital Corporation of America (HCA), 45

Hospitalist model: of clinical integration, 186–87; definition of, 186

Hospital outpatient departments (HOPDs), 83

Hospital-owned group practices, 183, 186

Hospital Quality Alliance, 143

Hospitals: acquisitions of, 214–15, 216; churn rates in, 106; critical access, 137; cyber attacks and, 139; efficiency and size of, 88; as employers, 31; electronic medical record adoption model, 135, *136*; hospice care and, 207; independent, 82; Indian Health Service, 137; joint ventures and, 47–48; Leapfrog safety standards and, 232–33; medical groups purchased by, 186; Medicare payment reductions for, *229*; mergers of, 214, 215, 216; number and sizes of, 214; as physicians' employers, 179, 189; social media adoption and, 121; by specialty and ownership, *49*; US, by bed size, category, and year, *32*; US, by category, 2005–2014, *31*; value-based purchasing program measures, 2016, *230*; Veterans Health Administration, 136. *See also* Acute-care hospitals; For-profit hospitals; *names of specific hospitals*; Not-for-profit hospitals; Physician–hospital integration, potential structures for; Specialty hospitals

Hospital Safety Score, 232

Hospital Standardization Program, 236

Hospital websites: evaluating, 120–21

Hospital workforce: growth in, 84

Huerta, T. R., 121

Human and Molecular Genetics Center, Medical College of Wisconsin, 251

Human genome, sequencing of, 249, 250

Human resources: healthcare business planning and, *152,* 154–56

Iacocca, Lee, 64

Idealized influence: transformational leadership and, 64, 65

Identity thieves, 138

Incentives: defined, 31, 74, 229; pay-for-performance, 105–6

Income statements, 20, 158, *159*

Independent hospitals: system membership and, 82

Indian Health Service: hospitals, 137

Indirect marketing, 122–23; definition of, 122; word-of-mouth advertising, 123

Individualized consideration: transformational leadership and, 64, 65

Individualized medicine, 250–51; population health and, 252

Infrastructure, 31

Innovation: joint ventures and, 187

Inpatient rehabilitation facilities (IRFs), 198, 201–3, 209

Inspirational motivation: transformational leadership and, 64, 65

Institute for Healthcare Improvement (IHI): Triple Aim concept of, 252, 255, 257

Institute of Medicine (IOM), 34; *Crossing the Quality Chasm,* 41; *Envisioning the National Healthcare Quality Report,* 182; *To Err Is Human,* 239; *Unequal Treatment,* 84, 86

Integrated care: Affordable Care Act and, 104

Integrated delivery systems (IDSs), of healthcare, 214, 216–18, 222

Integrated Health Association, 231

Integrated physician model: of joint ventures, 190

Integrity: transformational leaders and, 70; trust and, 68

Intellectual stimulation: transformational leadership and, 64, 65

Interactive patient care, 257

Interest, as cost of capital component, 154

Internal data, 40

Internal motivation, 66

Internal rate of return (IRR), 161–62, 164

Internal Revenue Code, 45

Internal Revenue Service (IRS): 501(c)(3) organizations, 44; role of, 45

Internal rewards, 64, 74

International health systems, 221–22

International migration: US, healthcare and, 200

Internet, 115, 117; healthcare information resources, 140; marketing, 119, 120; medical tourism and, 124

Internists: average compensation for, 186

Interoperability: definition of, 131

Intranet, 170

Jargon: avoiding, 170

Jefferson, Thomas, 174

Jobs, Steve, 29, 171, 173

Johns Hopkins Medicine, 221

Johnson, Lyndon B., 73

Joint Commission, The, 236, 240, 242

Joint ventures, 46–48, 187–89, 190; accountable care organizations and, 81; advantages of, 90; creating, 187; definition of, 46; equity-based, 188–89; hospital-physician, *188*; initiatives and potential of, 187–88; integrated physician model of, 190; profitability of, 189; strategic planning by, 54–55

Jones, John Paul, 64

Julius Caesar, 174

Kaiser Family Foundation, 142

Kaiser Permanente, 45, 84, 235

Kennedy, John F., 64, 73

King, Martin Luther, Jr., 64

Larsson, L. S., 122

Law, Vern, 77

Leaders: transformational, 64

Leadership: for CEO succession planning, 37; competency models of, 32; definition of, 32; delegating style of, 66, *67*; directing style of, 66, *67*; effective, ten concepts for, *263*, 263–66; ethics of, 68; managerial, 63; participating style of, 66, *67*; physician positions of, 179; servant, 51; transactional, 62, 63, *63*. *See also* Transformational leadership

Leading Health Indicators: *Healthy People 2020*, 94, 95

Leapfrog Group, 232–33

Lewin, Kurt, 107

Life expectancy: in United States, 199

Lifelong learning, 80

LifePoint Hospitals, 45

Lighting: for presentations, 173

Linear regression, 163

LinkedIn, 121

Local marketing, 123

Local planning, 93

Long-term care hospitals (LTCHs), 198

Long-Term Care Minimum Data Set (Centers for Medicare & Medicaid Services), 144

Long-term care services: adult health daycare centers, 208–9; hospice, 205–6, 207–8; inpatient rehabilitation facilities, 198, 201–3, 209; skilled nursing facilities, 198, 199, 201, 203–4, 209

Long-term strategies: strategic plans and, 86, 89–90

Magazine advertising, 119

Magnet hospital designation, 39; transformational leadership and, 72–74

Magnet Recognition Program, 72–74, 241

Managed care organizations, 42–44

Managed care plans, 235

"Management by walking around," 265

Managerial leadership, 63

Marketing: digital, 120–22; indirect, 122–23; telehealth services, 132. *See also* Healthcare marketing

Marketing media trends, 118–23; digital media, 120–22; external information and, 118–19; indirect marketing, 122–23; print media, 119; radio and television media, 119–20

Marketing plan, 157; definition of, 116; focus of, 124; primary components of, 116

Massey, Jack, 45

Mayo, William J., 248

Mayo Clinic, 45, 103, 124, 216, 234; Center for Individualized Medicine, 251; telehealth kiosks at, 132; telemedicine and, 256

Meaningful use: definition and stages of, 131

Medicaid, 73, 153; administration of, 140, 141; adult health day care centers and, 208; Affordable Care Act and expansion of, 94; Electronic Health Record Incentive Program, 135; gender and eligibility for, 200–201; patient-centered medical home program and, 181, 182; reimbursement rates of, 87, 88; skilled nursing care reimbursement rate, 199

Medical errors: financial and human cost of, 228; preventing, coordinated care and, 183

Medical foundations: definition of, 185; opposition to, 185–86; physician–hospital integration and, 183, 185–86

Medical Group Management Association, 34

Medical group practices: hospital purchases of, 186

Medical home: Agency for Healthcare Research and Quality definition of, 182

Medical records: black market sales of, 138

Medical staff: cofiduciary concept and, 42; definition of, 41

Medical technology: clinical integration and access to, 180

Medical tourism, 124

Medicare, 73, 153, 180, 190; administration of, 140, 141; Affordable Care Act marketing and, 170; ambulatory surgery centers and, 83; Conditions of Participation, 201; diagnosis-related groups and, 232; Electronic Health Record Incentive Program, 135; fee-for-service (FFS) expenditures, 184; hospice benefit, 206; inpatient rehabilitation reimbursement by, 203; Part A, 199, 230; Part B, 230; pay-for-performance initiatives of, 229–31; payment reductions for hospitals, *229*; patient-centered medical home model, primary care payment increases, and, 182; post-acute care coverage by, 198, 199, 209; reimbursement penalties, 181; reimbursement rates of, 87, 105; Shared Savings Program, 43, 184; skilled nursing facilities expenditures by, 204; skilled nursing facilities reimbursement by, 199; value-based purchasing and, 129

Medicare Health Support Chronic Disease Pilot, 231

Medicare Payment Advisory Commission (MedPAC), 82

Medicare Spending per Beneficiary (MSPB), 230

Mentoring, effective leadership and, 263, *263*

Mergers: acquisitions *vs.*, 215; horizontal, 220; of hospitals, 43, 56, 104, 214, 215, 216

Mission: definition of, 44, 56; relationship to strategic planning, 50, 51, 80, 95; transformational leaders and, 64, 66, 71

Mission statement: sample, 52

Mobile devices, 132, 133

Mobile health applications, 115

Morale, 66

Motivation: by transformational leaders, 65, 66; verbal presentation and, 171

Multiple regression analysis, 163

National Adult Services Association, 208

National Ambulatory Medical Care Survey, 142

National Center for Educational Statistics, 142

National Center for Healthcare Leadership (NCHL), 32, 34

National Center for Health Statistics (NCHS), 141–42

National Committee for Quality Assurance (NCQA), 236, 238, 254

National Federation of Independent Businesses v. Sebelius., 94

National Health Planning and Resources Development Act, 46, 47

National Patient Safety Goals (Joint Commission), 240

National planning, 94–95

National Quality Forum (NQF), 232

NationMaster, 140

Nebraska Health Information Initiative, 131

Net present value (NPV), 158–61, 164

Newspaper advertising, 119

New York: corporate practice of medicine doctrine in, 185

Nixon, Richard, 227

Nohria, Nitin, 168
Norway: adult health day care in, 208–9
Nosocomial infections, 91, 95n1
Not-for-profit health systems, 215, 216–17
Not-for-profit hospitals, 44–45; debt levels of, 87; definition of, 44; specialty, 48; strategic financial planning and, 53, 87; tax-exempt status of, 45
Nurses: retention of, 240
Nurse-sensitive patient outcomes, 241
Nurse staffing models, 40
Nurse-to-patient ratios: patient safety and, 89
Nursing home administrators: average annual compensation for, 204
Nursing Home Compare (Centers for Medicare & Medicaid Services), 144
Nursing homes, 209; palliative care programs and, 204; VistA and, 137

Obama, Barack, 64, 73, 137, 213, 229
Office of the National Coordinator for Health Information Technology (ONC), 131
Online Survey Certification & Reporting System database (Centers for Medicare & Medicaid Services), 144
Open-mindedness: effective leadership and, 263, 264
Operating margins, 53
Operating revenue, 157
Operational planning: strategic plans and, 91
Opportunities: definition of, 104; force field analysis and, 107, 110; in SWOT analysis, 102, 102, 104–6, 110
Organizational change: implementing, 55
Organizational culture: continuous quality improvement in, 34, 35; definition of, 50; as foundation for

strategic planning, 80; integrated delivery systems and, 130; servant leadership in, 51
Organizational goals: transformational leaders and, 69–70
Organizational surveys, 102
Organization for Economic Co-operation and Development, 140
Organizations: life cycle of, 48
Orthopedists: average compensation for, 186
Outcomes, in Donabedian framework, 234, 235
Outdoor advertising, 119
Outpatient services: increased use of, 53; palliative care programs and, 204
Outpatient surgery: rise of, 83
Ownership status: Not-for-profit hospitals: effect on strategic planning, 53–55, 56. See also For-profit hospitals

Pain management: hospice care and, 205, 206
Palliate, definition of, 204
Palliative care, 204–5, 206; definition of, 200; goals of, 204
Participating leadership style, 66, 67
Participative management: change and, 108
Password protection, 138
Patient-centered medical homes (PCMHs), 180–82, 190, 254–55
Patient centeredness: IOM definition of, 182
Patient demographics: healthcare marketing and, 117
Patient engagement, 241
Patient portals, 121–22; advantages with, 134; capabilities with, 133–34; definition of, 133
Patient safety, 239–40; high-performance work processes and, 63; nurse-to-

patient ratios and, 89; organizational culture and, 50; transformational leadership approach and, 67

Patient satisfaction: provider-patient communication and, 89

Patient stories: digital marketing and, 120

Patient-to-nurse ratios: improved patient outcomes and, 240

Payback period, 158, 161, 164; definition of, 158; projected physical therapy clinic, *160,* 160–61, *161*

Payer mix, 84

Payer relations, 38

Pay-for-performance (P4P) programs, 105–6, 231; commercial payer initiatives, 231; definition of, 228; incorporating into strategic plan, 233–34; physicians' attitudes about, 233; quality-related data and, 236; strategic planning and, 229

Pediatricians: average compensation for, 186

People: five Ps of healthcare marketing and, 117, *118*

Performance: continuous quality improvement and, 35

Performance evaluation, 91–93, 95

Personalized medicine, 137, 144, 250

Personnel management: strategic plans and, 86, 89

Pfizer kickbacks scandal, 68, 69

Pharmacogenomic testing, 251

Physician employment: advantages and disadvantages of, 189

Physician groups: joint ventures and, 47–48

Physician–hospital alignment: challenges in, 183

Physician–hospital integration, potential structures for, 183–90; accountable care organizations, 183–85; equity-based joint ventures, 188–89; hospi-talists, 186–87; hospital-owned group practices, 186; integrated physician model, 190; joint venture initiatives, 187–88; medical foundations, 185–86; physician employment, 189

Physician–hospital relationships: integrated physician model of, 179. *See also* Clinical integration

Physician-owned hospitals. *See* Specialty hospitals

Physicians: empowerment of, 190; in hospital-owned group practices, 186; pay for performance and, 233; range of work settings for, 179; referrals, 180; role in strategic planning, 41–42, 190; as stakeholders, 41, 42; total healthcare spending and spending on, 180

Piedmont Healthcare, Atlanta, Georgia, 33; board of directors, *35*

Pioneer accountable care organization model, 43

Place: five Ps of healthcare marketing and, 117, *118*

Pope Francis, 197

Population data, 1, 18–19

Population health, 251–54; definition of, 251; health disparities and, 94; individualized medicine and, 252; on island of Hispaniola, 165–66

Population health management (PHM), 129; implementing, steps in, 253–54

Post-acute care: definition of, 198

Post-acute care services, 209; network of, *202. See also* Long-term care services

PowerPoint presentations, 173

Precision medicine, 250

Preconception care, 108

Predictive human genomics, 249

Preferred provider organizations (PPOs), 42, 43

Prescription drugs, increased expenditures for, 31
Prezi, 173
Price: five Ps of healthcare marketing and, 117, *118*
Price analysis, annual, 87
Primary care physicians: average compensation for, 186; patient-centered medical home and, 182; telehealth and, 133
Print advertising, 117, 124
Print media: trends in, 119
Process, in Donabedian framework, 234, 235
Product: five Ps of healthcare marketing and, 117, *118*
Products and services mix: strategic plans and, 86, 90
Profitability: hospitalist model and, 187; joint ventures and, 189
Profit margin: definition of, 2
Profits: of hospitals, 42–43; relationship to ownership status, 53–55
Pro forma financial statements: definition of, 158; physical therapy clinic annual income statement, *159*
Promotion: five Ps of healthcare marketing and, 117, *118*
Prospective payment system (PPS): definition of, 203
Public Health Service Act: Title XVI, 4
Public health system: population health and, 252

Quality: accreditation and, 242; comparative outcomes and, 236; cost of, 227–29; defining, 235–36; Donabedian's definition of, 234; of healthcare, measurement of, 231; of healthcare, six aims of, 41; strategic plans and, 86, 88–89
Quality metrics, 236–40; systemwide tracking of, 130

Quality-related data: growing demand for, 236–39
Question-and-answer sessions: presentations and, 175

Radio advertising, 116, 117, 119, 124
Readmission rate, 30-day, 91, 95n2, 184
Reagan, Ronald, 64, 73
Referrals: to hospice programs, 206; to joint venture hospitals, 47–48; to specialty hospitals, 82; under Stark laws, 155
Refreezing, new attitudes, 108
Regional marketing, 123–24
Regional planning, 93–94
Regression analysis, 162–63, 164
Reimbursement: government, 87–88; managed care organizations, 42; medical foundations, 185
Replacement facilities, planning for, 156
Resource allocation: based on organizational culture, 80; definition of, 33; efficient, 31
Retreats, 50
Return on investment (ROI), 51
Rewards: effective leadership and, *263*, 265; external, 63, 74; internal, 64, 74
Riggio, Ronald E., 64
Robots: telemedicine, 257
Roosevelt, Eleanor, 64
Rounding: effective leadership and, *263*, 265
Rumsfeld, Donald, 149
Rural hospitals, virtual health systems and, 221

Safe harbors, 155
Safety. *See* Patient safety
Safety-net providers, 82
Salaries: physician, 186
Scorecards, balanced, 242
Scrushy, Richard M., 69

Search engine organization: digital marketing and, 121
Search engines, 132
Seating: for presentations, types of, 173
Securities and Exchange Commission (SEC), 69
Senior marketing executives, 40
Servant leadership, 51, *263,* 264
Service lines, 37
Shareholders, 45
Shaw, George Bernard, 168
Shimooka, Allison Cuff, 204
Silos, patient-centered medical home model, continuum of care, and, 181, *183*
Skilled nursing facilities (SNFs), 198, 201, 209; Medicare reimbursement, 199; trends in, 203–4
Small Business Administration (SBA): business planning resources, 150–51
Small Business Health Options Program exchanges, in states, 182
Smartphones, 120, 132, 133
Social media, 115; definition of, 121; marketing plan and, 116
Software: business planning, 162
Solutions orientation: effective leadership and, *263,* 266
Sony Pictures Entertainment, hacking incident, 138
Specialists: average compensation for, 186
Specialty hospitals, 48; impact of, 82
Specialty physicians: telehealth and, 133
St. Vincent's Healthcare (Florida): website for, 121
Stage charisma, 171
Stage 2 meaningful use: patient portals and, 121
Stakeholders: communicating strategic plan to, 171; definition of, 33; force field analysis and, 107; physicians as, 41, 42
Stark laws, 153–54, 155, 189

State Health Facts, 142
StateMaster, 142
Statement of operations, 158
Statement of purpose: healthcare business plan, 152, *152*
States: adult day healthcare in, 208; Affordable Care Act and Medicaid expansion in, 94; corporate practice of medicine doctrine in, 185; Small Business Health Options Program exchanges in, 182
Stock sales, by for-profit hospitals, 157
Strategic adaptation theory, 116
Strategic financial planning, 86–88
Strategic management theory, 116
Strategic planning, 50–51: as continuous activity, 91; critical success factors in, 80–81; definition of, 78, 95; diversity in workplace and, 86; efficiency and, 88; environment inside organization, analysis of, 79–81; environment outside organization, analysis of, 81–83; ethics as foundational in, 68–69; function of, 78; fundamentals of, 77–95; for healthcare value, 257; for health information technology, 137–39, 144; at health system level, 218–22; innovative, 78; leadership in, 35–41; long-term, 86, 89–90; model, *79;* ongoing process of, 50, 56; organizational objectives and, 33; ownership status and impact on, 53–55, 56; physicians' involvement in, 41–42, 190; planning areas, 86–91; primary aim of, 102; relationship to mission, vision, and values, 48, 50–52, 56, 80, 95; resource allocation function of, 31; transformational leaders and, 69–74. *See also* Culture; Leadership; Mission; SWOT analysis; Vision
Strategic plan presentations, 169–75; appearance, rehearsal, and arrange-

ment, 172, 175; audience engagement and, 173–74, 175; content and,
171–72; giving, *171*; maintaining
audience interest, 174; question-and-
answer session, 175; technology for,
173, 175; verbal communication
and, 170–71; written communication and, 169–70

Strategic plans: pay for performance
incorporated into, 233–34

Strengths: definition of, 103; force field
analysis and, 107, 110; in SWOT
analysis, 102, *102*, 103, 110

Structure, in Donabedian framework,
234, 235

Surveys, organizational, 102

SWOT analysis, 101–10, 257; definition of, 101; downstream revenue
and, 109, 110; force field analysis
and, 106–8, *107*, 110; gap analysis
and, 108–9, *109*, 110; matrix, *102*;
opportunities in, 102, *102*, 104–6,
110; steps in, 102–6; strengths in,
102, *102*, 103, 110; threats in, 102,
102, 106, 110; weaknesses in, 102,
102, 104, 110

Systems approach: to problem solving, 41

Tablet computers, 120, 132, 133

Target data breach, 138

Tax deduction, 46

Tax-exempt status, 45, 46

Teaching health centers: patient-centered
medical home model and, 182

Technology: for presentations, 173. *See
also* Health information technology

Telehealth, 135, 144; definition of, 132;
innovations in, 133

Telemedicine, 132, 255–57, 258; definition of, 255; innovations in, 256–57;
services, 255; virtual health systems
and, 221

Television advertising, 116, 117, 119, 124

Tenet Healthcare Corporation, 45

Texas: corporate practice of medicine doctrine in, 185

Therapeutic alliance, 241

Thirty-day readmission rate, 91, 95n2, 184

Threats: definition of, 106; force field
analysis and, 107, 110; in SWOT
analysis, 102, *102*, 106, 110

*To Err Is Human: Building a Safer Health
System* (Institute of Medicine), 239

Total cost, 88

Transactional leadership: definition of, 62;
transformational leadership *vs.*, *63*

Transformational leaders: ethical considerations of, 68–69; personality
characteristics of, *66*; strategies used
by, 70–72

Transformational leadership: components
of, 64; concepts of, 64–67; cultural
factors in, 67; definition of, 62; effect
on followers, 65–66, 74; hierarchical
model of, 66, *67*; high-performance
work processes and, 63; importance
of, 68; leadership team development
under, 72; Magnet designation and,
72–74; patient safety and, 67; in
strategic planning process, 69–74;
transactional leadership *vs.*, *63*

Transformational Leadership (Bass and
Riggio), 64

Transparency: of data, 242

Triple Aim (IHI), 252, 255, 257

Trust: integrity and, 68

Twitter, 121

Unequal Treatment (Institute of Medicine), 84, 86

Unfreezing, organizational perspective, 108

Uninsured population: safety-net providers and, 82

United Nations, 140

United States: fragmented healthcare system in, 190; healthcare spending in,

30–31, 78, 115, 227; life expectancy in, 199; trends in medical-budget spending for average family in, 2008 and 2013, 180, *181*

University of California at San Francisco, Philip R. Lee Institute for Health Policy Studies, 142

US Census Bureau, 81, 119, 141, 142

US Department of Defense (DoD), 46, 54, 137

US Department of Health and Human Services (HHS), 81, 105, 119, 140, 143, 239

US Department of Justice, 46, 69, 219

US Department of Veterans Affairs, 46, 84. *See also* Veterans Health Administration

US military: telemedicine and, 256

US Navy: Integrated Health Community Initiative, 252–53

US Office of Personnel Management: hacking incident, 138–39

US Public Health Service, 46

Value: definition of, 48, 89, 227; quality and, 88–89; relationship to strategic planning, 51, 56, 80, 95; strategic plans and, 86

Value-based purchasing, 105, 129, 229, 230, *230,* 231, 235, 242

Value-driven care episodes, 105

Value frontier, 227

Values statement: sample, 52

Variable cost, 88

Verbal communication: strategic plan presentation and, 169–70

Vertical integration, 152, 187, 216, 220

Veterans Health Administration, 54; electronic health record system of, 136–37; healthcare data warehouses of, 134

Videoconferences, 173

Virtual communities, 121

Virtual health systems, 221, 222

Vision: definition of, 48; relationship to strategic planning, 50, 51, 56, 80, 95; transformational leaders and, 64, 66

Vision statement: sample, 52

VistA (Veterans Health Information Systems and Technology Architecture), 136–37

VSee, 256

Vulnerable populations: healthcare for, 228

Walgreens, 130

"Walking the talk": transformational leadership and, 65

Walmart, 130

Waste, 228

Weaknesses: definition of, 104; force field analysis and, 107, 110; in SWOT analysis, 102, *102,* 104, 110

Webcasts, 173

Webinars, 173

WebMD, 121

Websites, hospital, evaluating, 120–21

Weighted average cost of capital, 160

Wellness: patient-centered medical home and, 181

Whiteboards, electronic, 173

Whole-genome sequencing, 250

Wireless technologies, 132

Women: healthcare and, 200; long-term care for, 201

Women, Infants, and Children program, 200

Word-of-mouth advertising, 123

Workforce: diversity of, 84, 86; impact on healthcare quality, 240–41

Workload projections: developing, 162–63

World Factbook, 140

Written communication: strategic plan presentation and, 169–70

Yelp, 121

ABOUT THE AUTHOR

Jeffrey P. Harrison, PhD, FACHE, is a professor of health administration at the University of North Florida (UNF) and chair of the Department of Public Health. As chair, he is responsible for the undergraduate and graduate programs in public health, the undergraduate and graduate programs in health administration, and the graduate program in clinical mental health counseling. He has faculty appointments at the UNF Brooks College of Health and the UNF Coggin College of Business, where he teaches healthcare finance, health information technology, and strategic planning.

Before joining academe full-time in 2002, Dr. Harrison held a wide range of managerial positions, including chief operating officer of a hospital, director of a large medical group, and leader at the health system level. He is the founder and president of Harrison Consulting Group, Inc., a healthcare consulting firm.

Dr. Harrison has a PhD in health services organization and research from Virginia Commonwealth University, a master's degree in business administration from the College of William and Mary, and a master's degree in health administration from the Medical College of Virginia. A Fellow of the American College of Healthcare Executives (ACHE), he is board certified in healthcare management.

Dr. Harrison has authored more than 40 articles and book chapters on healthcare management and strategic planning and has delivered national and international seminars on professional development to thousands of healthcare executives. He has been given numerous honors, including ACHE's Senior-Level Healthcare Executive Regent's Award for North Florida in 2008. He was selected one of the Top 100 health administration professors by *MHA Guide* in 2013. Additionally, he was named one of the most influential people in Jacksonville healthcare in 2013 by *Jacksonville Magazine*. He is a member of the Healthcare Financial Management Association, the Medical Group Management Association, and AcademyHealth and serves on the editorial board of *The Health Care Manager* magazine.

ABOUT THE CONTRIBUTORS

Debra A. Harrison, DNP, RN, is the chief nursing officer at Mayo Clinic in Jacksonville, Florida, and an assistant professor in nursing for the College of Medicine, Mayo Clinic. Her 40 years at Mayo include work as a bedside nurse, nurse manager, nursing education specialist, and nurse administrator.

Art Layne, MHA, was the president of Intellimed Corporation in Phoenix for ten years. Mr. Layne worked as an administrator and CEO at hospitals in North Carolina, South Carolina, Texas, and Arizona. He has served as the Executive in Residence for the Department of Health Administration at Virginia Commonwealth University (VCU). In 2013, he received the VCU School of Allied Health Professions Alumni Star award.

R. Timothy Stack, FACHE, was president and CEO of Piedmont Healthcare, a regional healthcare system based in Atlanta, Georgia. After becoming president in 2001, Mr. Stack helped expand the operation from $330 million in annual revenue to more than $1 billion. His previous positions include president and CEO of Borgess Health Alliance in Kalamazoo, Michigan, and president and CEO of South Side Healthcare System in Pittsburgh, Pennsylvania. His friends were saddened to learn that Mr. Stack passed away in 2010 at the age of 60. His long-standing contribution to this book is the Epilogue, which is necessary reading for any aspiring healthcare leader.